Health 5.0

This book presents a detailed explanation of the concepts, taxonomy, and challenges in Healthcare 4.0 and provides frameworks and architectures for the adaptation and fusion of emerging technologies under Healthcare 5.0. The healthcare industry requires technological upgrades to provide precise, accurate, and automatic remote health monitoring and diagnosis. This reference book offers an early opportunity to explore emerging technologies and understand current issues, problems, and concepts.

Health 5.0: Concepts, Challenges, and Solutions provides state-of-the-art research topics and opportunities of IoMT in personalized healthcare. It presents diversified IoMT applications for smart healthcare that supports lifestyle changes as a preventive measure and discusses health and care for all citizens to lead a good quality of life. The book illustrates the advancements of IoMT in augmented reality and AI and offers use-cases of edge computing for remote healthcare. The book also highlights the architectures, frameworks, and current research issues in IoMT and goes on to focus on sustainable healthcare for smart cities using edge computing, IoMT, and big data. The details of the development of advanced therapeutic instrumentation, along with the promotion of digital therapy, are also provided.

The primary audience for this book includes academicians, researcher scholars, IoMT developers, cloud-based health application designers, and medical practitioners who are engaged in providing healthcare services using recent technologies.

Prospects in Smart Technologies
Series Editor

Mohammad M. Banat
Jordan University of Science and Technology
Irbid, Jordan banat@just.edu.jo

Sara Paiva
Instituto Politécnico de Viana do Castelo
Viana do Castelo
Portugal sara.paiva@estg.ipvc.pt

Published Titles

Emerging Technologies for Sustainable and Smart Energy
Edited by Anirbid Sircar, Gautami Tripathi, Namrata Bist, Kashish Ara Shakil, and Mithileysh Sathiyanarayanan

CYBORG
Human and Machine Communication Paradigm
Kuldeep Singh Kaswan, Jagjit Singh Dhatterwal, Anupam Baliyan, and Shalli Rani

Emerging Technologies and the Application of WSN and IoT
Smart Surveillance, Public Security, and Safety Challenges
Edited by Shalli Rani and Himanshi Babbar

WSN and IoT
An Integrated Approach for Smart Applications
Edited by Shalli Rani and Ashu Taneja

Immersive Technologies
Navigating the Impacts, Challenges, and Opportunities
Sagaya Aurelia

Health 5.0
Concepts, Challenges, and Solutions
Hiren Kumar Thakkar, Chintan Bhatt, Victor C.M. Leung and Ilangko Balasingham

For more information on this series, please visit: https://www.routledge.com/Prospects-in-Smart-Technologies/book-series/CRCPST

Health 5.0

Concepts, Challenges, and Solutions

Edited by Hiren Kumar Thakkar,
Chintan Bhatt, Victor C.M. Leung, and
Ilangko Balasingham

CRC Press
Taylor & Francis Group
Boca Raton London New York

CRC Press is an imprint of the
Taylor & Francis Group, an **informa** business

Designed cover image: Getty Images

First edition published 2025
by CRC Press
2385 NW Executive Center Drive, Suite 320, Boca Raton FL 33431

and by CRC Press
4 Park Square, Milton Park, Abingdon, Oxon, OX14 4RN

CRC Press is an imprint of Taylor & Francis Group, LLC

ISBN: 978-1-032-49247-6 (hbk)
ISBN: 978-1-032-49378-7 (pbk)
ISBN: 978-1-003-39349-8 (ebk)

DOI: 10.1201/9781003393498

Typeset in Times
by Apex CoVantage, LLC

Contents

Part I Conventional Medicare, Health 5.0, and Next-Generation Internet of Medical Things (IoMT)

Part II Intelligent IoMT and New Age Computing: Principles and Perspective with AI and Edge Computing

Part IV AI-Enabled Smart Models and Algorithms for IoMT-Augmented Data Analysis

Preface

The recent advancements in embedded technologies have revolutionized remote healthcare monitoring and diagnosis using tiny, low-cost, and easy to wear Internet of Medical Things (IoMT) devices. With consistent advancements in Industry 4.0, the manufacturing industry has transformed healthcare monitoring into a state-of-the-art automation paradigm. On the foundation of Industry 4.0, an era of smart and e-connected healthcare monitoring cum diagnosis is touching new heights referred to as Healthcare 4.0. Healthcare 4.0 smartly utilizes the recent technologies such as Internet of Things, big data, and cloud computing to revolutionize the remote healthcare monitoring, diagnosis, and treatment strategies. Additionally, augmented reality has enabled the next generation healthcare applications and treatment possibilities with real-time access to data.

However, Healthcare 4.0 has limitations of processing and analyzing healthcare data. Usually, in Healthcare 4.0, the healthcare data is processed in cloud platforms using conventional statistical and machine learning approaches. However, conventional approaches are not suitable to analyze the IoMT data, which may not provide detailed insights. Moreover, cloud computing may not serve the purpose of real-time remote healthcare monitoring of patients due to severe latency issues. Therefore, artificial intelligence -enabled models are required, which can be further improved to suit the processing of healthcare data. Moreover, the IoMT collected data may come in diversified forms and accumulate over the period of time resulting in big data, which requires a specialized computing environment. To tackle the real-time data processing constraint of Healthcare 4.0, a paradigm shift to Health 5.0 with fog computing as the processing unit is required to analyze the data in an efficient manner. The fifth stage in Industry (Industry 5.0) recognizes the core role of customers (beyond the "customer is the king" mantra). Similarly, this book will explore the possibilities of fog/edge computing models, IoMT, 6G communications, and artificial intelligence to further advance the field of healthcare automation, i.e., digital wellness and support systems. The integrated AI and 6G communications for edge computing, together, may change the healthcare landscape and can revolutionize modern IoMT-based healthcare by enabling personalized, preventative, and collaborative forms of IoT care.

The main objective of this book is to illustrate new ideas, innovative research results, or systematic reviews in these areas. The emphasis of this book is also on using IoMT to respond to epidemic/pandemic situations and on the security aspect to keep the critical IoT infrastructure safe and running in states of emergency. The purpose of this book is to present the detailed explanation of the concepts, taxonomy, and challenges in current Healthcare 4.0 and to provide the frameworks and architectures for the adaptation of fusion of emerging technologies under Healthcare 5.0. The healthcare industry requires significant technological upgrades to provide precise, accurate, and automatic remote health monitoring and diagnosis. The seamless integration of the initial stage of 6G communications and fog commuting with AI models and IoMT devices requires novel architectures, frameworks, and models. In addition to seamless integration of technologies, Healthcare 5.0 needs to provide remote healthcare monitoring with minimum human intervention to provide state-of-the-art prediction for preventive diagnosis. This book will provide readers with early opportunities to these emerging technologies that help them understand the current issues, research problems, and concepts. This book will ensure lifelong partnerships with individual stakeholders in the healthcare sector.

The primary audience for the book includes academicians, researcher scholars, IoMT developers, cloud-based health application designers, and medical practitioners who are engaged in providing healthcare services using recent technologies.

About the Editors

Dr. Hiren Kumar Thakkar received his MTech in CSE from IIIT Bhubaneswar, India, in 2012 and a PhD degree from Chang Gung University, Taiwan, in 2018. Later, he worked as a postdoctoral fellow at the Motor Behavioral Research Lab (MBRL) at Chang Gung University, Taiwan. Before joining Pandit Deendayal Energy University (PDEU), he worked as Associate Professor at Nirma University, Ahmedabad. His research interest includes healthcare data analysis, cloud resource management, and opinion feature mining. He has published several SCI research papers in peer-reviewed journals and is a Senior member of IEEE.

Dr. Chintan Bhatt is Assistant Professor in the Department of Computer Science and Engineering (CSE), School of Technology, Pandit Deendayal Energy University (PDEU). Before joining PDEU, Dr. Bhatt served as an Assistant Professor in the CE department (CSPIT, CHARUSAT) for 11 years. Dr. Bhatt is the author and coauthor of 80-plus publications in the areas of computer vision, the Internet of Things, and fog computing. He has won several awards including the CSI Award and Best Paper Award for his CSI articles and conference publications.

Dr. Victor C.M. Leung is Emeritus Professor of Electrical and Computer Engineering at the University of British Columbia, Canada, and Distinguished Professor of Computer Science and Software Engineering at Shenzhen University, China. He has coauthored numerous refereed articles in the broad areas of wireless networks and mobile systems and is a Clarivate Analytics Highly Cited Researcher. Dr. Leung received the 2017 IEEE ComSoc Fred W. Ellersick Prize, the 2017 IEEE Systems Journal Best Paper Award, the 2017 Canadian Award for Telecommunications Research, the 2018 IEEE TCGCC Distinguished Technical Achievement Recognition Award, the 2018 IEEE CSIM Best Journal Paper Award, and the 2019 IEEE TCGCC Best Journal Paper Award, as well as several other awards. He is a Life Fellow of IEEE and a Fellow of the Royal Society of Canada, Canadian Academy of Engineering, and Engineering Institute of Canada.

Dr. Ilangko Balasingham received the Siv.Ing.(MSc) and Dr.Ing.(PhD) degrees, both in signal processing, from the Norwegian University of Science and Technology (NTNU), Trondheim, Norway, in 1993 and 1998, respectively. He did his Master's thesis at the University of California in Santa Barbara. From 1998 to 2002, he was employed as a research engineer developing video streaming solutions for mobile handheld devices at Fast Search & Transfer ASA, Oslo, Norway. Since 2002, he has been with the Intervention Center, Oslo University Hospital—Rikshospitalet, Oslo, Norway, as a Senior Research Scientist and Founder and Head of the Biomedical Sensor Network Research Group. He was appointed as Professor of Medical Signal Processing and Communications at NTNU in 2006. In 2017, he was promoted to Head of the Section for Medical ICT R&D at the Intervention Center. He was Professor by courtesy at the Frontier Institute, Nagoya Institute of Technology, Nagoya, Japan, during the academic year 2016–2017. His research interests include medical signal and image processing, wireless biomedical sensor networks for short-range sensing, imaging, localization, and communication, and multimedia patient record systems. Lately, he has been involved in nanoscale communication networks—molecular communications using biology and nanotechnology for intrabody applications, minimally invasive diagnosis, monitoring, and drug delivery.

Contributors

Apriandy Angdresey
Department of Informatics Engineering, Universitas Katolik De La Salle
Manado, Mandao, Indonesia

Aakash Bhandary
Department of Computer Science and Engineering, Pandit Deendayal Energy University
Gandhinagar, Gujarat, India

Alessandro Bruno
Department of Business, Economics, Law, Consumer Behaviour, IULM University
Milan, Milan, Italy

Chinmaya Dehury
Institute of Computer Science, University of Tartu
Tartu, Tartu, Estonia

Neel H. Dholakia
Department of Information Technology, Marwadi University
Rajkot, Gujarat, India

Vruti Dobariya
Department of Computer Science and Engineering, Pandit Deendayal Energy University
Gandhinagar, Gujarat, India

Prakhar Gupta
Department of Computer Science and Engineering, Pandit Deendayal Energy University
Gandhinagar, Gujarat, India

Devshree Jadeja
Department of Computer Science and Engineering, Pandit Deendayal Energy University
Gandhinagar, Gujarat, India

Rinkal Jain
Department of Computer Science and Engineering, Pandit Deendayal Energy University
Gandhinagar, Gujarat, India

V. Kakulapati
Sreenidhi Institute of Science and Technology
Hyderabad, Telangana, India

Jeet Khamar
Department of Computer Science and Engineering, Pandit Deendayal Energy University
Gandhinagar, Gujarat, India

Suraj Kothari
Department of Information Technology, Marwadi University
Rajkot, Gujarat, India

Vendra Durga Ratna Kumar
Department of Computer Science Engineering, SRM University
Mangalagiri, Guntur, India

Bhargav Limbasia
Department of Computer Science and Engineering, Pandit Deendayal Energy University
Gandhinagar, Gujarat, India

Saurav Mallik
Department of Pharmacology Toxicology, The University of Arizona
Tucson, Tucson, USA

Hemant Maravaniya
Department of Computer Science and Engineering, Pandit Deendayal Energy University
Gandhinagar, Gujarat, India

Abhijeetsingh Meena
Department of Computer Science and Engineering, Pandit Deendayal Energy University
Gandhinagar, Gujarat, India

Hiren Mewada
Electrical Engineering Department, Prince Mohammad Bin Fahd University
Al Khobar, Al Khobar, Kingdom of Saudi Arabia

Gone Neelakantam
Department of Computer Science Engineering, Ecole Centrale School of Engineering, Mahindra University (MU)
Hyderabad, Telangana, India

Ade Indra Onthoni
Institute of Population Health Sciences, National Health Research Institutes (NHRI)
Mioli, Mioli, Taiwan

Djeane Debora Onthoni
Institute of Population Health Sciences, National Health Research Institutes (NHRI)
Mioli, Mioli, Taiwan

Damodharan Palaniappan
Department of Computer Engineering, Marwadi University
Rajkot, Gujarat, India

Kumar Parmar
Department of Information Technology, Marwadi University
Rajkot, Gujarat, India

Jeet Patel
Department of Computer Science and Engineering, Pandit Deendayal Energy University
Gandhinagar, Gujarat, India

Shital Patel
Department of Information Technology, Ahmedabad Institute of Technology
Ahmedabad, Gujarat, India

Suyamoon Pathak
Department of Computer Science and Engineering, Pandit Deendayal Energy University
Gandhinagar, Gujarat, India

Bhumika Rupchandani
Department of Computer Science and Engineering, Pandit Deendayal Energy University
Gandhinagar, Gujarat, India

Ketan Sabale
Department of Computer Science and Engineering, Pandit Deendayal Energy University
Gandhinagar, Gujarat, India

Arvik Shah
Department of Computer Science and Engineering, Pandit Deendayal Energy University
Gandhinagar, Gujarat, India

Nabhi Shah
Department of Computer Science and Engineering, Pandit Deendayal Energy University
Gandhinagar, Gujarat, India

Priyanka Singh
Department of Computer Science Engineering, SRM University
Mangalagiri, Guntur, India

Hiren Kumar Thakkar
Department of Computer Science and Engineering, Pandit Deendayal Energy University
Gandhinagar, Gujarat, India

Kirtirajsinh Zala
Department of Information Technology, Marwadi University
Rajkot, Gujarat, India

Part I

Conventional Medicare, Health 5.0, and Next-Generation Internet of Medical Things (IoMT)

1 History, Concepts, and Conventional Medicare Technologies Using Artificial Intelligence

Jeet Khamar, Djeane Debora Onthoni, and Hiren Kumar Thakkar

1.1 INTRODUCTION

The unique field of artificial intelligence (AI) applications in conventional Medicare is discussed in this chapter. A generative sentence begins with, "In the days of high-tech innovations, the application of AI in healthcare has become one of the most essential breakthroughs." The impact of AI in the healthcare landscape is profound, heralding a new era of improved patient care, increased diagnostic accuracy, and overall greater efficiency. This chapter is dedicated to unraveling the theory of AI in medicine [1]. It lays out a comprehensive foundation on which AI-stimulated conventional medical technologies can be understood, as the chapter explores the history of AI in healthcare and the underlying fundamental concepts that have shaped it into such a transformative field over the past decades. The journey begins by looking back to analyze the evolution of AI in medicine and the core principles that have shaped its contemporary applications.

1.2 HISTORICAL PERSPECTIVE

1.2.1 Pre-AI Healthcare Landscape

The forms of AI in healthcare in both medical practice and the technological landscape were entirely different. Prior to the introduction of AI, mainstream diagnostic tools, along with medical expertise, relied heavily on manual methods for recording and retrieval in healthcare [1]. The technologies prevalent in healthcare during the mid-20th century had limited computational and data storage capabilities, leading to a significant dependence on human expertise for diagnosis and treatments.

DOI: 10.1201/9781003393498-2

1.2.2 Early AI Applications in Healthcare

The first occurrence of the use of AI in healthcare dates back a few decades to the late 1960s and early 1970s, a period marked by increased computer availability and advancements in the processing of medical information. Initial applications of AI were centered around rule-based expert systems developed as imitations of human ideals in clinical decision-making. These systems could provide diagnostic pointers and suggest treatment possibilities based on established medical knowledge [2]. While the impact of such systems was minimal, owing to the scarcity of medical data and limited computing power, this marked their initial entry into the field

Three remarkable milestones that mark the development of AI in Healthcare include visualization, dating back to the early 1970s, with the creation of an expert system for chemical mass spectrometry—Dendral. The work in this domain led to the emergence of rule-based artificial intelligence systems for medical diagnosis. In the 1980s, the expert system MYCIN for bacterial infection diagnosis served as an example of how AI can assist in medical decision-making support

By the 1990s, AI began to be implemented in medical imaging, contributing to the development of systems used to assist in the interpretation of radiological images such as magnetic resonance imaging (MRIs) and X-rays. This marked the establishment of new methods through which various medical problems could be diagnosed more rapidly and accurately

1.2.3 AI's Evolution in Healthcare

With improved techniques in Natural Language Processing (NLP), the available computational power saw the 21st century witness AI applications in genomics, drug discovery, and personalized medicine. Machine learning (ML) algorithms, especially deep learning (DL), have revolutionized the field by enabling AI systems to analyze vast datasets and identify new patterns that were previously unnoticed [3,4]. The integration of big data and AI has facilitated predictive analytics, early identification of diseases, and the development of improved treatment protocols for healthcare providers AI drives healthcare innovations that alleviate the strain on drug development, optimizing treatment efforts while enhancing the quality of client care and service delivery through telemedicine and home-monitoring establishments. This journey through history reveals the remarkable transformation of AI in the healthcare industry, from rule-based expert systems to today's era where it represents a paradigm shift for medicine itself. These milestones in AI healthcare research and development have paved the way for a future where AI can only continue to prove advantageous in enhancing the healthcare experience for patients and improving overall outcomes. The impact of AI in various aspects can be summarized in Table 1.1.

1.3 CONCEPTS OF ARTIFICIAL INTELLIGENCE IN HEALTHCARE

1.3.1 Machine Learning and Deep Learning

Machine learning (ML) and deep learning (DL) play an important role in healthcare by processing and analyzing vast and complex datasets. The overview of the ML and

DL techniques used in the field of healthcare can be found in Figure 1.1. In practice, ML algorithms are utilized for predicting disease outcomes, optimizing treatment plans, and identifying potential drug candidates. For example, they can analyze a patient's genetic profile to determine the diseases to which that individual is prone, facilitating the creation of customized healthcare interventions. On the other hand, DL excels at image recognition tasks. In medical imaging, DL algorithms rapidly and accurately identify abnormalities in X-rays, MRIs, and computed tomography (CT) scans. This capability reduces diagnosis durations and ensures quick intervention periods, thereby increasing the effectiveness of outcomes for patients [6].

TABLE 1.1
I Impact of AI in Various Healthcare Aspects

Aspect of Healthcare	Before AI	After AI
Diagnosis and treatment	Heavily reliant on human expertise	AI aids in diagnosis and treatment [1,2]
Electronic health records	Paper-based or fragmented	Centralized, digitized EHR systems [3]
Medical imaging [5]	Manual analysis of images.	AI assists in image analysis [2]
Telemedicine	Limited remote access	Widened telemedicine availability [2]
Drug discovery	Time-consuming and costly	AI accelerates drug discovery [2,3]
Administrative tasks	Manual scheduling and billing	AI automates administrative tasks [1,2]
Healthcare costs	Rising healthcare costs	AI helps control healthcare expenses [2]
Patient experience	Varied quality and access	Improved patient experience with AI [3]
Predictive analytics	Limited disease forecasting	AI enhances predictive analytics [1–3]

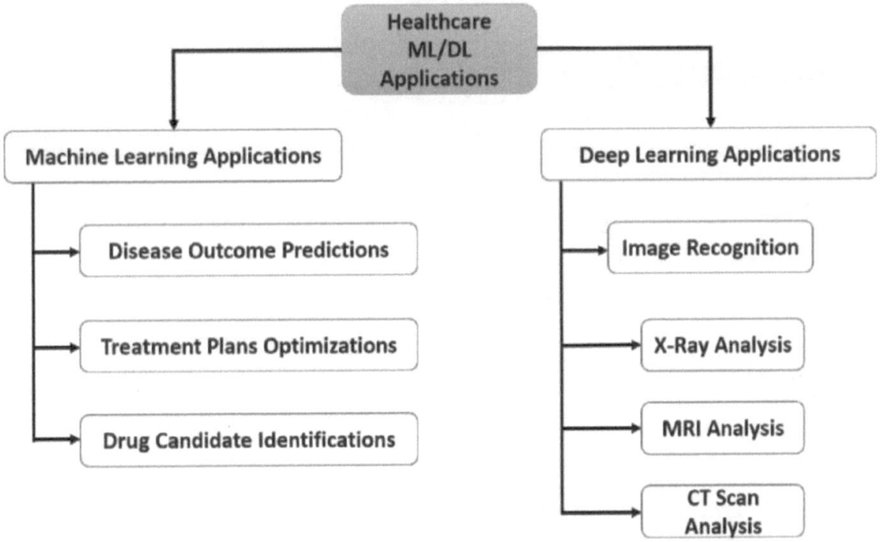

FIGURE 1.1 Overview of ML and DL techniques used in the field of healthcare.

1.3.2 Natural Language Processing

It is of high importance for management to handle vast amounts of unstructured text data existing in healthcare, such as medical records and research articles. Natural-language-processing- (NLP)-powered AI algorithms can extract valuable information from these sources, providing healthcare providers with ready access to relevant patient information and research findings. Another outcome of NLP is the creation of chatbots and virtual assistants that can answer queries, schedule appointments, and even assist in remote monitoring. NLP significantly contributes to better decision-making and enhanced patient care by enabling healthcare professionals to search and access data more effectively. Furthermore, it plays a crucial role in the development of clinical decision support systems, which advise and alert physicians based on data and medical guidelines [7]. Figure 1.2 shows the overview of NLP techniques used in Medicare.

1.3.3 Computer Vision

In healthcare, computer vision has emerged as a game-changer in medical imaging and diagnostics. The different ways of utilizing computer vision algorithms in analyzing medical images can be seen in Figure 1.3. Utilizing computer vision algorithms, AI systems can analyze medical images such as X-rays, MRIs, and CT scans. These systems rapidly and accurately identify anomalies, tumors, or other irregularities, aiding radiologists in the diagnostic process. This not only reduces the time taken to reach a diagnosis but also enhances accuracy. Moreover, computer vision enables the development of systems capable of detecting early symptoms of diseases like diabetic retinopathy by analyzing retina images, ensuring timely treatment for better recovery. Additionally, computer vision finds applications in robotic surgery, providing surgeons with improved vision and precision during operations [8].

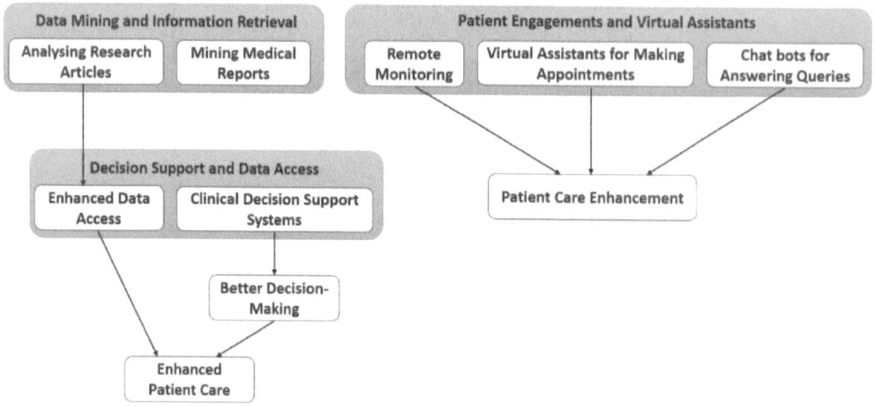

FIGURE 1.2 Overview of NLP techniques used in Medicare.

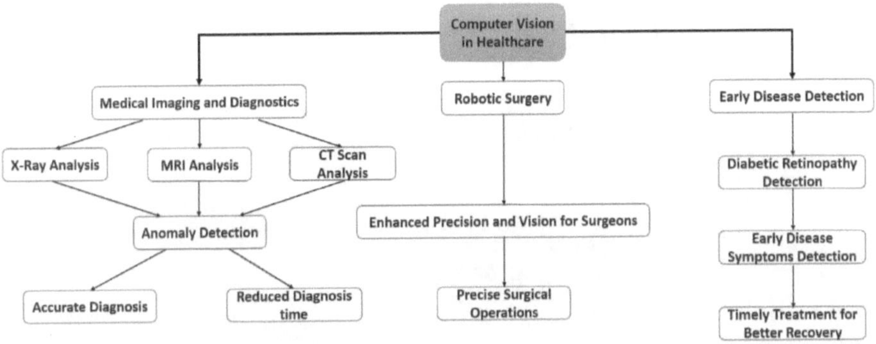

FIGURE 1.3 Different ways in which computer vision is applied in image analysis.

1.3.4 Expert Systems

Expert systems in healthcare simulate human expertise as virtual consultants for medical decision-making. They are designed to provide diagnostic support and treatment recommendations based on the average experiences observed in specific patients. Expert systems excel in offering credible, evidence-based counsel, particularly in situations where diseases are rare or challenging to diagnose. As shown in Figure 1.4, these systems use rules and algorithms to analyze either the symptoms or the history of a patient, aiding healthcare professionals in making more informed decisions. For example, an expert system may assist a general practice doctor by suggesting potential diagnoses based on patient symptoms or identifying the possibility of drug interactions within life-threatening medication regimens. This application of AI ensures that medical decisions are grounded in state-of-the-art research and best practices, ultimately improving patient care in the long run [9].

1.3.5 Predictive Analytics

Predictive analytics applies AI to predict trends in health and patient outcomes based on the study of recorded patient history. It identifies patterns and associations to enable early treatment of patients predisposed to certain conditions and develop directed care plans. For example, it can predict the likelihood of rehospitalization in chronic diseases, thereby necessitating mandatory preventive care among healthcare providers. In addition, predictive analytics optimizes the allocation of resources and ensures that the medical facilities have enough staff and supplies on-site. It is also helpful in monitoring diseases like epidemics through the examination of live data and the identification of potential centers [10]. Figure 1.5 shows the overview of different ways of applying predictive analysis in the Medicare industry.

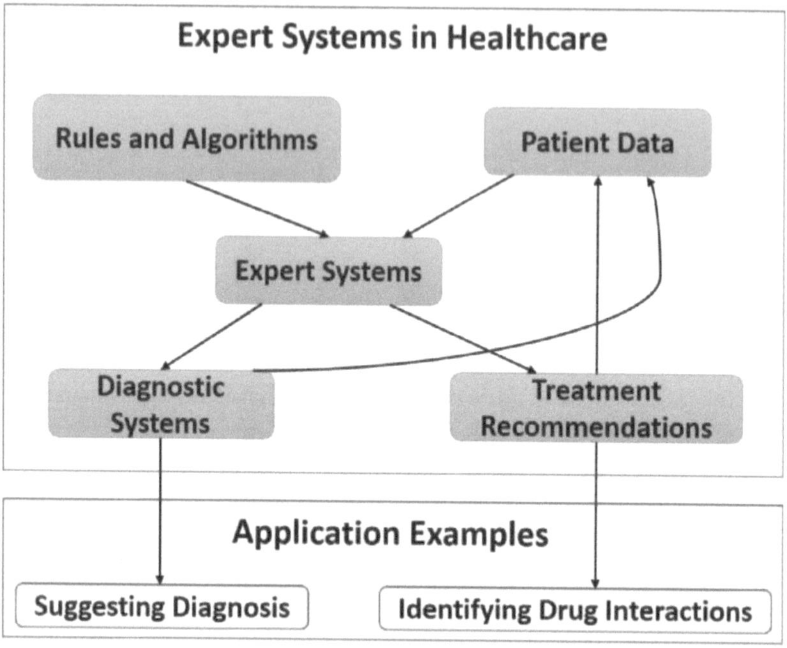

FIGURE 1.4 High-level overview of how expert systems work.

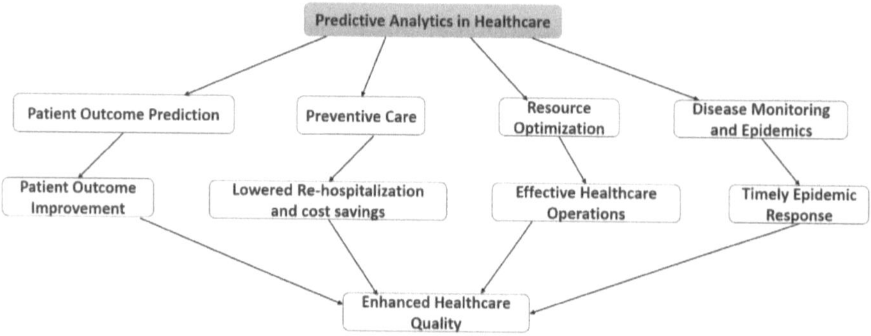

FIGURE 1.5 Different ways of applying predictive analysis in the Medicare industry.

1.3.6 Electronic Health Records (EHR) and Interoperability

The emergence of electronic health records (EHRs) has completely revolutionized the health-related records paradigm [11]. AI-enabled EHR systems systematize the process of acquiring information about patients in a simplified, easily retrievable, and secure format. If individuals provide information on paper forms, several problems can arise, which are familiar to anyone who has visited a hospital or walk-in clinic. Additionally, EHRs with AI algorithms can analyze patient records to identify potential drug–drug interactions or other clinical decision-support functions. Another key area in healthcare is interoperability, which helps ensure that different healthcare systems can communicate with one another. Through the standardization of data formats and protocols, AI makes it possible to share patient information easily among healthcare providers and the systems through which healthcare is accessed. This interoperability supports better coordination of patient care by minimizing duplication and enhances overall efficiency in the provision of healthcare services [12]. Figure 1.6 shows the conjunction of EHR with AI to provide advances in healthcare.

1.4 TYPES OF AI APPLICATIONS IN MEDICINE

In this section, types of AI applications in medicine are described. Figure 1.7 shows six types of AI applications: diagnosis of diseases and risk prediction, drug discovery and development, personalization of treatment, medical imaging and radiology, robotics in healthcare, and natural language processing for medical documentation.

The details of each applications can be found in Table 1.2.

1.4.1 Diagnosis of Diseases and Risk Prediction

AI is abundantly useful in the diagnosis of diseases and risk prediction. Some ML algorithms can analyze patient information such as genetics, medical history, and symptoms to identify the existence of diseases and predict individual risks. Prominent examples include IBM Watson for Oncology, which aids in making cancer treatment choices, and DeepMind by Google, which anticipates patient deterioration through an analysis of medical records [6].

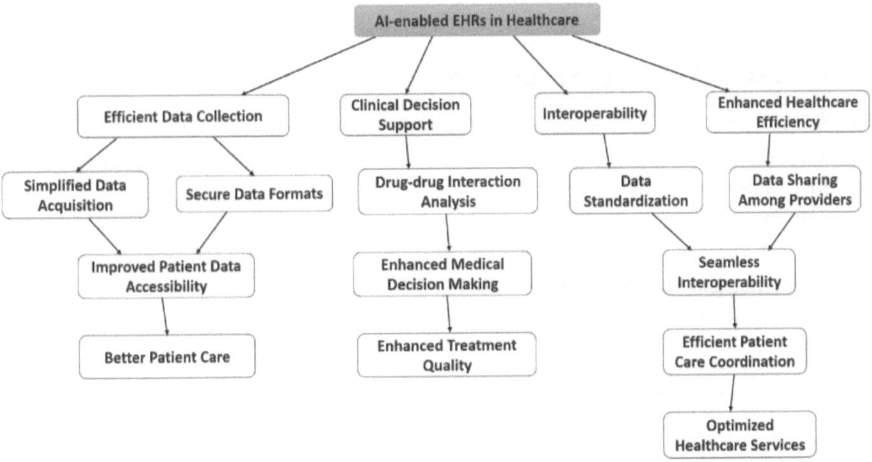

FIGURE 1.6 Conjunction of EHR with AI to provide advances in healthcare.

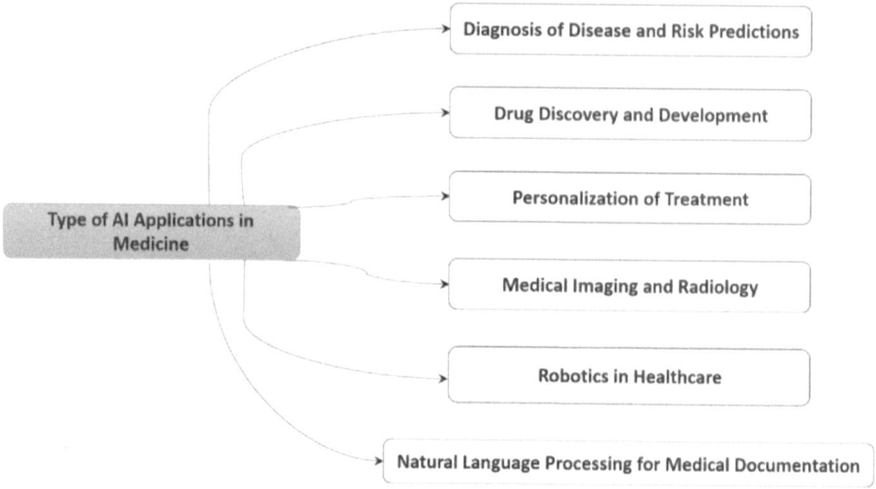

FIGURE 1.7 Applications of AI in the healthcare industry.

TABLE 1.2
Brief Overview of the Different Applications of AI in Healthcare

Application	Description
Diagnosis of diseases and risk prediction	AI aids in disease diagnosis and risk assessment [6].
Drug discovery and development	Accelerates drug research and development [7].
Personalization of treatment	Tailors medical interventions for individuals [12].
Medical imaging and radiology	Enhances image analysis for precise diagnoses [8].
Robotics in healthcare	Automates tasks and assists in medical procedures.
NLP for medical documentation	Streamlines medical data management [7].

1.4.2 Drug Discovery and Development

AI speeds up the process of drug discovery and development by analyzing massive datasets and simulating molecular interactions. This significantly reduces the time and cost implications of bringing new drugs to the market. For instance, Atomwise uses DL to screen billions of chemical compounds in search of suitable drug candidates. Another example is BenevolentAI, which employs AI to identify new drug targets for designing new drugs and even determines which existing drugs can be repurposed for treating other conditions [7].

1.4.3 Personalization of Treatment

AI facilitates personalized treatment plans by incorporating variations at an individual level, considering genetics, lifestyle, and medical history. In particular, oncologists can personalize cancer treatment using AI based on the genetic profile related to the tumor as well as the patient. Companies such as Tempus provide platforms that converge and analyze clinical and molecular data for use by oncologists, broadly enabling personalized treatment decision support [12].

1.4.4 Medical Imaging and Radiology

The technology employed by AI has truly revolutionized medical imaging. DL algorithms work by thoroughly examining X-rays, MRIs, and CT scans to identify anomalies, providing fast and accurate diagnoses. The Edison AI platform is one of GE Healthcare's recent solutions, utilizing AI technology to enhance the interpretation of medical images. Zebra Medical Vision's algorithms are capable of identifying diseases through image analysis, ranging from breast cancer to liver diseases [8]

1.4.5 Robotics in Healthcare

From surgical interventions and rehabilitation treatments to diagnostics and pathology, there is a very wide range of applications for robotics in healthcare. Surgical robots, such as the da Vinci Surgical System, assist surgeons in performing surgeries minimally and with a very high degree of precision. Apart from surgery, they are also used in patient care, including robotic exoskeletons that aid individuals with mobility problems. Additionally, robotic pharmacists work in hospitals for medicine dispensing.

1.4.6 Natural Language Processing for Medical Documentation

With NLP-powered AI algorithms, documentation and records management in the medical field are becoming much easier. The NLP accelerates the extraction of information from clinical notes and records, facilitating quicker access to data and analysis. For example, M*Modal NLP platform converts transcriptions of dictated spoken medical language into text. Beyond these applications, NLP is also helpful in automating coding and billing in healthcare, reducing administrative burdens and errors alike [7].

1.5 CHALLENGES AND ETHICAL CONSIDERATIONS

1.5.1 Data Privacy and Security

Data privacy and security issues take precedence over the incorporation of ethics in AI usage for healthcare. Over time, EHRs have flooded the health sector, making AI a prerequisite for managing the data. Therefore, protecting the confidentiality of patients is a major concern. A breach may lead to the exposure or misuse of a patient's data, making them victims of identity theft, fraudulent claims, as well as unauthorized access to sensitive medical records without their consent. Healthcare establishments should implement strong measures within every cybersecurity strategy and protection plan, including encryption, firewalls, and access controls to secure patient's data. Simultaneously, it is important to conduct regular security audits, ensuring compliance with data protection regulations such as HIPAA in the United States.

Moreover, clear and informed consent mechanisms around data use should be established so that patients have more power over how their data are used for AI applications. Thus effective patient education about the benefits of AI, along with a commitment to privacy, will be crucial in building faith and confidence on the part of the patients [13,14]. The types of data privacy and security can be seen in Figure 1.8.

1.5.2 Bias and Fairness

The ethical challenge of bias in AI healthcare algorithms is a significant issue. The data used to train an AI system may contain inherent bias, leading to the system generating inaccurate, unfair, or prejudiced results. This concern is particularly critical in healthcare, as biased algorithms could result in real-world, life-altering consequences. Ensuring fairness in AI algorithms goes beyond avoiding discrimination; it entails achieving equal and accurate performance across diverse population groups. Developers should utilize diversified and representative datasets that include a range of demographic groups, ensuring that their training data are not skewed toward any specific segment. Implementing bias detection mechanisms can help identify biases, allowing developers to take proactive measures to mitigate them during the development process.

Furthermore, transparency is a crucial requirement for accurately portraying the performance of AI systems across various demographic groups. Conducting regular audits of AI algorithms, specifically focusing on fairness and bias, is essential to address ethical concerns. This approach ensures that AI systems deliver fair performance across all categories of patients. By implementing these strategies and adhering to them, healthcare institutions can instill confidence in patients, healthcare providers, and regulatory bodies, thereby fostering ethical practices in AI healthcare [15].

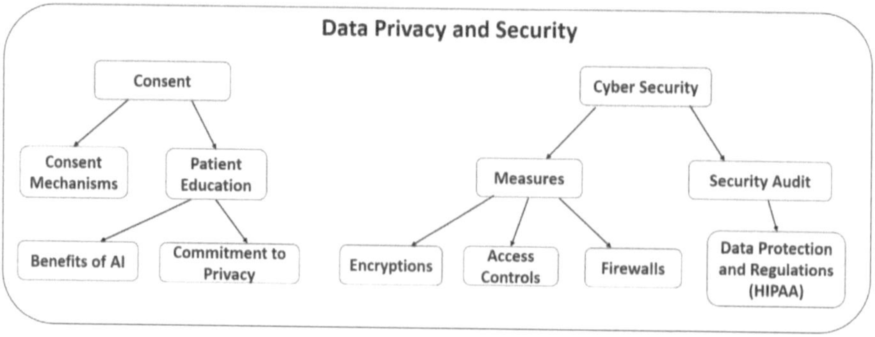

FIGURE 1.8 Advancing data privacy and security measures to protect individuals in the era of AI.

1.6 CASE STUDIES

1.6.1 PathAI: Enhancing Pathology Diagnostics

1. **Historical Context Pathology**: Pathology is a crucial element in medical diagnosis and treatment decisions. In the traditional context, pathologists identify various abnormalities and diseases through a manual review of tissue samples. The methodology behind this process involves complexity and subjectivity, making it time-consuming and susceptible to human errors. Against this backdrop, PathAI was launched in 2016, aiming to integrate AI into pathology diagnostics. Figure 1.9 shows a brief overview of how PathAI changed traditional pathology.
2. **Concepts Underlying AI Technologies**: PathAI's underlying concept revolves around assisting pathologists in making better and more effective use of AI for diagnostic decisions. Leveraging the latest in DL and computer vision algorithms, the platform analyzes high-resolution images of pathology slides. It achieves state-of-the-art levels of sensitivity, enabling the detection of even subtle abnormalities with a high degree of accuracy, identification of tissue structures, and classification of cell types. PathAI is designed to continuously learn from the massive volumes of data inputted into it, refining its diagnostic capabilities over time. Providing standardized reports with quantified information for pathologists means that it has the potential to result in more objective and consistent diagnoses.
3. **Impact on Healthcare**:

   Increase in Diagnosis Accuracy: The incorporation of AI in pathology allows pathologists to improve the accuracy of certain diagnoses, reducing the likelihood of error that may arise from misdiagnoses. This improvement contributes to enhanced healthcare outcomes and overall patient care.

   Efficiency and Speed: PathAI introduces speed into the diagnostic process. The software can rapidly process and analyze pathology slides much more quickly than a human could sift through them. This reduces waiting times for patients, which has a significant practical impact over time, enabling faster treatment decisions.

   Standardization and Objectivity: The implementation of AI in pathology leads to standardized and objective reports with quantifiable data. This minimizes subjectivity associated with the diagnosis procedures and ensures consistent standards in the quality of care.
4. **Challenges and Limitations**: Although AI integration in pathology diagnostics holds immense promise, it is also subject to multiple challenges. The quality and representativeness of training data are the key concepts requiring protection from biases and errors. Pathologists might need some time to adjust to working with AI systems, and the level of trust in AI recommendations may be a factor. In addition, the expenses associated with implementing AI technology within a clinic and ensuring compliance with no treatment neglected are real challenges that will persist. Moreover, ongoing

maintenance and updates are required to keep the system up-to-date and accurate.

The incorporation of AI in pathology diagnostics demonstrates the potential for significantly improving healthcare outcomes through enhanced diagnostic accuracy, efficiency, and objectivity. Challenges such as quality of data, trust, and regulatory compliance need to be addressed for continued success with AI in pathology and healthcare at large [16].

1.6.2 IBM Watson for Oncology

1. **Historical Context**: IBM Watson for Oncology represents a shining example of the actual implementation of AI in fundamental Medicare technologies. This system has been developed under conditions characterized by the increasing complexity of cancer care provision and the need for personalized treatment. Elaborate medical literature and clinical trials have always been used in traditional oncology practices to formulate the best treatment plan for a specific patient. However, it became challenging to keep pace with the rapid expansion of knowledge in oncology. The IBM Watson for Oncology was developed in 2013 to address the situation. The high-level view of IBM Watson for Oncology can be found in Figure 1.10.
2. **Underlying Concepts and AI Technologies**: In the case of IBM Watson for Oncology, the underlying concept is that the AI should provide precise recommendations and guidance based on evidence from the latest research, tailored to the specific history of the patient. It utilizes NLP and ML techniques to analyze vast amounts of clinical and research data, encompassing medical records, research papers, treatment guidelines, and patient histories.

   The system interprets such unstructured data, extracts valuable information, and offers personalized treatment recommendations. It aligns medical literature with patient-specific data, enabling oncologists to make rapid decisions. IBM Watson for Oncology also evolves, adapting to each interaction to continually enhance its advice.
3. **Impact on Healthcare**:

   Improved Treatment Decisions: Watson for Oncology enhances the quality and accuracy of treatments provided to oncologists based on evidence. This enables physicians to offer more precise and personalized treatments, ultimately influencing patient outcomes.

   Cost Efficiency: AI-powered systems such as Watson for Oncology, enable healthcare providers to fine-tune treatment plans, allowing for optimal treatments and avoiding unnecessary costs. This contributes to making the healthcare system more cost-efficient.

   Patient Experiences: Patients benefit from more individualized and successful treatment plans. They gain the ability to access the most current medical research, instilling trust in their caregivers and significantly enhancing their overall experiences on a larger scale.

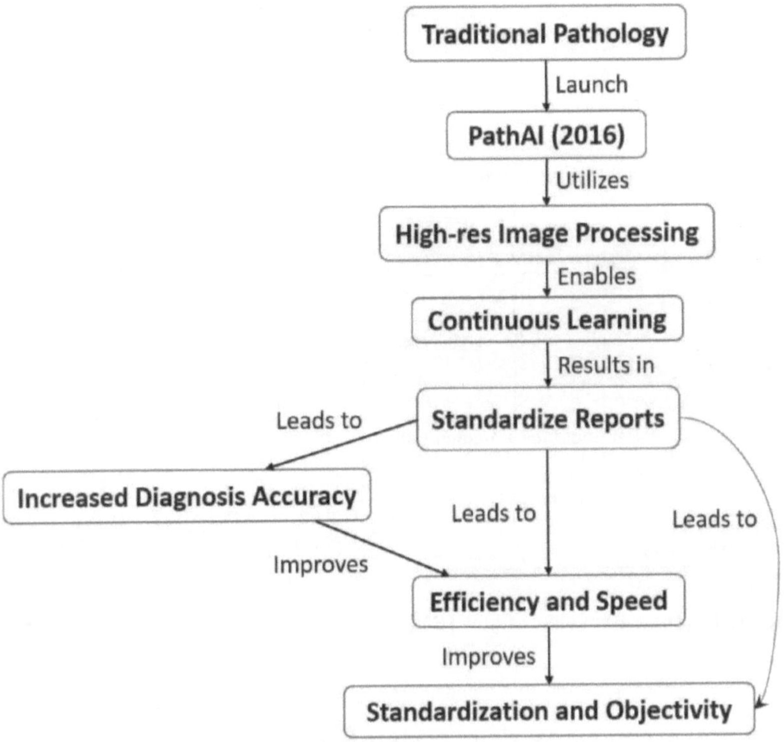

FIGURE 1.9 Brief overview of PathAI-changed traditional pathology.

4. **Challenges and Limitations**: However, the implementation of AI in healthcare through systems such as IBM Watson for Oncology also presents several challenges. Data privacy and security of the patient records must be guaranteed alongside these advantages. Consequently, there is a potential for bias in the AI algorithms that need continuous monitoring to prevent erroneous recommendations. Furthermore, the integration of AI systems into existing healthcare workflows and resistance from some healthcare providers to fully trust AI recommendations can be a significant hindering factors. Lastly, the initial substantial costs of implementing such systems, along with the pressing need for continued training, can pose considerable roadblocks.

   In summary, IBM Watson for Oncology serves as a testament to the successful integration of AI into Medicare technologies, enhancing the quality of healthcare outcomes delivery, cost-effectiveness, and overall patient experience. However, overcoming challenges such as data privacy and bias, integration hurdles, and the substantial costs involved are critical determinants for the continued success of AI advancement in healthcare [17].

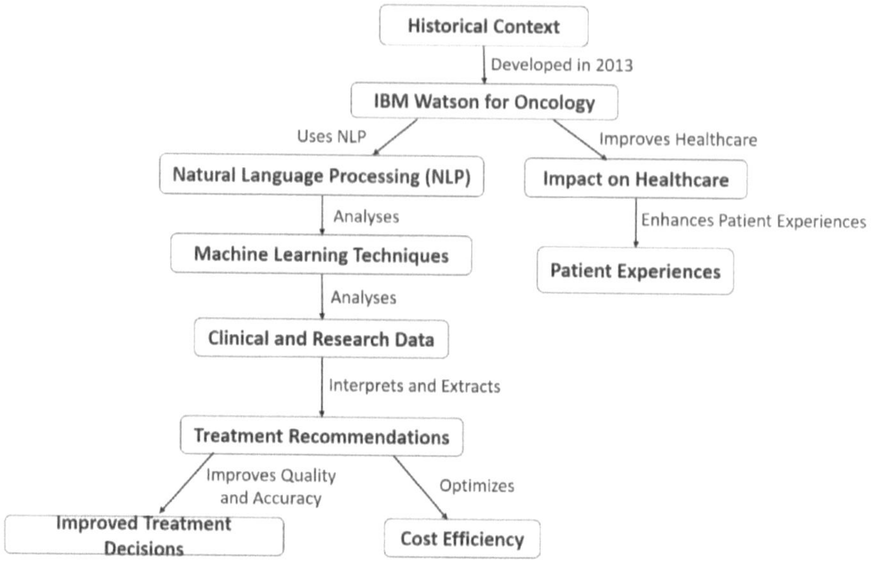

FIGURE 1.10 High-level view of how IBM Watson is used in the healthcare industry.
Source: Ref. [18].

1.7 CURRENT TRENDS AND FUTURE PROJECTS

1.7.1 Trends in the Recent Past in AI Application within Medicare

Within the recent past and with the immense improvement of technology, applications of AI have showcased dramatic trends and changes within the Medicare system. One trend dominating the field is the increased accuracy and efficiency in disease detection and subsequent diagnosis. DL algorithms for retinal images to predict cardiovascular risk factors are also available, using AI-powered diagnostic tools such as Google Health.

Another important trend is the movement toward personalization of treatment plans for individuals. AI, through analysis of patient information using ML algorithms, develops individualized medicines based on genetics, history of illnesses, and lifestyle, among other factors. This not only serves to improve the treatment results but also minimizes the side effects.

In addition, telemedicine and remote patient monitoring have grown significantly during the COVID-19 pandemic where AI is on the front line in facilitating access to healthcare remotely. The trends are expected to continue growing, making the accessibility of healthcare much easier and more convenient among patients [19].

1.7.2 Future Developments and Initiatives

AI is bound to have an even wider scope in the healthcare field in the days to come. Most notably, AI transforms drug discovery and development, potentially reducing the time and cost involved in deploying new drugs to the market. AI can aid researchers in identifying drug candidates and predicting the effectiveness of drugs against certain diseases to a certain extent, thus expanding access to novel treatments.

Anticipation by AI is further driven by predictive analytic integration in healthcare. Through the analysis of such patient data, providers could predict disease outbreaks, optimally allocate resources, and improve care delivery. This is anticipated to enhance both the quality of good health and resource utilization, as well as cost-effectiveness, respectively.

As AI continues to rise and transform the provision of healthcare, ethics and regulatory interventions become even more critical. The delicate balance between data privacy, bias mitigation, and transparent AI decision-making is crucial to placing patients at the forefront while ensuring the security and safety of their data. AI-powered decision support systems will also be integrated more deeply into the clinical workflows, providing real-time guidance to healthcare professionals and improving the quality of care while reducing the risks of medical errors. Hence, the major promise for the future lies in the impact of AI on shaping up the Medicare system and broader landscape of healthcare [20].

1.8 CONCLUSION

The integration of AI into healthcare is inevitable due to rapid technological advancements. From early applications to current use, AI, encompassing machine learning (ML), deep learning (DL), and natural language processing (NLP), has played a crucial role in diagnosing, treatment decisions, disease outcome prediction, treatment plan optimization, drug candidate identification, medical image analysis, and medical documentation processing. The case of PathAI for enhancing pathology diagnostics and IBM Watson for oncology are examined in detail in this chapter. While AI holds great promise for future Medicare, challenges such as data privacy, security, bias, and fairness must be addressed. Despite these challenges, the ongoing development of AI in healthcare is unstoppable. The aspiration is for the ongoing growth and transformation of AI in healthcare to significantly enhance professionals' capabilities in diagnoses, treatment plans, and other medical decision-making processes, particularly in the era of personalized and effective healthcare.

REFERENCES

[1] Jiang F, Jiang Y, Zhi H, et al. Artificial intelligence in healthcare: Past, present and future. *Stroke and Vascular Neurology*. 2017;2(4).

[2] Bohr A, Memarzadeh K. The rise of artificial intelligence in healthcare applications. In: *Artificial intelligence in healthcare*. Elsevier; 2020. pp. 25–60.

[3] Shortliffe EH, Shah NH. AI in medicine: Some pertinent history. In: *Intelligent systems in medicine and health: The role of AI*. Springer; 2022. pp. 21–50.

[4] Thakkar HK, Chowdhury SR, Bhoi AK, et al. Applications of wearable technologies in healthcare: An analytical study. In: *5G IoT and edge computing for smart healthcare*. Elsevier; 2022. pp. 279–299.

[5] Singh P, Devi KJ, Thakkar HK, et al. Region-based hybrid medical image watermarking scheme for robust and secured transmission in IoMT. *IEEE Access*. 2022;10:8974–8993.

[6] Garg A, Venkataramani VV, Karthikeyan A, et al. Modern AI/ML methods for healthcare: Opportunities and challenges. In: *International conference on distributed computing and internet technology*. Springer; 2022. pp. 3–25.

[7] Locke S, Bashall A, Al-Adely S, et al. Natural language processing in medicine: A review. *Trends in Anaesthesia and Critical Care*. 2021;38:4–9.

[8] Pun T, Gerig G, Ratib O. Image analysis and computer vision in medicine. *Computerized Medical Imaging and Graphics*. 1994;18(2):85–96.

[9] Zhou L, Sordo M. Chapter 5—Expert systems in medicine. In: Xing L, Giger ML, Min JK, editors. *Artificial intelligence in medicine*. Academic Press; 2021. pp. 75–100. Available from: https://www.sciencedirect.com/science/article/pii/B9780128212592000053.

[10] Janke AT, Overbeek DL, Kocher KE, et al. Exploring the potential of predictive analytics and big data in emergency care. *Annals of Emergency Medicine*. 2016;67(2):227–236.

[11] Zala K, Thakkar HK, Jadeja R, et al. On the design of secured and reliable dynamic access control scheme of patient e-healthcare records in cloud environment. *Computational Intelligence and Neuroscience*. 2022:3804553.

[12] Jardim SV. The electronic health record and its contribution to healthcare information systems interoperability. *Procedia Technology*. 2013;9:940–948.

[13] Blobel B, Lopez D, Gonzalez C. Patient privacy and security concerns on big data for personalized medicine. *Health and Technology*. 2016;6:75–81.

[14] Devi KJ, Singh P, Dash JK, et al. Secure transmission of medical images in multi-cloud e-healthcare applications using data hiding scheme. *Journal of Information Security and Applications*. 2023;79:103655.

[15] Chen RJ, Wang JJ, Williamson DF, et al. Algorithmic fairness in artificial intelligence for medicine and healthcare. *Nature Biomedical Engineering*. 2023;7(6):719–742.

[16] Bera K, Schalper KA, Rimm DL, et al. Artificial intelligence in digital pathology—new tools for diagnosis and precision oncology. *Nature Reviews Clinical Oncology*. 2019;16(11):703–715.

[17] Hamilton JG, Genoff Garzon M, Westerman JS, et al. "A tool, not a crutch": Patient perspectives about IBM Watson for Oncology trained by Memorial Sloan Kettering. *Journal of Oncology Practice*. 2019;15(4):e277–e288.

[18] Kohn MS, Sun J, Knoop S, et al. IBM's health analytics and clinical decision support. *Yearbook of Medical Informatics*. 2014;23(1):154–162.

[19] Parikh D, Armstrong G, Liou V, et al. Advances in telemedicine in ophthalmology. In: *Seminars in ophthalmology*; Vol. 35. Taylor & Francis; 2020. pp. 210–215.

[20] Kumar K, Kumar P, Deb D, et al. Artificial intelligence and machine learning based intervention in medical infrastructure: A review and future trends. In: *Healthcare*; Vol. 11. MDPI; 2023. p. 207.

2 Recent Advancements and Issues in AI for Health 5.0

Nabhi Shah, Shital Patel, Rinkal Jain, and Alessandro Bruno

2.1 INTRODUCTION

AI-powered Healthcare 5.0 has the potential to revolutionize the healthcare industry. In the future, technology, including artificial intelligence, must be made accessible, understandable, and affordable to meet patient demands. Collectively, the case studies highlight the significance of adopting AI-driven solutions while continually enhancing and customizing them to match the needs of the healthcare business, eventually resulting in improved patient care and results. Health 5.0 differs from earlier versions, such as Health 4.0, in that it supports the concept of providing customized and personalized treatments. To support personalized treatments, Health 5.0 AI models must consider the various aspects of the patient's data such as medical history, age, gender, geographical location, etc. Such personalized treatment is expected to be more effective in generic treatment, and at the same time it is expected to reduce the financial burden by eliminating the unnecessary checkups and test.

Health 5.0 AI models are expected to continue the legacy of healthcare services and has enabled real-time virtual patient monitoring as well as sensor-based data gathering through smart wearable devices.

Healthcare practitioners are immediately notified of abnormalities or deviations from baseline health data, ensuring quick action in urgent cases. Patients, especially those with chronic diseases, benefit from additional security because of this real-time monitoring.

In addition to providing therapy and diagnostics, Health 5.0 simplifies hospital procedures. AI-driven solutions automate routine administrative chores like arranging appointments, managing electronic health records, and billing, giving healthcare workers more time to focus on providing direct patient care. By decreasing wait times, lowering mistakes, and improving the entire patient experience, this enhanced efficiency is a win–win for patients and healthcare professionals. In short, by incorporating artificial intelligence into every aspect of the healthcare sector, Health 5.0 is positioned to transform the industry entirely. Precision, customization, and efficiency combine to build a healthcare system that genuinely places the patient at its center. Figure 2.1 illustrates a few other applications of AI. We cannot limit these applications to a number; hence imagination is the limit when it comes to applying AI in healthcare.

DOI: 10.1201/9781003393498-3

2.1.1 Obstacles of AI in Healthcare

However, several obstacles and other ethical considerations are linked to the use of artificial intelligence (AI) in Healthcare 5.0. Usually, the AI models need to be trained on a large pool of sensitive patient's data for reliability. However, it is very challenging to provide data security and the privacy of the patient's data against unauthorized access. Moreover, the trained AI model may generate biased outputs if not trained on a diversified and well-balanced dataset. Therefore, it is essential to consider these suggestions and ethical considerations while designing a robust AI model for efficient healthcare service delivery.

The solutions to these challenges required elaboration and discussion across the scientific communities and researchers. It is observed that researchers are working on the major obstacles of the AI in healthcare to provide reliable as well as efficient remedies.

The rest of the chapter is organized as follows: We first discuss the recent advancements observed in AI that reflect advantageous applications in Health 5.0. We then discuss some of the significant concerns that AI and its applications raise. The chapter concludes after we discuss some real applications of AI, with a discussion on the feasibility of AI applications to healthcare, specifically in the 5.0 era.

2.2 LATEST ADVANCEMENTS OF AI FOR HEALTH 5.0

2.2.1 Prediction Analysis

Predictive analytics in healthcare is analyzing historical healthcare data to identify patterns and trends that may predict future events. Predictive analytics in healthcare can predict the likelihood of particular health conditions, clinical decisions, trends, and even disease spread.

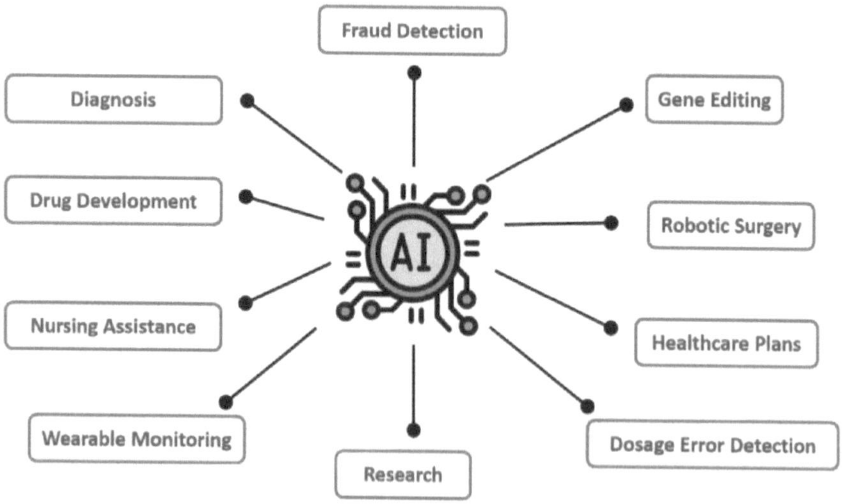

FIGURE 2.1 Applications of AI in healthcare.

The benefits of predictive analytics in healthcare are as follows:

1. **Enhanced Patient Care and Outcomes**: Using historical and current data, predictive analytics in healthcare enhances patient care and outcomes by identifying high-risk individuals and assisting in the early detection of diseases like cancer or heart disease. The possibility of survival rises, and timely interventions are made possible.
2. **Cost Reduction and Efficiency Improvements**: In the healthcare industry, predictive analytics facilitates targeted discharge planning and follow-up care, predicts patient readmissions, and efficiently manages inventory to ensure resource efficiency and minimize waste.
3. **Enhanced Disease Management**: By tracking health data from wearables and electronic records, predictive analytics improves the management of chronic diseases while reducing the overall hospitalization rates. Moreover, it improves the activities of the daily living of the patients and ensures improved quality of life.
4. **Personalized Medicine**: The predictive AI models likely analyzes the various parameters, such as lifestyle, habits, sleeping patterns, weather and conditions, and may provide personalized medication schedules with customized treatment plans.
5. **Improved Health Insurance Models**: The incorporation of predictive analytics is likely to assist the health insurance companies to improvize their medical service delivery by providing customized health insurance plans that may reduce the overall premium and saves millions of dollars for companies.

Figure 2.2 shows the four-step process of predictive analysis such as data gathering, data scrutiny and analysis, model designing, and applications. Each step may have different implications based on the data type and use-case.

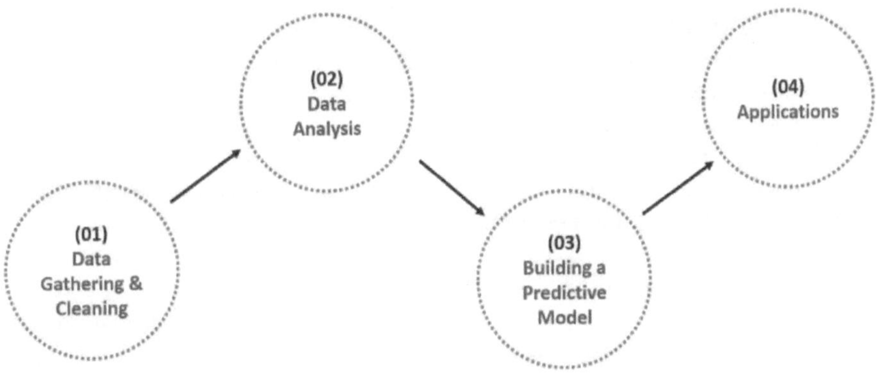

FIGURE 2.2 Four-step process to predictive analysis.

2.2.2 Explainable AI (XAI) in Healthcare

Explainable AI (XAI) is a set of methods, architecture, and processes that help the machine learning engineer to understand the reasoning behind the AI model's decision-making process. The primary concern of AI models is the opacity of its result generation and lack of model's interpretability [1]. However, the use of XAI in healthcare-related AI applications tries to mitigate the challenges of accountability and interpretability. It is to be noted that in the XAI domain, the terms "explainable" and "interpretable" are used interchangeably. Usually, the explainable models use post hoc analysis to support the predictions made. On the contrary, interpretable models generate the outputs that humans can easily understand. The very purpose of XAI is to make users understand the objective and rationale behind the decision-making process of the AI models. The information obtained can be used further as follows.

1. To improve the accuracy of the model
2. To identify and address the undesirable behaviors of the models such as biased decision-making
3. To assist in the interpretation of various AI models in healthcare domains such as medical imaging
4. To build trust and confidence in AI models for further deployment into production

The following are the few applications in healthcare using XAI:

- **XAI for Decision-Making**: Generally, the fundamental idea behind engaging XAI is to facilitate understanding about how the AI models make decisions. Such understanding eventually helps the healthcare professionals to make an informed decision and comprehend the underlying concepts behind decision-making. The role of XAI becomes crucial in areas where the decision is solely made by the AI models and not by the healthcare professional.
- **XAI to Detect Biased AI Models**: The XAI-obtained understanding of the AI models significantly helps to identify the biasness in AI models. Bias identification is crucial as it may produce erroneous results, leading to incorrect diagnosis and treatment.
- **XAI for Transparency**: The use of XAI results in more confidence in the model's output generation and therefore provide transparency, which will help the healthcare professional to summarize the decision-making process. This results in greater acceptance of the models in the healthcare industry.
- **XAI to Generate New AI Systems**: The interpretability of XAI may assist in designing new AI systems from the existing ones, which is likely to further improvize prediction accuracy with more reliability.

Figure 2.3 shows the comparison between black box AI and white box XAI.

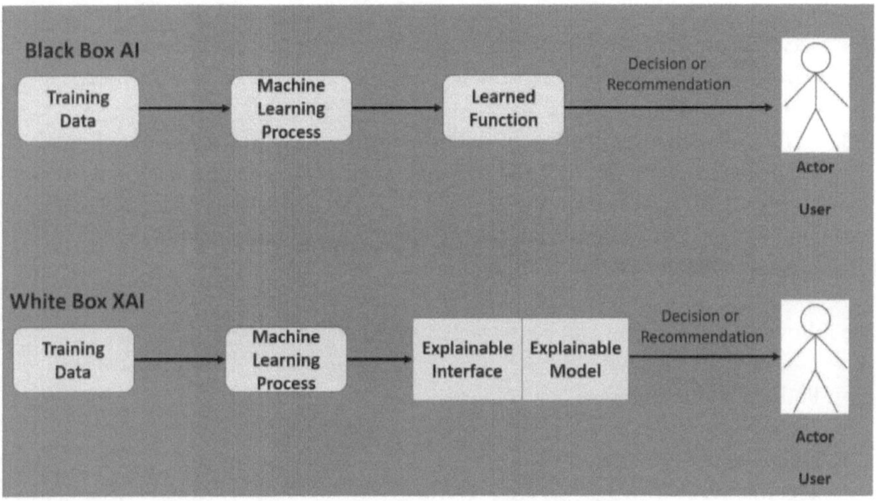

FIGURE 2.3 Black box AI vs. white box XAI.

In black box AI systems, the AI model merely provides the decision or recommendation. However, it does not explain how the model reaches a certain decision. On the contrary, white box XAI models provide the explainable model rather than the AI model with the explainable interface, along with the decision and recommendation.

2.2.3 Use of Natural Language Processing (NLP) in Healthcare

Natural language processing (NLP) is a subfield in computer science and deals with the way humans and machines interact in a natural manner. The emergence of novel NLP models made it more applicable to various healthcare applications. For instance, the NLP can be engaged to decipher the meaning of the clinical notes of the doctors and obtain the insights to form assistive feedbacks. Moreover, the ability of the NLP to identify and bridge the context among the words in a sentence allows us to interpret the patient–doctor conversion in a meaningful manner with improved reliability. The natural engagement of NLP helps healthcare practitioners to manage healthcare data for clinical testing, treatment places and follow-ups for improved healthcare services.

The following are the advantages of engaging the NLP in the healthcare domain:

1. Overall improvement in the way patient interacts with the healthcare service provider. NLP likely bridges the knowledge gap among the complex medical jargons and ease the overall communication among the various stakeholders. We can increase patient health literacy by using machine learning models to interpret patient health data.
2. Improvement in overall healthcare service quality with effective evaluation.

3. Robust NLP algorithms trained on sufficiently large and diversified datasets can produce detailed insights about the patient's conditions and help doctors prepare a robust treatment plan for complicated and challenging patient conditions.
4. NLP tools can effectively deal with the unstructured nature of the clinical records written by doctors and patients. Such comments are insightful and constructive. However, in the absence of the NLP methods, these notes are not helpful. Therefore NLP tools are engaged to comprehend the challenging nature of unstructured clinical notes.

The following information can be extracted by NLP algorithms.

- Patient demographics
- Symptoms
- Diagnoses
- Treatments
- Medications
- Allergies
- Social history
- Family history

This information is crucial and help make the improved diagnosis plan and treatment procedure. Careful and meaningful use of this information from NLP can likely help identify the person with a greater risk of a certain disease. Moreover, it also helps us understand the effectiveness of certain treatment procedures and therapy. In several cases, NLP bridges the gap between patients and doctors from diversified backgrounds by supporting and designing a multilingual systems for translation purposes.

For instance, in [2], NLP models have demonstrated the successful extraction of terms related to "smoking" from unstructured multilingual electronic health records (EHRs). Usually, electronic health records contain details about the medical history of the patients along with the current health condition. In Figure 2.4, an approach is suggested on how NLP models work on the unstructured nature of the EHRs including in Korean, Chinese, and English. The method is intended to extract smoking-related keywords from multilingual electronic health records (EHRs) in both Korean and English.

In order to identify all the terms related to "smoking," a novel strategy was employed called shifted positive point mutual information (SPPMI), [2] as shown in Figure 2.4. There are three primary phases: data preprocessing, seed keyword generation, and term extraction with similarity metrics. Leveraging SPPMI methods coupled with machine learning models significantly increases the accuracy of the keyword identification and subsequent categorization.

2.2.4 LLM-Assisted Health 5.0

In the evolution of the healthcare industry from Healthcare 1.0 to Healthcare 5.0, Healthcare 5.0 uses state-of-the-art intelligent tools and devises healthcare strategies

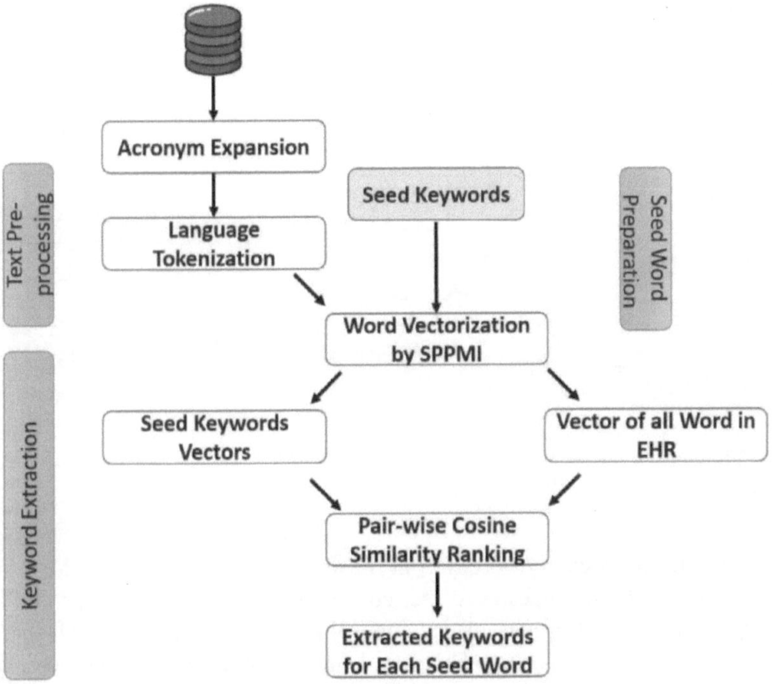

FIGURE 2.4 Step-by-step method for SPPMI technique.

considering the patient centered on the patient. Several advanced technologies are used in Healthcare 5.0. However, large language models (LLMs) are highly useful and play a pivotal role for further advancement. For instance, a recently released model called Med-PaLM 2 from Google, generated high-quality responses to medical questions. Their proficiency in analyzing large amounts of data, drawing conclusions, and crafting human-grade writing results in advancements in the medical field. LLMs have the potential to change many aspects of healthcare, and in this chapter, we'll see how they can make healthcare better for patients, researchers, and doctors. Figure 2.5 illustrates various uses of LLM in Healthcare.

The very capability of LLMs to rapidly read the tons of input medical data and to process it provides an opportunity to the doctors to make patient-centric decisions in a quick manner. LLMS may be engaged to diagnose rare diseases that are difficult to diagnose manually. Moreover, it also helps plan possible alternative treatment plans generation and may generate warnings for certain medical conditions. On the other hand, LLM also suggests customized and personalized medicine based on specific patient-centric medical parameters such as age, gender, habits, test results etc. These advantages put LLM at the forefront of Healthcare 5.0 with better suggestions for therapies with fewer side effects.

It is observed that the LLMs are efficient in reading, deciphering, and understanding written human language. Therefore, LLMs are considered helpful to doctors in noting down patients' medical conditions and keeping patients' records while

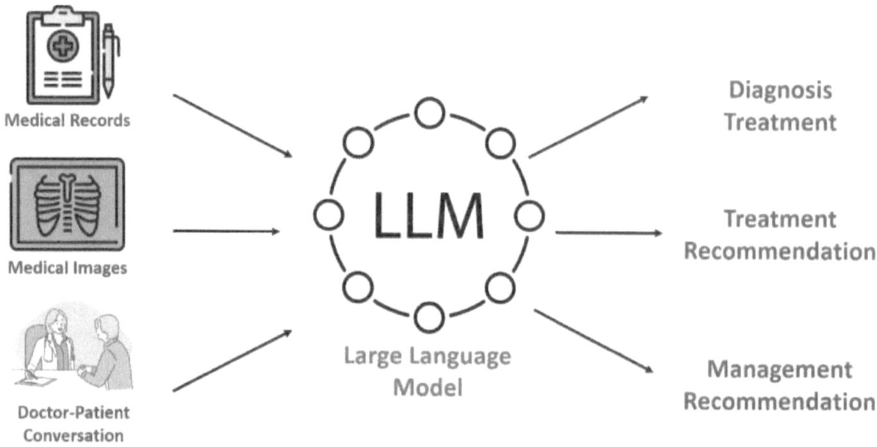

FIGURE 2.5 LLMs use in healthcare.

interacting with the doctors. Moreover, in the area of drug research, LLMs process tons of medical data to suggest a further course of action. In some areas, the LLM models may suggest preliminary drug composition and the set of chemicals that may work for producing certain drugs. This way, LLM can make the entire process faster for new drug discovery and reduce the overall cost. Additionally, new trends are emerging to engage LLMs for designing chatbots and virtual helpers. However, such robo chatbots are in the preliminary stage, and they assist the patients with basic tasks such as talking with patients, answering basic queries, and making appointments.

Table 2.1 lists the potential use-cases of engagement of LLMs with respect to assistance to the doctor and patients.

2.3 CONCERNS OF AI IN HEALTHCARE

2.3.1 Disadvantages of AI in Healthcare

The disadvantages of the use of AI in healthcare can be described in detail as follows:

- **Diagnosis Bias**: The AI models are usually trained on a large pool of real-world data, which is comprised of diversified parameters such as gender, age, habits, and financial status, and therefore the trained models are highly likely to be biased if data is skewed and not properly balanced. Moreover, the models need to be trained on data that represents the generic behavior of the population and must capture the trend rather overfitting the given data [3].
- **Transparency**: AI models must be explainable, and the results they produce must be simple to understand and provide the underlying reasoning for the given set of predictions. AI models merely providing the output without explainability may complicate the diagnosis process [4]. The transparent model helps practitioners to comprehend the results and improves trust in it.

TABLE 2.1
Different Use-Cases of Large Language Models (LLMs) in Healthcare

Sr. No.	Use-Cases for Healthcare Professionals (Doctors)	Use-Cases for Patients
1.	**Documentation**: LLMs may help the professional to generate the reliable and detailed reports for better understanding. LLMs can potentially help convert the speech to text and generate the automated clinical documents.	**Health Assistant**: LLMs can help patients in the following manner. • Maintain health records • Symptoms tracking • Alerts and reminders • Personalized recommendations
2.	**Medical Investigation**: Articulate the research document. Provide up-to-date information on the current topics. Provide scientific backgrounds.	**Health Knowledge Discovery**: Patients may utilize LLMs as follows: • Obtain reliable and easy to understand health information. • Explain medical jargons in report in a simple layman language.
3.	**Diagnosis**: LLMs can assist as follows: Disease diagnosis Provide symptomatic analysis. Provide the medical background and history of a patient. Suggest alternative diagnosis methods. Suggest potential alternative tests to be conducted.	**Symptom Checker**: Symptoms analyzers Make symptom-based recommendations.
4	**Telemedicine**: Doctors can use LLMs for: • Remote virtual consultations. • Telemedicine • Virtual visits.	**Virtual Doctor Visits**: Patients can take the help of LLMs in the following manner: • Conduct virtual doctor visits. • Virtual consultations for non-emergency assistance. • Follow-up appointments for medical assistance.
5.	**Medical Transcription**: Transcribe the interaction of doctor and patient.	**Medication Management**: Keep track of medication schedules. Provide medication information and timely alerts for compliance.
6.	**Workflow Optimization**: LLMs can assist as follows: • Optimizing healthcare workflows • Streamlining administrative tasks • Appointment scheduling • Resource allocations such as consultation slots, operation theaters, etc.	**Health Monitoring**: Patients with chronic conditions can use LLMs as follows: • Health monitoring • Intimation for abnormal readings
7.	**Medical Coding**: LLMs can assist in assigning accurate medical codes for billing and insurance purposes, reducing billing errors.	**Insurance and Billing Assistance**: Patients can use LLMs to understand insurance claims, medical billing, and explanations of benefits, ensuring they are correctly charged for healthcare services.
8.	**Drug Interactions**: Doctors can use LLMs to check for potential drug interactions and contraindications when prescribing medications.	**Medication Interaction Checker**: Patients can verify possible interactions between their drugs and those prescribed by healthcare providers.

- **Privacy**: Because AI usage in healthcare needs data privacy as it uses the patient's data whose identity must not be revealed. The AI models must be designed in a way that can provide the results without revealing the personal identity as it is considered a sensitive medical record [5]. AI models designed to predict the heart disease may access sensitive medical information about the patients, which raises the potential challenge of safeguarding the medical data.
- **Mass Layoffs**: Recent advanced AI models based on natural language processing can automate human tasks to a certain extent and therefore are considered potential risk of the mass layoffs in the healthcare sectors. The AI-powered chatbots such as Alexa may answer basic patients' questions about their health.
- **Ethical Consequences**: The application of AI in healthcare may create severe societal impacts by mass layoffs and health disparities. The biased AI model for a certain population or region is more dangerous and may jeopardize overall health service delivery.
- **Data Security**: Inadequate security measure for patient data storage may provide an opportunity to the hacker for data theft and AI models' manipulation.
- **Interoperability**: Since each hospital and healthcare data collection center may collect data in a different way with different parameter names, it is highly complicated task to make the AI models interoperable across hospitals. Therefore, it is very important to have standardization in order to deal with heterogeneous systems [6].

These are only a few possible drawbacks to employing AI in Healthcare 5.0. Before applying AI solutions in healthcare, it is critical to assess these dangers thoroughly. However, keep in mind that AI has the potential to significantly enhance healthcare by making it more efficient, accurate, and accessible. The idea is to employ AI responsibly and ethically while also addressing the issues it presents.

2.4 CASE STUDIES

1. A Human-Centered Evaluation of a Deep Learning System Deployed in Clinics for the Detection of Diabetic Retinopathy—Google

To detect the condition known as diabetic retinopathy in people's eyes, Google developed a clever computer system. Although the technology performed well in tests, it could have performed better [7] when it was used in actual clinics in Thailand. The issue was that the way the technology was tested was different from how it was utilized in the clinics. The internet quality in specific clinics could have been better, and the quality of the nurses' photographs could have been improved for the system. Patients were displeased as a result of the delays.

The study concluded that new technology like this must match the actual world and its users. The researchers discovered that more than simply having a solid idea is required; you also need to consider that it will work in the real world.

TABLE 2.2
Recent Examples of Healthcare Chatbots

Chatbot Name	Description	Key Features
Healthily	Helps patients diagnose diseases based on symptoms and offers appointment booking and diagnosis center information.	Symptom-based diagnosis, appointment booking
Ada Health	Diagnoses diseases using patient symptoms, asks questions and connects patients with local healthcare experts.	Symptom-based diagnosis, medical condition information
Sensely	Collects user symptoms through text and voice, connects to Mayo Clinic info, and syncs with health devices.	Symptom collection, connection to healthcare experts
Babylon Health	Connects patients with virtual doctors based on symptoms and utilizes speech recognition and NLP for relevant results.	Direct connection to doctors, speech recognition
Buoy Health	Uses clinical data from medical journals, matches patient inputs with evidence-based data, and provides detailed symptom information.	Evidence-based data matching, symptom details
Forksy	Helps users track calorie intake, suggests healthy diet choices, and advises avoiding health risks.	Calorie tracking, diet suggestions
Cancer Chatbot	Provides comprehensive information on cancer, including research, clinical trials, and treatment options.	Cancer-related information, clinical trials

2. Various Healthcare Chatbots

Healthcare chatbots have proven highly effective in diagnostics, mental health, and patient engagement beyond medical facilities. A few examples have been shown in Table 2.2. Numerous research studies suggest a promising future for healthcare chatbots [8].

3. Arterys Cardio AI

Arterys Cardio AI [9] is advanced software for cardiac MRI (magnetic resonance imaging) analysis. The following are the prominent features of the system.

Critical Features of Arterys Cardio AI

1. **Efficient Workflow**: It saves MRI investigation time using deep learning and computing resources.
2. **Detailed Analysis**: It utilizes multisliced velocity-encoded MR images from multiple phases to analyze the heart and arteries.
3. **Clinically Relevant Data**: It provides measurable data to identify potential heart anomalies to aid health experts.
4. **Validation**: It is highly reliable as it has been validated for 1.5T and 3.0T MR images.

5. **Healthcare Professional Support**: It greatly aids the healthcare professional by providing interpretation of the images and data. However, it is not designed for standalone diagnosis.
6. **Training Data**: Thorough training on the huge collection of MR images was conducted along with domain experts' suggestion for increased accuracy.
7. **Performance Information**: It provides detailed performance results such as variance with respect to ground truth, the rate of detection, and DICE score.

Arterys Cardio AI is an intelligent technology that aids healthcare practitioners in swiftly and precisely analyzing cardiac MRI images, perhaps leading to faster and more exact diagnoses of heart-related diseases.

2.5 CONCLUSION

The case studies show how artificial intelligence transforms healthcare, particularly in Healthcare 5.0. These studies highlight the need to integrate and adapt new technologies to meet the complex real world's d ever-changing healthcare demands of the rare 5.0 driven by AI, which can potentially transform the healthcare business. Technology, especially artificial intelligence, must be adaptive to fulfil patient requests and real-world conditions in the future. Collectively, the case studies emphasize the need to implement AI-driven solutions while continuously improving and customizing them to meet the demands of the healthcare company, resulting in enhanced patient care and outcomes.

With this report, we realized that artificial intelligence (AI) is rapidly transforming the healthcare industry. AI-powered solutions are being used to improve patient care, expedite processes, and improve outcomes. However, several obstacles and ethical considerations are also linked with using artificial intelligence in healthcare.

Despite these challenges, the AI in healthcare provides significant advantages as follows.

- AI in healthcare likely enhances the detection accuracy of the diagnosis.
- It provides the customized healthcare with respect to the patient's condition.
- It helps automate the diagnosis and therefore may decrease cost.
- It likely improves the patient's safety by aiding the doctors and professionals.
- It potentially eases access to healthcare services.

AI in healthcare plays a pivotal role for the gradual advancement of the healthcare industry. However, it is vital to consider that the use of AI in healthcare does not violate the safety of the patients and that it is used ethically following all standard operating procedures. The following are general suggestions and recommendations for the ethical usage of AI in healthcare to minimize the potential challenge that may arise:

- **Healthcare Data Privacy**: The patient's data privacy is the most important aspect and must not be revealed at any stage.

- **Healthcare Data Security**: Healthcare data must be stored in a safe and secure manner to protect against identity theft.
- **AI Algorithmic Bias**: The AI algorithm must be trained on balanced data to provide the algorithm a generic view of the underlying condition rather than learning a biased condition.
- **Job Layoffs**: AI in healthcare must be used as an assistive tool rather than replacement of the healthcare professional in order to avoid job layoffs and provide reliable healthcare services.
- **Responsible Services**: The responsible use of AI must be used according to norms and mandated by government laws to protect patients from undesirable side effects.

These suggestions are not exhaustive and can be expanded as and when AI usage in healthcare evolves. The suggestions followed in their true spirit can realize AI usage in healthcare to its full potential.

REFERENCES

[1] Praveen, S., & Joshi, K. (2022). Explainable Artificial Intelligence in Health Care: How XAI Improves User Trust in High-Risk Decisions. In *Explainable Edge AI: A Futuristic Computing Perspective.* Studies in Computational Intelligence (Volume 1072). Cham: Springer International Publishing.

[2] Bae, Y. S., Kim, K. H., Kim, H. K., Choi, S. W., Ko, T., Seo, H. H., Lee, H. Y., & Jeon, H. (2021). Keyword Extraction Algorithm for Classifying Smoking Status from Unstructured Bilingual Electronic Health Records Based on Natural Language Processing. *Applied Sciences, 11*(19), 8812. https://doi.org/10.3390/app11198812

[3] Nazer, L. H., Zatarah, R., Waldrip, S., Ke, J. X., Moukheiber, M., Khanna, A. K., Hicklen, R. S., Moukheiber, L., Moukheiber, D., Ma, H., & Mathur, P. (2023). Bias in Artificial Intelligence Algorithms and Recommendations for Mitigation. *PLOS Digital Health, 2.*

[4] Bernal, J., & Mazo, C. (2022). Transparency of Artificial Intelligence in Healthcare: Insights from Professionals in Computing and Healthcare Worldwide. *Applied Sciences, 12*(20), 10228.

[5] Naresh, V. S., Thamarai, M., & Allavarpu, V. V. (2023). Privacy-Preserving Deep Learning in Medical Informatics: Applications, Challenges, and Solutions. *Artificial Intelligence Review, 56*, 1199–1241.

[6] Jain, S., Subzwari, S. W. A, & Subzwari, S. A. A. (2022). Generative AI for Healthcare Engineering and Technology Challenges. In *International Working Conference on Transfer and Diffusion of IT (TDIT)* (pp. 68–80). Springer Nature Switzerland.

[7] https://techcrunch.com/2020/04/27/google-medical-researchers-humbled-when-ai-screening-tool-falls-short-in-real-life-testing/

[8] https://www.smatbot.com/blog/healthcare-chatbots

[9] https://www.medical-xprt.com/software/arterys-version-cardio-ai-assisted-cardiac-mri-software-751790

3 Smart Healthcare and IoMT

Best Practices and Perspectives of AI and ML

Aakash Bhandary, Ade Indra Onthoni, and Hiren Kumar Thakkar

3.1 INTRODUCTION

Smart healthcare refers to the pivotal integration of technology, data, and digital elements into the healthcare sector to improve healthcare services, help patients with better experiences, and streamline healthcare operations. Smart healthcare is an umbrella term encompassing various key enabling technologies, including but not limited to telemedicine, wearable devices and the Internet of Things (IoT), artificial intelligence (AI), and big dataanalytics (BDA). All these key technologies are utilized in the healthcare sector using the concept of the Internet of Medical Things (IoMT) [1,2].

IoMT systems are IoT systems that encompass the use of various smart and interconnected devices, sensors, and medical equipment to collect, transmit, and analyze patient health data [3], as described in Table 3.1. IoMT systems are tailored specifically to cater to the needs of the healthcare sector. These systems enable new services such as continuous remote patient monitoring, real-time data on health conditions, improved healthcare delivery times, and they help minimize hospital readmissions, alleviate the cost burden of healthcare on individuals, and deliver timely interventions in emergency situations. Some key elements of IoMT systems are summarized in Table 3.1.

AI and machine learning (ML), when integrated with IoMT, emerge as a transformative concept [5]. AI and ML algorithms can be harnessed to analyze the vast amounts of data collected using IoMT systems. This enables predictive analysis, early disease detection, personalized recommender systems, personalized treatment plans, and similar applications. AI and ML can be used to empower healthcare professionals to make informed, data-driven decisions when it comes to patient care. Analysis of the collected data aids professionals in their work by providing more in-depth insights into patterns of patient data signatures. AI and ML prove to be important aspects of smart healthcare, contributing to the improvement of the quality of healthcare services and to the efficient allocation of healthcare resources.

 DOI: 10.1201/9781003393498-4

TABLE 3.1
Key Elements of IoMT Systems

Element	Description
Wearable devices [4]	These include smart watches, trackers, and various other devices to collect and analyze data related to vital signs, physical activity, etc.
Medical sensors	These sensors are implanted in the body of patients or into smart wearables that monitor specific parameters such as blood sugar level, heart rate, blood pressure, etc.
Remote patient monitoring	Through the use of the internet and interconnectivity, patient data collected from sensors and devices can be transmitted to enable remote monitoring and intervention.
Interconnected medical equipment	Modern equipment like ventilators and defibrillators can be connected to networks, enabling the collection of and access to data for healthcare professionals. It also enables timely maintenance of this equipment.
Healthcare facility management	Data gathered and analyzed using IoMT systems can be used to optimize various aspects of a healthcare facility, such as equipment maintenance and the flow of patients.
Telemedicine	Remote consultations are made possible due to IoMT, allowing doctors to diagnose patients using remote access to data and using video conferencing.
Data analysis and decision-making	The data collected using IoMT systems can be analyzed using AI systems to help professionals make better informed decisions.

Figure 3.1 shows the schematic flowchart for the decision-making process by incorporating AI/ML into IoMT systems. A simplified workflow for a patient monitoring system integrating IoMT with a cloud infrastructure is given in Figure 3.3. The cloud infrastructure can house the components and applications used for analytics, processing, and storage of the data generated in the IoMT network (see Figure 3.4).

In the coming sections, the best practices and perspectives of AI and ML in smart healthcare using IoMT are discussed through a comprehensive description of implemented systems.

3.2 SOME IMPACTFUL APPLICATIONS OF AI-ML IN IOMT SYSTEMS

IoMT systems integrated with AI-ML are helpful in a lot of applications for smart healthcare, however some very impactful applications are discussed below. These applications are traditionally highly resource-intensive, requiring a high level of human intervention and decision-making.

3.2.1 AI-ML-Enabled Cardiovascular Monitoring

Cardiovascular disease (CVD), simply known as heart disease, is a leading cause of death worldwide. Since it is so widespread, effective detection strategies have become necessary to mitigate its impact globally. The use of machine learning approaches

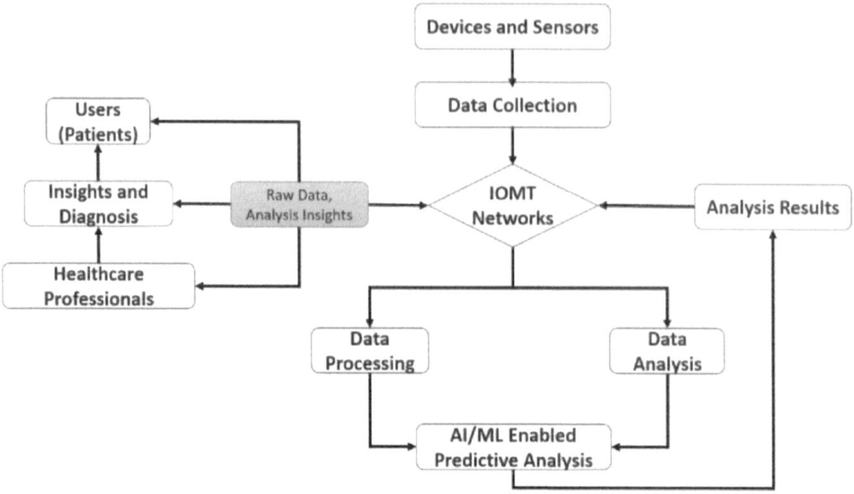

FIGURE 3.1 Decision-making flowchart for IoMT systems.

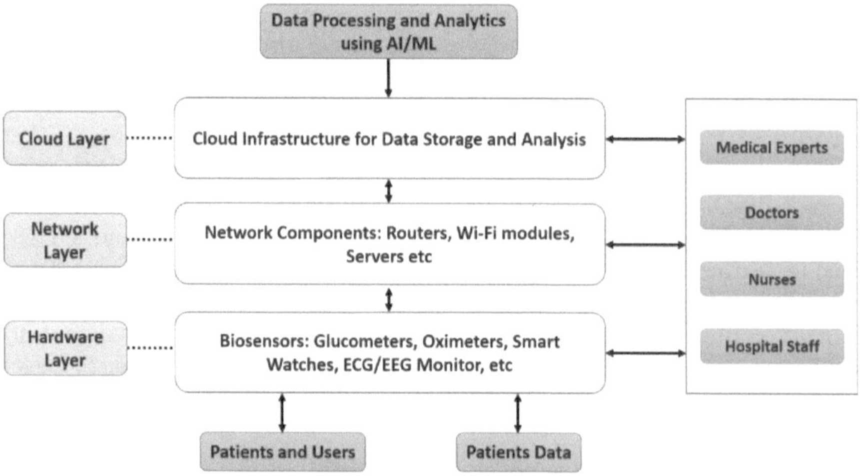

FIGURE 3.2 IoMT reference model.

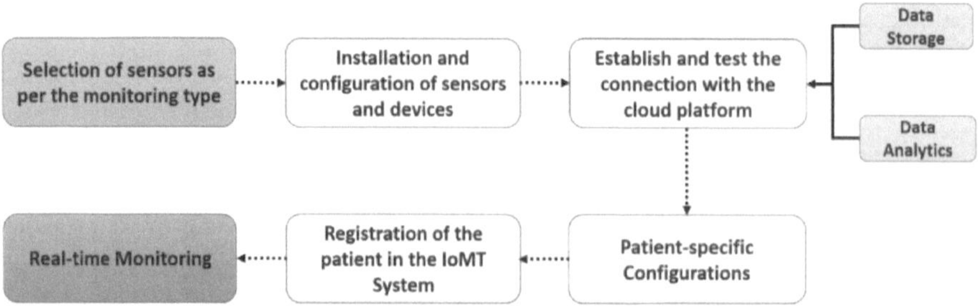

FIGURE 3.3 Simplified workflow for real-time patient monitoring.

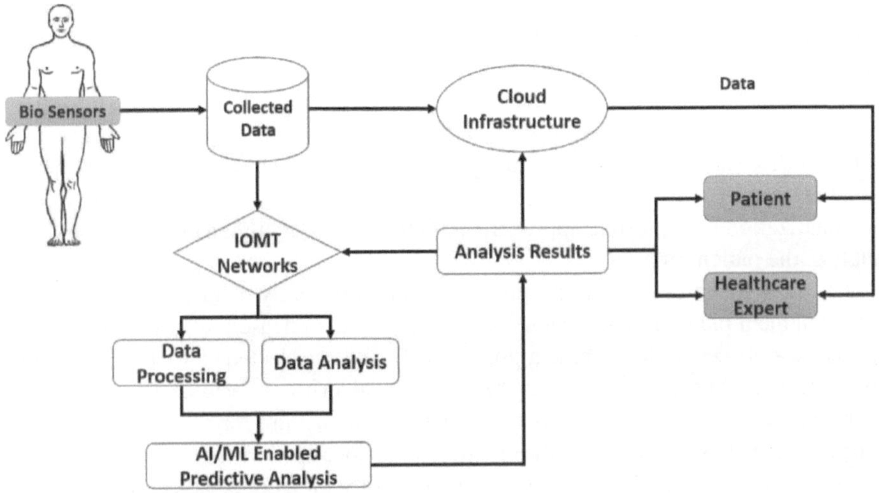

FIGURE 3.4. Use of biosensors and cloud infrastructure to store and process patient data. This workflow is a generalized representation of the procedure implemented in IoMT systems discussed in Section 3.2 of this chapter.

has been proven, promising to aid heart disease detection strategies, helping reduce human overhead, and perform diagnosis in the early stages of the disease [6].

Heart ailments are monitored using several tools and machines, including computed tomography (CT) scans, electrocardiograms (ECGs), stress test devices, and blood pressure monitoring devices. Stress is one of the significant factors involved in the development of cardiovascular conditions and needs to be monitored effectively. All these metrics can be monitored using biosensors and can provide a cost-effective remote monitoring method using IoMT networks [7]. The data collected using biosensors can be analyzed using ML algorithms, and predictive analysis can be conducted for the early detection of CVD. These algorithms can also be used to build personalized care plans for individuals with CVD that cater specifically to their needs, requirements, and tolerances. Moreover, images captured using magnetic resonance imaging (MRI) scans can also be analyzed using deep learning (DL)—a subset of ML—algorithms for the identification of sensitive areas in the patient's body. This can be used to precisely detect cardiovascular anomalies. This not only enhances the diagnosis accuracy but also streamlines the process, potentially reducing waiting times and stress/anxiety for the patients.

AI-ML algorithms offer a promising addition to IoMT systems for the early detection of heart disease and help reduce human overhead, reduce the chance of human error, and help save costs by implementing remote sensing and monitoring.

3.2.2 AI-ML-Enabled Cancer Treatment

Cancer is the uncontrolled division and growth of abnormal cells in the human body, which is a formidable ailment for healthcare. It can affect people of all ages and backgrounds and can affect every part of the human body, giving rise to difficulty in diagnosis. Moreover, cancer is very difficult to diagnose in its early stages as serious symptoms start showing only in the later stages. Hence cancer treatment is primarily conducted using reactive measures instead of proactive measures. Reactive measures refer to such treatments as the chemotherapy and radiation therapy given to cancer patients after the disease has been diagnosed in the later stages. Also, cancer, a complex disease that can affect all body parts along with variations in each person's genetics. makes it very difficult to develop a treatment plan that fits everyone. Hence personalization is a plausible approach, but it takes a lot of human effort to study and analyze the patient first.

AI-ML algorithms emerge as a powerful tool for the early diagnosis and personalized treatment plan for cancer patients [8]. Cancer data released by governments and hospitals is utilized to train these algorithms. The data collected using IoMT systems for patients is then analyzed using these trained algorithms for detection and treatment plan creation. Vast amounts of available data account for a variety of patient types and genetics, allowing for the creation of personalized treatment schemes while reducing human effort. Furthermore, cellular information collected can be analyzed to detect cancer before traditional methods can. This involves sensor data such as blood samples, breathing patterns, ECG signals, etc. Moreover, images generated using MRIs and CT scans can be analyzed using DL algorithms to detect malignancies that a human may miss. Convolutional neural networks (CNNs) can be used for cancer detection using images. The workflow for this has been described in Figure 3.5.

After undergoing treatment, the patient can be monitored continuously and in an automated manner using real-time sensor data and IoMT networks. Their equipment and medicine flow can be monitored and modified as per the patient's response to certain previous changes. Hence, AI-ML helps not only in the early diagnosis of cancer but also reduces human overhead and helps simplify the inherent complexities involved in cancer care.

3.2.3 AI-ML-Enabled Drug Development

The development of new and better medical drugs and remedies is a time- and resource-intensive procedure. Scientists need to identify a potential candidate for

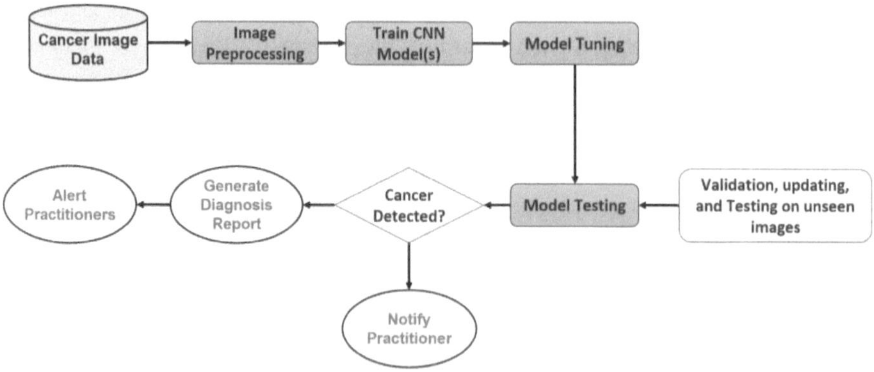

FIGURE 3.5 CNN workflow for cancer detection using images.

improvement or new development, acquire approval from regulatory authorities, and then acquire the materials needed for research and development, which are often hard to come by. Once a new drug is developed, it is often tested on animals such as rats, or human trials are conducted, especially in the case of vaccines. These trials are not only a time-consuming and laborious process but also face the risk of safety and efficacy, as there has to be a waiting period before efficacy can be ensured. Moreover, clinical trials often lack reliability as there is a high dropout rate of test subjects, as well as a lack of biomarkers to test responses to the treatment. This accounts for high costs and delays in delivering improved medication.

AI-ML can be used to analyze datasets of chemical compounds and predict their potential as drug candidates by comparing their structural similarity to existing medicines [9]. These algorithms can help identify the necessary biomarkers and new targets associated with certain diseases. AI-driven simulations can help predict the behavior of a new drug in the human body, enabling fast identification of candidates with higher success chances. ML algorithms can help identify eligible candidates for clinical trials by studying their medical history and vital signatures. AI-ML algorithms can also assist in predicting patient responses to certain treatments, helping reduce anomalies during trials. Through IoMT systems, real-time patient monitoring can ensure that side effects or adversities are quickly detected and addressed by alarming healthcare professionals, improving the safety and efficiency of clinical trials.

Through IoMT systems, real-time monitoring of patients during clinical trials has become much more feasible. Various sensors, such as ECGs, glucose monitors, wearable devices, respiration sensors, and oximeters collect a lot of data. This data can be processed and analyzed rapidly, enabling faster detection of adverse or side effects. Healthcare professionals can be alerted instantly, ensuring that the patients' safety is prioritized and any new issues are promptly addressed, ultimately improving the efficiency and safety of clinical trials.

3.2.4 AI-ML-Enabled Target Treatment Delivery

Surgical procedures, simply referred to as surgeries, require a high amount of human expertise and precision. The integration of AI-ML into surgeries enable highly precise and efficient outcomes. One of the ways AI can be integrated is through the use of algorithms that identify the specific areas where treatment is required, for example, detecting cracks in bones using computer vision algorithms. The results from these algorithms can then be used to devise highly precise surgical strategies.

Electroencephalogram (EEG) comes into the picture here [10]. EEG is the signal reading of brain activity. When the human body receives inputs or generates certain outputs, the brain generates signals for these responses, which can be read using an EEG machine. ML models can be trained on various signal data features such as signal vector amplitude (SVA) or the like. Moreover, models can study the trend in certain signals and associate it with a condition they have seen during the training phase. These trained models can then be used to classify the EEG signals and associate them with certain diseases. Automated IoMT systems can then be utilized to activate certain actuators installed in the patient's body to release the required medicine at the exact target location, thus helping minimize side effects.

However, the models need to be chosen, trained, and tested very carefully before deployment. These models need to be highly accurate and not perform misdiagnoses, which can lead to adverse effects. Hence a large amount of training data is required for these models. Figure 3.6 presents a generalized implementation workflow for this proposition. Some examples of implementations of AI-ML algorithms for disease detection tasks have been summarized in Table 3.2.

3.2.5 AI-ML-Enabled Surgical Procedures

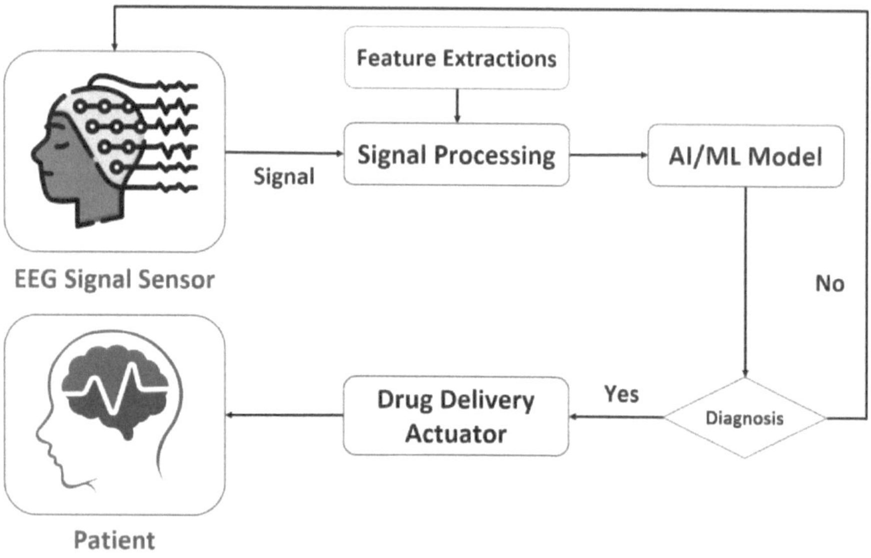

FIGURE 3.6 Targeted drug delivery workflow.

TABLE 3.2
Algorithms Implemented in Smart Healthcare IoMT Systems

Application	AI-ML Algorithms Used
Chronic kidney disease diagnosis [11]	Random forest (RF), support vector machine (SVM)
Cancer detection [12,13]	Artificial neural network (ANN), convolutional neural network (CNN), SVM
Heart disease detection and monitoring [14–16]	RF, K-nearest neighbors (KNN), SVM
Helping in surgery [17]	SVM, ANN, decision tree (DT)
Monitoring glucose [18]	KNN, DT, SVM, logistic regression (LR)
Healthcare resource management [19]	LR, KNN, ANN, SVM, naïve Bayes (NB)
Generalized monitoring system [20]	DT, RF, KNN
Disease diagnosis using images [21]	ANN, CNN

3.3 CHALLENGES ASSOCIATED WITH IMPLEMENTATION OF IOMT SYSTEMS

AI-ML proves to be a valuable asset for addition to IoMT systems; however, IoMT systems themselves have to overcome a few challenges before complete integration into traditional healthcare systems.

First, these approaches are sophisticated and require a lot of technological equipment. Professionals using these systems need to be trained to use them. This will incur costs for healthcare providers aiming to implement IoMT, in addition to other IoMT equipment such as sensors and network equipment. Moreover, connectivity needs to be ensured within the system, indicating the need for robust internet connectivity. Loss of internet connectivity would lead to loss of vital patient monitoring data. One potential solution to the connectivity loss issue could be having a storage system that stores some of the data locally near the point of recording before sending it into the IoMT network. This signifies additional storage systems that need to be deployed.

One major concern regarding the implementation of IoMT is the security and privacy of the patients being monitored. Their data is being collected and sent into a network of devices over the internet. These networks are often prone to external attacks and data theft. IoMT networks need to be robust enough to prevent these attacks from happening. Moreover, security measures implemented have to be reliable enough for the patients themselves to trust the data shown by these systems.

Also, since a vast amount of data being collected every moment, it is being referred to as big data. This prompts the need for the implementation of sophisticated systems that go beyond the capabilities of traditional AI-ML algorithms in terms of processing power and hardware requirements.

In conclusion, IoMT along with AI-ML integration can prove to be revolutionary in the field of smart healthcare. Many practitioners prefer these systems over traditional methods for diagnoses owing to their reliability and accuracy. Moreover, much research is being encouraged and conducted in this domain which will help improve accessibility to reliable and cost-effective healthcare in the near future.

3.4 CONCLUSION

In conclusion, the integration of AI and ML technologies with IoMT devices or data offers a significant pathway for advancing healthcare. This strategic amalgamation promises an enhanced level of sophistication, marking a decisive step forward in the trajectory of smart healthcare advancements. This integration of AI and ML not only advances smart healthcare but also proves instrumental in reducing the time, human intervention, and resources required in the healthcare sector. As discussed earlier, it streamlines processes such as drug development, cutting down on trial and error. Additionally, it simplifies health treatment procedures and enhances early disease detection. In summary, this approach represents a significant leap in the progression of smart healthcare, simultaneously optimizing efficiency and resource utilization.

REFERENCES

[1] Manickam P, Mariappan SA, Murugesan SM, et al. Artificial intelligence (AI) and Internet of Medical Things (IoMT) assisted biomedical systems for intelligent healthcare. *Biosensors*. 2022;12(8):562.

[2] Singh P, Devi KJ, Thakkar HK, et al. Region-based hybrid medical image watermarking scheme for robust and secured transmission in IoMT. *IEEE Access*. 2022;10:8974–8993.

[3] Adeniyi EA, Ogundokun RO, Awotunde JB. IoMT-based wearable body sensors network healthcare monitoring system. *IoT in Healthcare and Ambient Assisted Living*. 2021:103–121.

[4] Thakkar HK, Chowdhury SR, Bhoi AK, et al. Applications of wearable technologies in healthcare: An analytical study. In: *5G IoT and edge computing for smart healthcare*. Elsevier; 2022. pp. 279–299.

[5] Devi KJ, Singh P, Thakkar HK. Dual secured reversible medical image watermarking for Internet of Medical Things. In: *Connected e-health: Integrated IoT and cloud computing*. Springer; 2022. pp. 457–473.

[6] Rai D, Thakkar HK, Singh D, et al. Machine learning assisted automatic annotation of isovolumic movement and aortic valve closure using seismocardiogram signals. In: *2020 IEEE 17th India Council International Conference (INDICON)*. IEEE; 2020. pp. 1–6.

[7] Divya K, Sirohi A, Pande S, et al. An IoMT assisted heart disease diagnostic system using machine learning techniques. *Cognitive Internet of Medical Things for Smart Healthcare: Services and Applications*. 2021:145–161.

[8] Khan SU, Islam N, Jan Z, et al. An e-health care services framework for the detection and classification of breast cancer in breast cytology images as an IoMT application. *Future Generation Computer Systems*. 2019;98:286–296.

[9] Boehme P, Hansen A, Roubenoff R, et al. How soon will digital endpoints become a cornerstone for future drug development? *Drug Discovery Today*. 2019;24(1):16–19.

[10] Jain S, Nehra M, Kumar R, et al. Internet of Medical Things (IoMT)-integrated biosensors for point-of-care testing of infectious diseases. *Biosensors and Bioelectronics*. 2021;179:113074.

[11] Swain D, Mehta U, Bhatt A, et al. A robust chronic kidney disease classifier using machine learning. *Electronics*. 2023;12(1):212.

[12] Gardezi SJS, Elazab A, Lei B, et al. Breast cancer detection and diagnosis using mammographic data: Systematic review. *Journal of Medical Internet Research*. 2019;21(7):e14464.

[13] Alakwaa W, Nassef M, Badr A. Lung cancer detection and classification with 3D convolutional neural network (3D-CNN). *International Journal of Advanced Computer Science and Applications*. 2017;8(8).

[14] Mohan S, Thirumalai C, Srivastava G. Effective heart disease prediction using hybrid machine learning techniques. *IEEE Access*. 2019;7:81542–81554.

[15] Deekshatulu B, Chandra P, et al. Classification of heart disease using k-nearest neighbor and genetic algorithm. *Procedia Technology*. 2013;10:85–94.

[16] Sahoo PK, Thakkar HK, Lee MY. A cardiac early warning system with multi channel SCG and ECG monitoring for mobile health. *Sensors*. 2017;17(4):711.

[17] Chang M, Canseco JA, Nicholson KJ, et al. The role of machine learning in spine surgery: The future is now. *Frontiers in Surgery*. 2020;7:54.

[18] Shokrekhodaei M, Cistola DP, Roberts RC, et al. Non-invasive glucose monitoring using optical sensor and machine learning techniques for diabetes applications. *IEEE Access*. 2021;9:73029–73045.

[19] Kaushik AK, Dhau JS, Gohel H, et al. Electrochemical SARS-CoV-2 sensing at point-of-care and artificial intelligence for intelligent COVID-19 management. *ACS Applied Bio Materials*. 2020;3(11):7306–7325.

[20] Kaur P, Kumar R, Kumar M. A healthcare monitoring system using random forest and Internet of Things (IoT). *Multimedia Tools and Applications*. 2019;78:19905–19916.

[21] Muhaba KA, Dese K, Aga TM, Zewdu FT, Simegn GL. Automatic skin disease diagnosis using deep learning from clinical image and patient information. *Skin Health and Disease*. 2022;2(1):e81.

Part II

Intelligent IoMT and New Age Computing

Principles and Perspective with AI and Edge Computing

4 Issues and Challenges of Intelligent IoMT for Edge Computing

V. Kakulapati and Prakhar Gupta

4.1 INTRODUCTION

IoMT can process intricate data; however it may need significant processing resources. Artificial intelligence and edge computing can intelligently examine this data, providing sophisticated healthcare services. Nevertheless, prior research has failed to examine the aspects of the architecture, authentication, security, sensor type, and devices of edge computing. Converting urban regions into smart cities requires further investigation and financial resources. Deploying these technologies in metropolitan areas may enhance healthcare services [1].

The healthcare sector is quickly growing, with an emphasis on delivering crucial services and income. The incorporation of IoMT-edge cloud technologies may enhance facilities and infrastructure. This chapter describes a smart city healthcare monitoring system based on edge computing and the IoMT that may improve facilities, provide timely patient treatment, and improve health infrastructure during pandemics. The system suggests an end-to-end network slice for healthcare services, effective patient scheduling, and resource allocation [2].

The healthcare sector is quickly growing, with an emphasis on delivering crucial services and income. The incorporation of IoMT-edge cloud technologies may enhance facilities and infrastructure. A smart city healthcare monitoring system based on edge computing and IoMT may improve facilities, provide timely patient treatment, and improve health infrastructure during pandemics. The improved IoMT system is expected to suggest an end-to-end network of components for quality healthcare such as effective patient scheduling, and better resource allocation.

The core challenges in the government and public sectors are chronic illness in patients, disaster management, and dangerous hazards such as COVID-19, cholera, etc. However, IoMT devices are being designed to support the goal of engaging to identify disease in its early stages. The fundamental constraint of handling the huge number of IoMT devices is their constrained computational and storage capacities. To alleviate the constraint, the use of the cloud computing was suggested. However, cloud computing faces the challenges of network delay and congestions [3]. The entire field of IoT healthcare research, also called IoMT, is primarily comprised of multiple domains such as network engineering, device design, security, etc. After

DOI: 10.1201/9781003393498-6

the COVID-19 pandemic, the potential of IoMT is realized in the field of e-health, telemedicine. However, IoMT-based healthcare systems are still in their early stages and require further research to improvise the methodologies and models considering the novel field. There is a lack of professional researchers in the field of IoMT, which poses an obstacle for its application in the healthcare sector. In this chapter, we examine the interoperability of data in the Internet of Medical Things (IoMT), its product design issues, industry acceptance, and other prominent issues [4].

In the past few decades, there has been exponential growth in medical data generation, which has rendered the use of the centralized models inoperative and ineffective. However, the healthcare data growth and its processing issues can be alleviated by engaging the IoMT and edge computing with limited resources. In this study of IoMT with edge computing, we attempt to investigate the impact of intelligent edge computing on IoMT systems with respect to fairness in healthcare.

Edge computing platforms have arisen as a remedy to network-constrained cloud computing technology. Edge computing facilitates computing capabilities and IT services close to the edge of the IoMT network, and therefore it mitigate the problem of network delay [5].

The Internet of Medical Things (IoMT) engages the numerous sensors to capture the data from different sources and sends it to the nearest edge device to perform computationally demanding tasks within the healthcare boundary. However, edge devices are equipped with sufficient computational power, which often generate results in a time-bound manner.

4.1.1 IoMT Revolution

In the recent past, healthcare facilities have seen the emergence of notable issues in dealing with the Internet of Things (IoMT), such as performance, operations, network infrastructure, etc. To tackle these challenges, the models require the interconnected infrastructure such as WiFi, Bluetooth, barcodes, and security sensors.

One of the best revolutions in IoMT is the wearable healthcare technology, with the design and development of novel IoMT devices such as heart monitors and smartwatches. These tiny and low-cost electronic gadgets help to monitor health metrics and establish connections, which minimizes the need for repeated checkups. Moreover, it also helps to notify the patients for various conditions [6]. The fundamental idea behind the wearable devices is to assist patients in monitoring activities such as standing, walking, medication intake, dietary choices, and appointment scheduling. The potential of wearable healthcare is truly realized due to network connectivity and processing in edge devices. For instance, the wearable devices that monitor heart rate and ECG have been significantly impacted positively by providing continuous monitoring of heart activities. Similarly, the personal wearable glucose monitors are revolutionizing the lives of individuals with diabetes using uninterrupted monitoring and abnormal notifications.

A design for implementing edge computing technologies is suggested [7] to facilitate the provision of healthcare services on a broad scale. Their solution exhibits an average latency of 0.5 second and consumes 0.003 kilowatt-hour of electricity for a user base of 150,000 individuals using 50 cloudlets. The primary objective of this system is to assist public health personnel in identifying patterns and trends related to diseases. Nevertheless, these studies fail to adequately address the specific requirements of a vast medical community. Edge-enabled healthcare systems may mitigate the discrepancy between current infrastructure and hospital needs for concurrent record storage and patient monitoring.

Extensive healthcare systems need substantial data for analysis and security purposes. Edge mining approaches mitigate the amount of data sent to cloud services. However, in the case of prolonged and uninterrupted data gathering from medical sensors, more reduction is necessary. Large volumes of data often need analysis using novel approaches that use data characteristics.

Healthcare devices with edge computing capabilities improve patients' quality of life and generate money for both healthcare providers and 5G network operators. Nevertheless, apprehensions over the confidentiality of patient information escalate with the implementation of extensive deployments. Current HIPAA regulations are inadequate for monitoring systems that use edge computing technology, and any unauthorized access to data might result in legal consequences for both healthcare providers and network operators. Italy and Germany have no regulations or limitations regarding data breaches. Existing policies prioritize the protection of personal information; however, [8] that demonstrates that identifiable data has the potential to become personal. To ensure patients' ownership and control over their medical data obtained from IoT devices, it is necessary to implement authorization techniques that rely on patient consent, such as blockchain-based mobile edge computing (MEC) frameworks. Large-scale healthcare systems need sophisticated privacy and anonymization structures. However, the use of computationally costly cryptographic approaches may undermine both computing efficiency and anonymization risk.

The existing network installations are inadequate to support extensive dispersed sensor-based medical monitoring and reporting. The convergence of telecommunications and IT services from a centralized cloud platform to the edge is crucial, but it relies on the successful implementation of many enabling technologies [9]. Virtualization approaches, such as virtual machines (VMs) and containers, enable edge computing devices by providing efficient virtualization solutions on consumer devices. Network function virtualization (NFV) separates network operations and services from exclusive hardware, enabling the placement of numerous service instances on a single virtual machine (VM). Software-defined networks (SDNs) enable the control of network connections and services across diverse multi-ethernet platforms (MEC). Network slicing is the division of a network into numerous instances that are specifically tailored for certain purposes. The implementation of 5G is crucial for the widespread establishment of healthcare infrastructure based on mobile edge computing (MEC). However, the incorporation of artificial intelligence (AI) is necessary to provide prompt service delivery. Advancements in machine learning, namely deep learning, have recently led to improvements in facial recognition, medical diagnosis, and natural language processing [10–12]. Nevertheless, these operations need intricate processing of vast datasets in both centralized and distant data centers, demanding substantial storage capacity and computational capabilities. In [13], it is observed that the neural networks, such as autoencoders

(AEs) and generative adversarial networks (GANs) are highly recommended for the implementation in mobile edge computing (MEC).

IoMT-enabled AI models consider the vital signs of patients such as age, gender, and medical problems while predicting the outcome [14] followed by detailed analysis of anomalous readings for accurate classifications. Therefore, the implementation of such a health system that considers patients' vital signs is essential for achieving individualized outcomes. In this regard, the researchers should prioritize the development of decentralized training models with low latency on edge devices, using a wide range of input data from health sensors [15]. Another aspect of improvisation is the integration of edge computing with the 5G network, which can promptly record, diagnose, and monitor the health status of patients in real time and assist early intervention in emergencies [16,17].

4.1.2 Benefits

4.1.2.1 Monitoring and Timely Interventions

The foremost benefit of IoMT devices is continuous monitoring of vital parameters for easy healthcare access. Such easy access to the information helps the professional healthcare provider make informed decisions in early interventions. Such real-time data is extremely valuable to make alternative treatment plan and to take critical decisions.

4.1.2.2 Enhanced Data Processing and Analysis

Usually, in edge computing, data processing is carried out at the source of data generation. This reduces the time for healthcare data processing and subsequent analysis and generates insights in real-time. The reduced predictive analytics due to edge computing enhances healthcare service delivery with improved quality.

4.1.2.3 Improved Quality of Service (QOS)

The prompt predictive analytics supported by IoMT and edge computing facilitates the healthcare professional to make quick informed decisions and therefore expedites service delivery. The doctors can make more accurate and patient-centric treatment plan using AI models for timely recovery.

4.1.2.4 Data Privacy and Security

Considering the unsecured connection between the IoMT devices and edge computing resources, the data security and privacy is the prominent issue. To ensure the confidentiality and integrity of patient data, processing data at the edge without letting the data cross the network boundary may mitigate the risk of data breaches.

4.1.2.5 Interoperability and Standardization

Concerns about interoperability are common in the healthcare industry due to lack of standardization across countries. The quick and sustainable solution to address interoperability is to bring all the collaborators onto the same platform and design standardized protocols that promote data sharing and system compatibility across different devices.

4.1.2.6 Regulatory Compliance

Considering the sensitive nature of the healthcare data and the risk of data breach in the absence of robust data security protocols, it is imperative to enforce regulation compliance in order to protect the patient's data with the use of IoMT devices. To ensure compliance with this legislation and build strong data governance frameworks, healthcare providers must collaborate with legislators.

In this study, the challenges relate to presenting informative case studies and examples that demonstrate the implementations of IoMT for Edge Computing within the healthcare sector. Furthermore, it provides recommendations for both research purposes and practical applications. In conclusion, the report underscores the benefits of IoMT for Edge Computing, in enhancing healthcare services while emphasizing the need to address associated challenges to guarantee its effective deployment. Section 4.2 delves into the existing literature on smart healthcare systems, and Section 4.3 discusses Intelligent IoMT for Edge Computing. Section 4.4 elaborates on the issues and challenges in IOMT, and Section 4.5 emphasizes possible solutions and strategies for overcoming challenges. Section 4.6 discusses the use-cases and examples associated with the application of edge computing and IoMT in healthcare. Section 4.7 explores the applications, and Section 4.8 provides concluding remarks followed by future enhancement.

4.2 LITERATURE SURVEY

IoMT technology significantly reduced the spread of COVID-19 by enabling remote patient detection, diagnosis, monitoring, and treatment. It collected and analyzed patient data, storing results in the cloud for quick knowledge extraction. This smart healthcare system improved traditional systems by allowing caregivers to service multiple patients simultaneously, addressing the growing patient population [18].

Healthcare is leveraging IT to create smart systems that improve health diagnosis and treatment. These systems, which include intelligent health surveillance frameworks and automated medical diagnosis systems, are employed in a variety of environments such as hospitals, offices, and residences. These methods minimize doctor visits while improving patient care quality. The global adoption of healthcare IoT devices, which is expected to exceed 162 billion by 2020, has had a tremendous influence on the healthcare sector [19].

Wireless body sensors frequently gather data from the same user base, resulting in data redundancy at local edge nodes. When DL models are retrained or updated, they become poorly fitted or overfitted. Because distributed deep learning (DL) models must be retrained and updated regularly, the demanding computation is frequently offloaded to the cloud [20]. To overcome this issue, academics have proposed new IoT designs and ideas, such as distributed deep networks, which may be utilized to create point-to-point topologies. Research suggested a distributed deep network using local edge nodes, employing a basic neural network and weight interchange to train nodes in a distributed way [21]. Researchers have suggested distributed training for DL models and ML algorithms at the edge layer to decentralize classification tasks, which might solve data distribution difficulties in IoT-based healthcare systems. This method can also solve covariate shift concerns by segmentation at the edge nodes [22].

Smart healthcare systems use IoM cloud services, giving patients smart devices for finding hospitals and managing electronic health information. With the exponential rise of the Internet of Things, these apps may manage individuals' private health information internationally. However, security and privacy concerns must be addressed [23]. The IoT application market is also expanding, with wearable sensor devices available for a variety of healthcare applications. Noninvasive glucose sensing technologies, such as glucose-level sensing, rely on IoM to continuously monitor blood glucose levels. The 5G network has reignited interest in multiaccess edge computing (MEC), which depends on data producers and consumers to minimize latency, enhance transmission speed, and monitor power. This enables primary illness diagnosis at the edge and cloud-based supervision [24,25].

4.3 INTELLIGENT IOMT FOR EDGE COMPUTING

The Internet of Medical Things (IoMT) for Edge Computing is a state-of-the-art technological paradigm that combines the capabilities of edge computing with the fields of medical data processing, analysis, and gathering seamlessly. A thorough definition of this complex idea is discussed next.

Intelligent IoMT for Edge Computing is used to describe a sophisticated, integrated framework that uses edge computing, artificial intelligence, and the Internet of Things (IoT) to enable extremely effective, real-time patient monitoring, diagnosis, and treatment. Intelligent IoMT is fundamentally an ecosystem of wearable sensors and medical devices that are specifically engineered to record and transfer a wide range of critical medical data, from vital signs to complex diagnostics like electrocardiograms and glucose levels [26].

The symbiotic interaction between these intelligent IoMT devices and edge computing platforms is the innovation's key component. In the context of healthcare settings, edge computing is a distributed computing approach that best places processing and data storage power close to the actual sources of data collection. Without the need for centralized cloud-based infrastructure, this tactical location makes it easier to analyze and analyze medical data instantly.

4.4 ISSUES AND CHALLENGES OF INTELLIGENT IOMT FOR EDGE COMPUTING

4.4.1 Issues of IoMT for Edge Computing

4.4.1.1 Security and Privacy Concerns

There are several issues with the use of IoMT systems for healthcare service delivery. The IoMT devices gather patient's health data and later transmit these enormous amounts of critical health-related data to the servers for further analytics. However, the lack of sophisticated security protocols may compromise the data and expose the patient's identity. Such data compromise may erodes the public confidence from the medical systems, and therefore proposed IoMT systems must address security and privacy concerns as well.

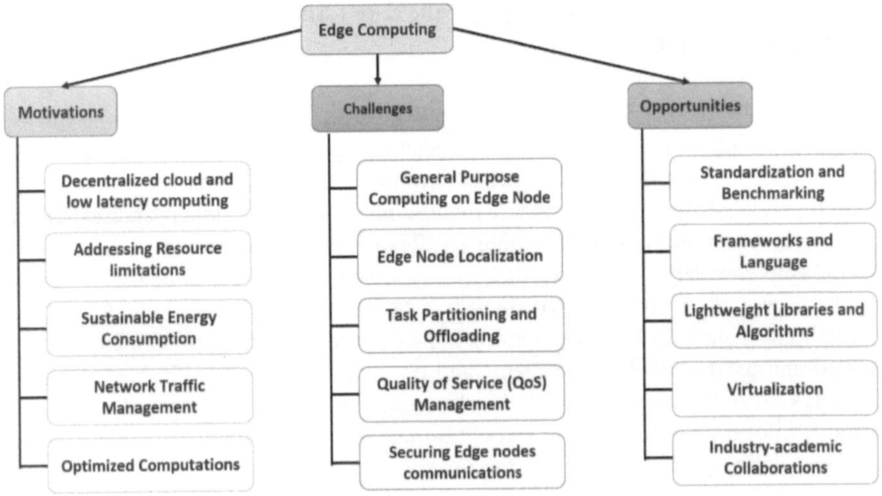

FIGURE 4.1 Edge computing challenges and opportunities [27].

4.4.1.2 Latency and Bandwidth Issues

The idea behind the lower latency in edge computing is to process the data very close to its generation. IoMT devices are producing an increasing amount of data, which can put pressure on network capacity and cause latency problems when processing data in real-time.

Critical medical decisions and interventions might be postponed by latency concerns, particularly in emergency scenarios. Inadequate data processing speed can result in delayed or missed diagnoses.

4.4.1.3 Storage and Computation Intensity at Every Edge Device

Large volumes of data are produced by intelligent IoMT devices, necessitating processing and storage capacity at each edge device. Edge devices may struggle to manage this load. Data loss, poor processing efficiency, and a decline in the responsiveness of real-time healthcare services can all result from inadequate computing and storage resources.

4.4.1.4 Lack of Standardization

The lack of standardized data formats, communication protocols, and interfaces in the IoMT sector may make it more difficult for various systems and devices to work together. In the absence of the standards, compatibility problems may arise, which make it very difficult to connect with IoMT devices resulting in poor IoMT systems.

4.4.1.5 Integration with Existing Healthcare Systems

The introduction of IoMT system must be inexpensive, and therefore it must be able to be flawlessly integrated with the existing healthcare system. The researchers must ensure that IoMT protocol design adapts the data formats and interfaces with the existing legacy healthcare systems.

4.4.1.6 Funding and Resource Constraints

The introduction of novel IoMT-enabled edge computing system will require new staff trained on the IoMT devices, it also requires a new set of hardwares and software. It may be difficult for healthcare institutions with small budgets and resources to implement and maintain this technology. Resource constraints may cause inequities in healthcare services and restricted access to cutting-edge healthcare technologies by slowing down the deployment of Intelligent IoMT for Edge Computing.

Intelligent IoMT for Edge Computing in healthcare cannot be successfully implemented and used until these problems and obstacles are resolved. Robust security measures, standardized protocol development, network capacity optimization, resource allocation optimization, and obtaining sufficient funds for implementation are some strategies that may be used to mitigate these issues.

4.4.2 Challenges

4.4.2.1 Massive Amounts of Electronic Healthcare Systems

Large-scale healthcare infrastructures are based on 50 cloudlets and have a half-second latency and 0.003 kilowatt-hour power usage per 150,000 users. These tools might assist public health officials in detecting disease transmission patterns. However, these studies do not address the demands of major medical communities with many patients. Edge-enabled healthcare systems can eliminate infrastructure disparities while improving record storage and patient monitoring [28].

4.4.2.2 Patient Privacy

Edge-enabled healthcare devices improve patients' quality of life while also generating cash for healthcare providers and 5G network operators. Concerns for patient information privacy arise when large-scale deployments take place. Existing HIPAA regulations are insufficient for edge-enabled monitoring systems, and data breaches may result in legal ramifications for health providers and network operators. Countries such as Italy and Germany have no limitations on data leaks. As patients acquire and control their medical data via IoT devices, patient permission-based authorization solutions, such as blockchain-based MEC frameworks, are required. Large-scale healthcare systems require sophisticated privacy and anonymization structures, and computationally intensive cryptography approaches can reduce computing performance. The allocation of workloads across sensor nodes and edge computing platforms while maintaining privacy and security remains a difficulty [29,30].

4.4.2.3 Integrating AI

Artificial intelligence (AI) is being incorporated into large-scale MEC-based healthcare infrastructure to ensure that consumers receive timely services. AI uses elements such as user mobility, device usage, patient monitoring information, and medical conditions to provide accurate health diagnoses. Recent discoveries in machine learning, particularly deep learning, have allowed for improvements in facial recognition, medical diagnosis, and natural language processing. However, these necessitate the complicated processing of big datasets in centralized and distant data centers, which necessitates massive storage and computer capacity [31]. AI-integrated 5G infrastructure for a distributed healthcare system might incorporate supervised learning, unsupervised learning, and reinforcement learning. Neural networks such as autoencoders and generative adversarial networks are more suited to MEC implementation. AI implementation at the edge may be achieved by a helper-device split, which allows each device to create a learning model from local data and send it to a helper [32].

4.4.2.4 Availability

Medical facilities should prioritize real-time patient care to avoid misdiagnosis and probable worsening of medical problems, utilizing ultra-reliable low latency (URLL) services, since fast diagnosis can prevent condition worsening and its consequences.

4.4.2.5 Budget Friendly

Healthcare services should be economical, necessitating the integration of cost-effective equipment and solutions into e-health systems to assure the projected cost of medical treatments.

4.4.2.6 Fairness

Healthcare services are tailored to each patient's specific needs, principles, and desires.

4.4.2.7 Appropriate Medical Treatment

E-health services should be based on scientific evidence, such as laboratory testing, clinical research, and epidemiological studies, and should have interfaces and linkages to medical facilities for monitoring.

4.5 SOLUTIONS AND STRATEGIES FOR OVERCOMING CHALLENGES

4.5.1 Edge Computing and Fog Computing

By processing data closer to the point of data generation, edge computing and fog computing paradigms can greatly reduce latency and bandwidth constraints. Data is examined locally, lightening the load on central cloud resources and improving real-time processing by dispersing computing and data processing among edge nodes and fog layers. This method optimizes data delivery while reducing latency.

4.5.2 Data Processing on Network Nodes and Layers

It is possible to reduce the storage- and computation-intensive demands on individual devices by implementing data processing on network nodes and layers instead of just on edge devices. The strain on the edge devices can be reduced by careful allocation of data processing responsibilities across the network. This way, the IoMT system ensures that data-intensive jobs get priority, and overall system response time increases.

4.5.3 Standardization of Protocols and Interfaces

The standardization of the IoMT protocol and user interface is one of the essential tasks that needs more attention. Standardization ensures the interoperability of various components, devices, and platforms for unified task processing. It help improvise the overall IoMT ecosystem and generate a flawless system usage.

4.5.4 Collaboration among Stakeholders

The key aspect to overcoming the financial and resource constraint challenges is collaboration among academia, research centers, government, and private industry. The meaningful collaboration among these stakeholders bring novel concepts and ideas for further improvisation with more funding and representations.

4.5.5 Regulatory Frameworks and Policies

The IoMT systems faces the challenges of data privacy and security. By the time protocols are designed and implemented, the regulatory frameworks and policies need to be put in place to restrict unauthorized access to the critical patient's data.

4.6 CASE STUDIES AND EXAMPLES

4.6.1 Real-World Examples of Intelligent IoMT in Healthcare

4.6.1.1 Remote Patient Monitoring

Remote patient monitoring is essential to reduce cost for chronic disease patients. Therefore, the IoMT domain heavily relies on wearable devices to monitor their vital signs for real-time analysis. In the event of irregularities, healthcare providers are immediately notified for prompt intervention. The quality of life of patients can be greatly improvised with a reduced number of hospital admissions with the help of remote patient monitoring.

4.6.1.2 Predictive Maintenance

With the continuous use of the medical equipment, its maintenance on a regular basis is essential. Large network hospitals can continuously track the medical equipment using sensor-based devices for overall system robustness.

4.6.1.3 Personalized Medicine

Each patient condition differs based on the severity of the illness, and therefore each patient requires personalized medicinal support in terms of dosage. IoMT captured data can be transferred to the AI algorithms to analyze the patient data in order to formulate individualized treatment plans. With the use of personalized medicine, treatment strategy can be made more effective and can improve patient conditions.

4.6.1.4 Emergency Response

The strategic use of the IoMT devices can keep a watch on patients' vital parameters and notify all the stakeholders in the event of an emergency situation. For instance, an ambulance can be equipped with IoMT devices for continuous patient monitoring when travelling to the nearest hospital. In the event of an emergency, quick action can prevent the unforeseen fatalities in life-threatening circumstances.

4.6.1.5 Clinical Trials

Using Intelligent IoMT for Edge Computing, a pharmaceutical company carries out clinical trials. Trial participants wear Internet of Medical Things (IoMT) devices that gather health data in real-time. Clinical researchers can gain insights from edge devices that process this data. The discovery of novel therapies is accelerated by the increased efficiency and information provided by clinical trials.

4.6.2 Success Stories and Best Practices

4.6.2.1 Improved Patient Outcomes

In several cardiology departments across the country, the emerging technologies such as Intelligent IoMT for Edge Computing is introduced. Early identification of cardiac disorders was made possible by ongoing monitoring and real-time analysis of patients' cardiac data. This resulted in 15% reduction in hospital admissions connected to cardiac problems. The advantage of IoMT-enabled edge computing is improved patient outcomes and reduced healthcare expenditures using early intervention and routine monitoring.

4.6.2.2 Reduced Healthcare Costs

Usually, post-operative patients monitoring incur a sizable cost. However, monitoring of the post-operative patients using IoMT-enabled edge computing technology eliminates the need for the physical presence of attendants, and therefore it reduces the significant cost as well. Engaging IoMT and edge computing results in shorter hospital stays as real-time data analytics identifies the problems at an early stage. It is observed that with the introduction of these technologies, the hospital expenses are reduced by nearly 20% as a result.

4.6.2.3 Increased Efficiency

The design and development of standardized IoMT protocols require a group of researchers and healthcare providers to collaborate. Such standardized IoMT protocols are expected to improve the healthcare coordination and efficiency by 25% with interoperability among the diversified IoMT devices for seamless integration. It is noticed that healthcare services greatly improve and become accessible with IoMT standardization.

4.6.3 Lessons Learned

4.6.3.1 Importance of Collaboration

For an effective development of IoMT systems, the collaboration among stakeholders from multiple channels, such as healthcare providers, technology vendors, legislators, and patients, is essential. Collaboration from foreign researchers also provides opportunities for state-of-the-art development of IoMT systems.

4.6.3.2 Need for Standardization

The high compatibility and interoperability among the diversified system resources and devices require standardization and protocol development. Moreover, the standardized interfaces are also essential for smooth functioning. It is observed that system standardization makes the overall system integration easier and promotes a harmonious healthcare ecosystem.

4.6.3.3 Challenges of Funding and Resource Constraints

It is observed that novel IoMT systems require a significant amount of resources and funding that makes intelligent IoMT adoption a rapid success. However, it requires significant support from government, as well as budget spending from public–private partnerships.

4.7 APPLICATIONS AND USE-CASE OF INTELLIGENT IOMT FOR EDGE COMPUTING IN HEALTHCARE

The set of relevant applications of IoMT for edge computing in the healthcare domain is discussed next.

4.7.1 Strategies of Intelligent IoMT for Edge Computing in Healthcare

4.7.1.1 Virtual Patient Monitoring

One of the important applications of IoMT using edge computing is remote patient monitoring. In this feature, the vital body signs of the patients are monitored continuously and remotely for patient diagnosis and follow-up treatments. The vital signs may include body temperature, weight, height, BMI index, etc. Remote patient monitoring facilitates an improved health outcome with reduced cost, and it saves time for the patient. Real-time patient monitoring may also result in improved activities of daily living and fewer hospital admissions.

4.7.1.2 Chronic Disease Management

IoMT coupled with edge computing in healthcare may also benefit patients with long-term conditions such as diabetes, heart disease, and asthma through continuous monitoring of vital parameters using edge devices. Using real-time monitored vital signs and parameters, healthcare professionals may proceed for detailed data analysis and insights, which are highly useful in making informed decisions. IoMT-supported healthcare also provides an opportunity for remote patient monitoring, and therefore it facilitates customized treatment planning and quality healthcare service delivery.

4.7.1.3 Telemedicine

Usually, in the case of disease or bodily problems, patients have to visit the nearby hospital and meet their doctors in person. However, with the introduction of telemedicine, the very need of in-person visits to doctors can be eliminated using a virtual doctor cosultation. Such virtual consultations through IoMT-supported healthcare delivery help both the stakeholders and save time. With proper infrastructure in place, access to healthcare services can be greatly improvised in remote underserved rural areas with reduced healthcare cost.

4.7.1.4 Wearable Technology for Predictive Analytics

Wearable devices, such as smart watches, fitness trackers, and heart monitoring belts, form the core components of data acquisition for Intelligent IoMT enables edge computing. These wearable devices facilitate the continuous monitoring of the vital bodily parameters and provide customized health suggestions to patients in real time in the form of the alert notifications. Such informed alerts are generated based on the predictive analytics of the collected data over a period of time, which are personalized and based on the patient's historical as well as current health conditions. Predictive analytics also help to know the illness development and the risk level associated with specific disorder, and they also help modify the corresponding treatment plans.

4.7.1.5 Clinical Trials and Decision Support

Usually, data collection plays an important role for any patient's effective diagnosis and treatment. In medical science, IoMT-enabled devices greatly eases the cumbersome process of clinical trial data collection in real time. In several instances, IoMT devices offer an efficient alternative and make clinical trials more efficient and closer to real time for treatment efficacy while reducing the possible side effects with improved patient health. Moreover, IoMT devices collect data and can be coupled with AI to support healthcare providers in making well-informed decisions and providing enhanced care.

4.7.1.6 Emergency Response

The one of the important aspects of quality healthcare services is to provide timely interventions to the patients and doctors. The fundamental aspects of IoMT devices is to detect emergencies such as heart attacks or strokes and to generate warning alerts in real time to keep all stakeholders informed. Such real-time responses may save lives in critical situations and provide prompt and appropriate care to the patients.

IoMT for Edge Computing opens the range of opportunities and has several use-cases with applications in the healthcare industry, including but not limited to wearable technology, clinical decision support, emergency response, remote patient monitoring, and disease management.

4.7.2 Use-Cases for Edge Computing in Healthcare

Edge computing enables the local processing of healthcare data and facilitates its prompt computing data analytics. In recent years, due to the emergence of edge computing, the healthcare industry has seen a tremendous transformation by employing remote patient monitoring, telemedicine, and detecting abnormal heart rhythms and strokes. Usually, the healthcare industry was facing a challenge of delay in data transfer, and edge computing has mitigated the delay problem and has improvised the ability of the pharmaceutical drug manufacturing and supply chain to guard against disruption. Edge computing, coupled with the blockchain technology, can accurately identify, track, and trace the risk associated with the drug manufacturing, temperature control, etc. Moreover, the integration of the edge computing with IoMT produces the robust AI models that help robots in surgical procedure, virtual assistance, etc. Additionally, the integration of 5G technology with edge computing facilitates the real-time monitoring of health status and remote operation.

With the emergence of edge computing, improved data transfer becomes the norm when coupled with faster device reaction times, which optimize the use of virtual reality in medical operations and training for improved outcomes. Such virtual training will likely revolutionize the way healthcare practitioners obtain their knowledge and conduct their practices. Rapid and quick response is essential for providing emergency healthcare services. Technologies such as edge computing incorporated with AI and IoMT facilitate diagnosis and predictive analytics.

Accelerating the transmission of patient information is crucial for hospitals, since latency difficulties, sluggish processing, and unstable networks may hinder emergency assistance. Utilizing edge networks to decentralize data aligns with data sovereignty requirements and mitigates data breaches by thwarting hackers' ability to infiltrate whole systems via a single access point. Akamai's inventive methods of providing assistance and ensuring the safety of healthcare and life sciences enterprises at all stages of growth are crucial for this advancement [33].

The Internet of Things (IoMT) can transform healthcare by delivering up-to-the-minute, precise, and safeguarded medical data. However, in certain cases, the overall cost of the entity becomes an obstacle to its popular implementation. Usually, several cost components are associated with the implementation of the infrastructure and IoMT configurations such as sensors, networks, and fog computing technologies associated with medical devices. Moreover, cloud computing technology helps to certain extent. However, the delay in the data transfer is prominent, and therefore it is not widely accepted. To mitigate the problems, researchers are designing novel deployment configurations that reduce overall maintenance costs while ensuring consistent IoMT deployment.

On the contrary, data security and privacy help form the secured IoMT system, which is of paramount importance in sustainable and secured system design. The vulnerability of public networks and their unsecured sensors deployment increase the chances of potential breaches of the system, which result in the transfer by hostile intruders of compromised data. To address these concerns, it is essential to design robust authentication and verification methods supported with advanced encryption techniques coupled with state-of-the-art blockchain technology. One example of secured system design is smartcard-based telemedicine systems, which safeguard the patient's data against unauthorized access to the system.

The precision of IoMT data is essential in any healthcare service delivery. However, for such high precision, it is essential that healthcare systems remain consistent and produce reliable results with accepted accuracy over repeated applications. In such situations, the intelligent model designed as a backbone to the proposed healthcare system potentially serves as a remedy. However, the fundamental challenges of engaging intelligent models is the lack of ability of limited computer-powered IoMT devices to carry out complex computations.

The design and development of sustainable medical devices that effectively provide reliable healthcare service and also generate power is crucial to promote Internet of Medical Things (IoMT) systems [34].

The market for wearable technology connected to pregnancy has shown substantial growth, with devices such as fetal monitors and health screening equipment being used to track maternal health indicators. IoT and AI technologies are being suggested to enhance maternal healthcare to decrease maternal death rates, such as an Internet of Things (IoT) platform using wearable sensors [35] created for fog computing and cloud analytics. In contrast, an IoT and artificial intelligence (AI) system [36] was introduced that monitors maternal vital signs and delivers immediate alarms. Li et al. introduced an advanced Internet of Medical Things (IoMT) platform designed [37] specifically for maternal medical services. This platform allows for the efficient and accurate monitoring of vital signs in real time, ensuring the dependable management of maternal health data.

Edge computing is essential for healthcare applications because it enables the connection of the Internet of Medical Things (IoMT) devices with high-processing machines, resulting in minimal network latencies. The Internet of Medical Things (IoMT) has transformed healthcare by enabling intelligent home-based monitoring and diagnosis for older individuals suffering from chronic illnesses. Internet of Medical Things (IoMT) devices collect live medical data, which decreases the need for hospital trips and stays and which enables prompt monitoring and diagnosis in smart homes. Continuous monitoring enhances the efficient use of hospital resources and alleviates the fiscal load associated with the aged population. The rise in popularity of 5G mobile technology has expedited the transition of the conventional medical business to intelligent and wireless healthcare [38] Nevertheless, the current state of the medical data monitoring and diagnostic approach, which relies on IoMT and cloud computing, is still in its early stages and requires substantial computational and communication resources. The objective of an edge-assisted Internet of Medical Things (IoMT) smart-home monitoring system is to accomplish localized medical data diagnosis and swift communication by using edge and fog computing.

The Internet of Things (IoMT) has truly revolutionized healthcare service delivery by engaging novel services such as remote patient monitoring. Additionally, IoMT has also been a successful case study for remote patient monitoring for those patients suffering from dementia based on the illness stage and diagnosis without physical presence of the medical officer. It is to note that timely identification of dementia using the Internet of Medical Things (IoMT) is basic for improved therapy and medication. IoMT systems coupled with AI can help identify the dementia at an early stage, which makes it possible for more effective surveillance and therapy. In this context, a recent example is Demencare, which is a novel concept that utilizes IoT and edge computing for remote monitoring of dementia patients, and it also provides crucial information about both the patients and their caretakers. Although there is currently no remedy for dementia, Demencare may assist patients in expressing their requirements and effectively managing their disease. The sector offers extensive opportunities to use IoT and sensors to enhance the lives of dementia sufferers by creating a technologically advanced environment that improves convenience [39].

4.7.3 Edge Computing Contributes to Resilient and Secure Healthcare Data Systems

Smaller private physicians' offices have specific difficulties when it comes to implementing digitization since they lack specialized IT personnel and struggle with adhering to data standards. Edge databases serve as repositories for storing data locally, whilst tablets such as iPads are used for gathering and monitoring data. Nevertheless, it is inadvisable to keep data in a centralized cloud server due to the heightened risk of data breaches and the regulatory problems it poses. Cloud-based configurations need uninterrupted internet connectivity [40].

Edge computing facilitates the reliable operation of digital healthcare apps, enabling ambulance crews and physicians to promptly provide optimal treatment. This technology will reduce friction, optimize operational procedures, and expedite treatment time by syncing pertinent information with corresponding healthcare units.

Interoperability and data security are essential for the proper operation of the Internet of Medical Things (IoMT). An innovative approach is required to integrate digital amenities with medical services. Prospective studies should prioritize investigating clinical reasoning, differential diagnosis, joint and soft tissue evaluation, high-resolution digital methods for muscle stretching, thoracic manipulation, effective strategies for spine locking, and cloud data-based prescription for spine training [41].

Major Roles of IoMT in Covid Era

- Proactive orthopedic therapy
- Cost savings
- Urgent medical attention
- Teleorthopedics
- Health surveillance and monitoring
- Surveillance implemented on the policyholder to prevent any fraudulent activities, enhancing the transparency of the claims, facilities, and other related aspects
- Enabling the computation of medication storage and use by connecting various devices
- Assisting orthopedic surgeons in efficiently overseeing their responsibilities in both clinical and hospital settings by providing comprehensive administrative and clinical capabilities

The use of remote telemedicine enables the feasibility of conducting consultations. The IoMT can serve as a useful tool in hospital management through various means:

1. Tracking and monitoring valuable assets such as expensive medical instruments and implants
2. Efficiently managing inventory
3. Enhancing the management of patient flow within the hospital and identifying any issues
4. Measuring staff productivity and efficiency, among other benefits

The use of the Internet of Things (IoMT) technology in healthcare faces a set of challenges such as data security, data privacy, data vulnerabilities, data interoperability, data scalability, and trust preservation. However, data vulnerability in healthcare also faces significant cyber threats and causes tsignificant issues. Data interoperability is also essential to pursue noticeable insights with meaningful clinical outcomes. However, regulatory certification is essential and requires the clearance for medical devices to meet clinical standards. Usually, IoMT IT infrastructure, cloud computing, and the high expenses associated with infrastructure are the foremost challenge for the implementation of IoMT. Another fundamental challenge is the lack of standardization, which restricts data scalability and increases time to the market. Gradually, these challenges impact interoperability and reduce the applicability of the Internet of Medical Things (IoMT). A further challenge is the high level of strain on networks among the hospitals. A proper network infrastructure is necessary to support a full deployment of an IoMT system. Ensuring a high level of confidence is essential for healthcare companies to effectively provide the smooth usage of data to avoid the potential damage for advantageous data accessibility [42].

4.8 CONCLUSION

The study explores the potential of Intelligent IoMT (Internet of Medical Things) for Edge Computing in the healthcare industry, highlighting its potential for improved patient outcomes, reduced healthcare costs, and increased operational efficiency. However, challenges such as security, privacy, latency, and interoperability exist. The study suggests that IoMT integration could revolutionize smart city healthcare services, improving patient care, cost savings, and operational efficiency. Real-time monitoring, predictive maintenance, and personalized medicine can improve patient outcomes and early diagnosis. The technology can also lower operating expenses by reducing hospital stays and equipment downtime. The study emphasizes the need for continuous research, cooperation, and a strong regulatory framework to fully realize IoMT's potential in smart cities.

4.9 FUTURE DIRECTIONS

In the future, the Intelligent IoMT for Edge Computing in healthcare has the potential to revolutionize the industry by improving patient outcomes, reducing costs, and increasing productivity. Collaboration among technology suppliers, legislators, patients, and healthcare providers is crucial for its success. Funding for research and development, policies, and regulatory frameworks are necessary to ensure compliance, safety, and security. Standardization of protocols and interfaces is also necessary for interoperability. Blockchain and AI can provide transparent patient data management, while telemedicine expansion will enhance healthcare accessibility in smart cities. Patient involvement in healthcare can increase as IoMT devices become more accessible and networked.

REFERENCES

[1] Kamruzzaman MM, Alrashdi I, Alqazzaz A. New opportunities, challenges, and applications of Edge-AI for connected healthcare in Internet of Medical Things for smart cities. *J Healthc Eng.* 2022:2950699. https://doi.org/10.1155/2022/2950699. Retraction in: *J Healthc Eng.* 2023:9823658.

[2] Alrazgan M. Internet of Medical Things and edge computing for improving healthcare in smart cities. *Math Probl Eng.* 2022;2022: Article ID 5776954, 10 pages. https://doi.org/10.1155/2022/5776954

[3] Awad AI, Fouda MM, Khashaba MM, Mohamed ER, Hosny KM. Utilization of mobile edge computing on the Internet of Medical Things: A survey. *ICT Express.* 2023;9(3):473–485, ISSN 2405-9595. https://doi.org/10.1016/j.icte.2022.05.006.

[4] Kakhi K, Alizadehsani R, Khosravi A, Nahavandi S, Islam SMS. Challenges of Internet of Medical Things for electronic healthcare. In: *2021 IEEE 4th International Conference and Workshop Óbuda on Electrical and Power Engineering (CANDO-EPE).* Budapest, Hungary, 2021, pp. 19–24. https://doi.org/10.1109/CANDO-EPE54223.2021.9667929

[5] Gyamfi, E, Ansere, JA, Kamal, M. Network security system in mobile edge computing-to-IoMT networks using distributed approach. In: Srivastava G, Ghosh U, Lin JCW (eds.). *Security and Risk Analysis for Intelligent Edge Computing.* Advances in Information Security, Vol. 103. Springer, Cham;2023. https://doi.org/10.1007/978-3-031-28150-1_9

[6] https://ieeexplore.ieee.org/stamp/stamp.jsp?tp=&arnumber=9254501, accessed on January 31, 2024

[7] Althebyan Q, Yaseen Q, Jararweh Y, Al-Ayyoub M. Cloud support for large-scale e-healthcare systems. *Ann Telecommun.* 2016;71(9–10):503–515.

[8] Cavoukian A, Fisher A, Killen S, Hoffman DA. Remote home health care technologies: How to ensure privacy? Build it in privacy by design. *Identity Inf Soc.* 2010;3(2):363–378. https://doi.org/10.1007/s12394-010-0054-y

[9] Bernardos CJ, de la Oliva A, Serrano P, et al. An architecture for software-defined wireless networking. *IEEE Wirel Commun.* 2014;21(3):52–61. https://doi.org/10.1109/MWC.2014.6845049

[10] Cetinkaya S, Hashmi US, Imran A. What user-cell association algorithms will perform best in mmWave massive MIMO ultra-dense HetNets? Paper presented at. In: *2017 IEEE 28th Annual International Symposium on Personal, Indoor, and Mobile Radio Communications (PIMRC).* Montreal, Canada, 2017.

[11] Bai T, Heath RW. Coverage and rate analysis for millimeter-wave cellular networks. *IEEE Trans Wirel Commun.* 2015;14(2):1100–1114. https://doi.org/10.1109/TWC.2014.2364267.

[12] Andrews JG, Bai T, Kulkarni MN, Alkhateeb A, Gupta AK, Heath RW. Modeling and analyzing millimeter wave cellular systems. *IEEE Trans Commun.* 2017;65(1):403–430. https://doi.org/10.1109/TCOMM.2016.2618794.

[13] Rappaport TS, Gutierrez F, Ben-Dor E, Murdock JN, Qiao Y, Tamir JI. Broadband millimeter-wave propagation measurements and models using adaptive-beam antennas for outdoor urban cellular communications. *IEEE Trans Antennas Propag.* 2013; 61(4):1850–1859. https://doi.org/10.1109/TAP.2012.2235056

[14] Park J, Samarakoon S, Bennis M, Debbah M. Wireless network intelligence at the edge. *CoRR.* 2018. https://arxiv.org/abs/1812.02858.

[15] Goodfellow I, Bengio Y, Courville A. *Deep Learning.* Cambridge, MA: MIT Press, 2016. http://www.deeplearningbook.org

[16] Dean J, Corrado GS, Monga R, et al. Large-scale distributed deep networks. In: *Advances in Neural Information Processing Systems 25*, Vol. 1, pp. 1223–1231, Curran Associates Inc, Red Hook, New York; 2012.

[17] Jin P, Yuan Q, Iandola F, Keutzer K. How to scale distributed deep learning? *CoRR.* 2016. http://arxiv.org/abs/1611.04581.

[18] Javaid M, Khan IH. Internet of Things (IoT) enabled healthcare helps to take the challenges of COVID-19 pandemic. *J. Oral Biol. Craniofacial Res.* 2021;11(2):209–214.

[19] Akmandor AO, Jha NK. Smart health care: An edge-side computing perspective. *IEEE Consum Electron Mag.* 2018;7(1):29–37.

[20] Poniszewska-Maranda A, Kaczmarek D, Kryvinska N, Xhafa F. Studying usability of AI in the IoT systems/paradigm through embedding NN techniques into mobile smart service system. *Computing.* 2019;101(11):1661–1685.

[21] Chung K, Yoo H. Edge computing health model using P2P-based deep neural networks. *Peer Peer Netw Appl.* 2022;13(2):694–703.

[22] Park J, Samarakoon S, Bennis M, Debbah M. Wireless network intelligence at the edge. *Proc. IEEE.* 2019;107(11):2204–2239.

[23] Muhammed T, Mehmood R, Albeshri A, Katib I. UbeHealth: A personalized ubiquitous cloud and edge-enabled networked healthcare system for smart cities. *IEEE Access.* 2018;6:32258–32285.

[24] Jaiswal K, Anand V, A survey on IoT-based healthcare system: Potential applications, issues, and challenges. In: *Advances in Biomedical Engineering and Technology*, pp. 459–471, Springer, New York, US;2021.

[25] Barik RK, Dubey H, Misra C, Mishra P, Das H, Mankodiya K. Fog assisted cloud computing in the era of big data and internet-of-things: Systems, architectures, and applications. In: *Cloud Computing for Optimization: Foundations, Applications, and Challenges*, pp. 367–394, Springer, New York, US;2018.

[26] Guo Y, Zhao Z, Zhao R, et al. Intelligent offloading strategy design for relaying mobile edge computing networks. *IEEE Access.* 2020;8:35127–35135.

[27] https://www.canva.com/design/DAFxziYFw0U/lFk8Gmd2NTugEVjKI-t3obg/edit?utm_content=DAFxziYFw0U&utm_campaign=designshare&utm_medium=link2&utm_source=sharebutton.

[28] Althebyan R, Yaseen Q, Jararweh Y, Al-Ayyoub M. Cloud support for large scale e-healthcare systems. *Ann Telecommun.* 2016;71(9–10):503–515.

[29] Casola V, Castiglione A, Choo KR, Esposito C. Healthcare-related data in the cloud: Challenges and opportunities. *IEEE Cloud Comput.* 2016;3(6):10–14. https://doi.org/10.1109/MCC.2016.139.

[30] Cavoukian A, Fisher A, Killen S, Hoffman DA. Remote home health care technologies: How to ensure privacy? Build it in privacy by design. *Identity Inf Soc.* 2010;3(2):363–378. https://doi.org/10.1007/s12394-010-0054-y

[31] Chung K, Park RC. Cloud-based u-healthcare network with QoS guarantee for mobile health service. *Cluster Computing.* 2017. https://doi.org/10.1007/s10586-017-1120-0

[32] Varshney U. Pervasive healthcare and wireless health monitoring. *Mob Netw Appl.* 2007;12(2–3):113–127. https://doi.org/10.1007/s11036- 007-0017-1 17
[33] https://www.akamai.com/blog/security/how-edge-computing-transforming-healthcare
[34] Niu Q, Li H, Liu Y, Qin Z, Zhang L-b, Chen J, Lyu Z. Toward the Internet of Medical Things: Architecture, trends, and challenges. *Math Biosci Eng.* 2024;21(1):650–678. https://doi.org/10.3934/mbe.2024028
[35] Venkatasubramanian S. Ambulatory monitoring of maternal and fetal using deep convolution generative adversarial network for smart health care IoT system. *Int J Adv Comput Sci Appl.* 2022;13:214–222. https://doi.org/10.14569/IJACSA.2022.0130126
[36] Vemuri PK, Kunta A, Challagulla R, Bodiga S, Veeravilli S, Bodiga VL, et al. Artificial intelligence and Internet of Medical Things based health-care system for real-time maternal stress-strategies to reduce maternal mortality rate. *Drug Invent Today.* 2020;13:1126–1129. http://doi.org/10.6084/m9.figshare.13213631
[37] Li X, Lu Y, Fu X, Qi Y. Building the Internet of Things platform for smart maternal healthcare services with wearable devices and cloud computing, future gener. *Comput Syst.* 2021;118:282–296. https://doi.org/10.1016/j.future.2021.01.016
[38] Wang X, Song Y, Edge-assisted IoMT-based smart-home monitoring system for the elderly with chronic diseases. *IEEE Sensors Letters.* 2023;7(2):1–4, Art no. 7500204, https://doi.org/10.1109/LSENS.2023.3240670. Keywords: {Medical diagnostic imaging;Older adults;Diseases;Edgecomputing;Monitoring;Real-timesystems;Hospitals;Sensornetworks; Edge computing;Fog computing;Internet of Medical Things (IoMT);Smart-home monitoring},
[39] Juneja S, Dhiman G, Kautish S, Viriyasitavat W, Yadav K. A Perspective roadmap for IoMT-based early detection and care of the neural disorder, dementia. *J Healthc Eng.* 2021;2021:6712424. https://doi.org/10.1155/2021/6712424. PMID: 34880977; PMCID: PMC8648455.
[40] https://objectbox.io/iot-edge-computing-and-digitalization-in-healthcare/
[41] https://www.journal-cot.com/article/S0976-5662(20)30179-X.
[42] https://cifs.health/backgrounds/internet-of-medical-things-challenges-and-adoptions/.

5 Data Generation, Storage, and AI-Enabled Processing of IoMT Healthcare Data in Edge Computing

Vruti Dobariya, Gone Neelakantam, and Hiren Kumar Thakkar

5.1 INTRODUCTION

Internet of Medical Things (IoMT), edge computing, and artificial intelligence (AI) have revolutionized medicine by unveiling the modern age in healthcare delivery. As a result, a great volume of health data has been generated, stored, and processed due to this integration, leading to unforeseen opportunities for improving patients' services, saving costs, and streamlining organizational performance management. With the expansion of the Internet of Healthcare Things (IoHT), the industry faces an explosion of healthcare information that needs new technologies for edge analytics as described by the authors in [1] and [2].

This report looks at the complicated connections among IoMT, edge computing, and AI inside the healthcare data environment, which involve how AI works with health data that is generated by IoMT and stored by edge computing. Edge computing helps to process data near its origin; this reduces latency and is cost-effective since data can be processed instantaneously for real-time insight with quick response intervention. At the same time, AI plays an important part in the auditing of complex datasets, looking for patterns and providing relevant data for personalized healthcare delivery and predictive maintenance.

The current study intends to offer an in-depth investigation into problems and prospects regarding the integration of IoMT, edge computing, and artificial intelligence, as shown in Figure 5.1. First, it aims at bringing out the impact that this union can have on changing patient follow-up, chronic disease control, and the healthcare service provision system as a whole. This report also looks at the issues related to the security of data and personal information, as well as the legislative requirements that are needed to ensure the security of sensitive health-related information in this era of technological revolution.

DOI: 10.1201/9781003393498-7

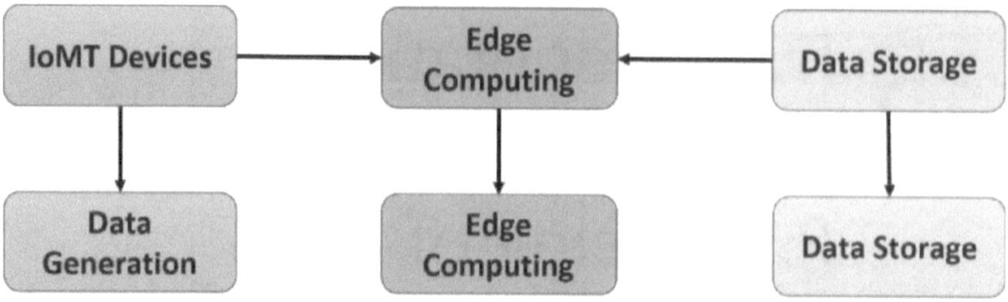

FIGURE 5.1 Integration of Internet of Medical Things, edge computing, and AI.

This study aims at adding value to the discussion about healthcare system development, which relies on advanced technologies with the aim of achieving patient-centered care. The analysis intends to enrich healthcare providers, scientists, policymakers, and developers of the IoMT, edge computing, and AI to achieve an effective, reliable, and responsive health system.

This is a detailed description of how IoMT interacts with edge computing and AI within the universe of healthcare data. Second, it explains different types of IoMT data including patient-generated data, clinical data, and sensor data, which must be generated in real time for better healthcare and surveillance services. This chapter then considers options for storing IoMT healthcare data such as cloud storage, on-premises storage, and hybrid approaches while ensuring compliance and data integrity in medical care. Furthermore, it examines the role of AI in managing IoMT healthcare information's confidentiality and enhancing precautionary medicine, diagnostic accuracy, and specific treatment procedures for each patient. Last, other issues concerning IoMT data security and privacy such as loopholes and breaches of the Health Insurance Portability and Accountability Act (HIPAA)/General Data Protection Regulation (GDPR) are also examined in this chapter. Lastly, this work offers hands-on tips for applying safe and effective information technology (IT) usage in patient serving healthcare systems to healthcare stakeholders.

5.2 RELATED WORK

The next part of the report comprises some outstanding pieces of work carried out on IoMT-based healthcare systems. These studies demonstrate numerous ways in which IoMT can be applied. These include patient tracking and monitoring using a Holter device, noncontact detection of COVID-19 and fever or disease, and physiological anomaly detection in real time. In addition, the investigations of the mentioned research reveal the importance of remote health monitoring, fall detection systems, and daily health tracking through data gathered at home about movement and soundness. This report is aimed at providing a context for this present-day research against the background of leading study papers in the field of IoMT, highlighting major strides and future perspectives on healthcare provision models and patient practice management.

The summarized study in Table 5.1 shows us the use of IoMT and its effect on patients' health management in medical care and hospitals for detection of a patient's

TABLE 5.1
Studies on IoMT-Based Healthcare System

Study	Objectives	Methodology
[3]	Tracking and monitoring of patients using a Holter device at home	Indoor tracking with the use of accelerometers and Wi-Fi networks
[4]	Monitoring of heart pulse rate and body temperature	Remote health monitoring facilitated through cloud services
[5]	Daily health monitoring through the collection of motion and audio signals at home	Collection of medical data through environmental and wearable sensors at home
[6]	Noncontact detection of COVID-19, fever, and cyanosis	Real-time detection and segmentation of forehead and lip regions, along with temperature estimation via infrared camera images
[7]	Real-time anomaly detection in physiological parameters	Implementation of an edge stream computing architecture with a distributed HTM algorithm for anomaly detection
[8]	Monitoring of cardiovascular and diabetes patients for a fall detection system	Implementation of a fall detection system

condition and disease finding. However, the first generation of such works was essential for present-day health monitoring systems, which rely on timely data gathering, remote surveillance, and noninvasive diagnostics. A review of a few notable research studies is presented here so as to assess the existing position of scientific probes in IoMT. The article further emphasizes the role played by technology in redefining a patient's care and health management. The fact that the achievements demonstrate this implies that IoMT can improve healthcare services. Additionally, such an environment enables greater innovation.

5.3 DATA GENERATION IN IOMT

5.3.1 Overview of the Types of Data Generated in IoMT, Including Patient-Generated Data, Clinical Data, and Sensor Data

- **Patient-Generated Data**: Such data comprises daily activities, vital signs, adherence to medications, and patient-reported symptoms that come from the wearable devices or healthcare apps used by the patients.
- **Clinical Data**: These include EHRs, medical imaging, laboratory test outcomes, and other disease-related data obtained by medical personnel during observation, diagnosis, and treatment of a patient.
- **Sensor Data**: This encompasses sensor information derived from medical instruments, such as heart rate monitoring, glucose meters, blood pressure cuffs, etc., and remote health care monitoring equipment. The sensors continuously record actual physiological and surrounding information and ensure regular monitoring of the patient's condition.

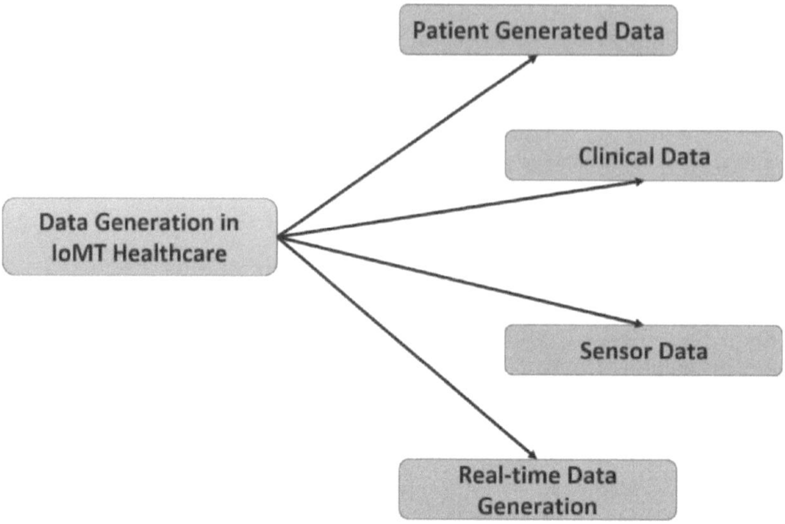

FIGURE 5.2 Data generation in IoMT healthcare.

The techniques associated with generating real-time information for patients' data in IoMT has expanded and now accommodates many types of modern technologies for effective health monitoring data management systems, as described in Table 5.2. Wearable sensors are very important in obtaining real-time information about vital health aspects that are critical in enabling an environment for proactive health monitoring and personalized care approaches. Moreover, mobile health applications have proved to be effective as user-friendly means for patients to generate data on symptoms and medication adherence. Such apps promote interaction with patients, enabling them to become better partners in their healthcare management; hence the health delivery outcomes are better. Second, remote patient monitoring systems are used in transferring patient data for the timely detection of medical problems and in providing remote healthcare to patientsm as illustrated in Figure 5.2. In addition, electronic health records make it easy for accessing and accurate data, thus streamlining data management and complete information on patients toward healthcare providers according to the studies in [9] and [10].

5.3.2 Importance of Real-Time Data Generation and Its Impact on Patient Care and Monitoring

IoMT generates critical information about a patient's health status that healthcare providers can use to make timely decisions and draft personalized treatment plans. Monitoring of the patient's vital signs, drug adherence, and even other important DM indicators in real-time mode enhances the effectiveness of treatment results and DM itself. Immediate access to data during an emergency scenario is critical since it gives time for decision-making by medical professionals. In addition, instant data enable healthcare personnel to take lifesaving measures or improve the quality of service.

TABLE 5.2
Data Generation Method

Data Generation Method	Description	Benefits
Wearable sensors [11]	Devices with sensors for real-time monitoring of vital health parameters like heart rate and physical activity	Facilitates proactive health monitoring and personalized care.
Mobile health apps	User-friendly apps for patients to input symptoms and medication adherence data	Encourages patient engagement and self-management.
Remote patient monitoring	Systems using connected devices for real-time tracking and transmission of patient data	Enables early detection of health issues and supports remote healthcare services.
Electronic health records	Digital platforms for comprehensive patient records accessible to healthcare providers	Streamlines data management and ensures accurate information availability.

5.3.3 Challenges Related to Data Quality, Security, and Privacy in IoMT Data Generation

- **Data Quality**: The correctness, credibility, and adequacy of the IoMT data are necessary for making appropriate treatment decisions. Healthcare information may be corrupted by a number of factors, including device failure, data transmission errors, inconsistent measurements, and incorrect recordkeeping. These instances often lead to misdiagnosis or inappropriate clinical decision-making.
- **Security**: The security of patient information is vital in IoMT and includes protecting data from hackers, intruders, and information theft. Medical device interconnectivity combined with health data transmission through networks increases exposure to security vulnerabilities that require strong encryption and authentication protocols as well as restricted access to patients' information.
- **Privacy**: Data generation in IoMT calls for protection compliance regarding patients' privacy and data. Privacy must be protected through strict guidelines, confidentiality of personal information and patient data, and consent with the patient before his or her data are shared, as illustrated in Figure 5.3.

5.4 STORAGE SOLUTIONS FOR IOMT HEALTHCARE DATA

5.4.1 Analysis of the Various Storage Options for Healthcare Data in Edge Computing, Including Cloud Storage, On-Premises Storage, and Hybrid Storage Solutions

- **Cloud Storage**: This entails healthcare data storage on distant servers available over the internet. Scalable, cost-effective, and convenient cloud storage give medical institutions the possibility of accessing medical data irrespective of location or time period.

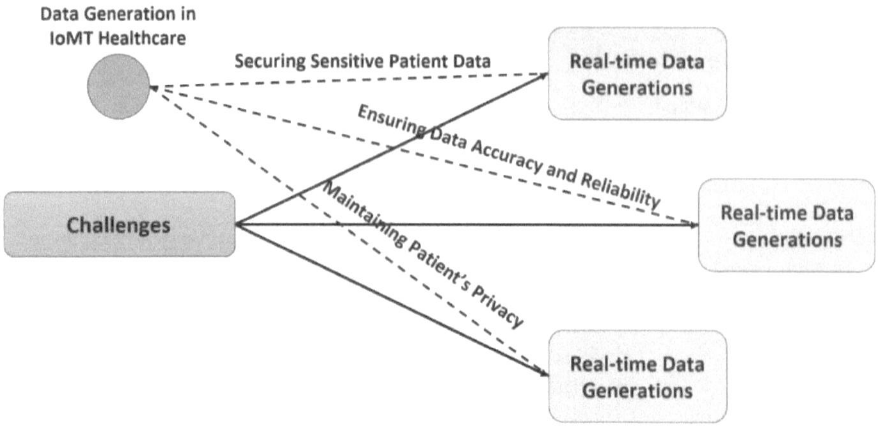

FIGURE 5.3 Challenges faced in IoMT healthcare.

- **On-Premises Storage**: On-premises storage allows healthcare organizations to maintain exclusive possession of their data as they store it on their local server within their premises. The strategy is more secure and complies with the required regulations for patient data that require tight regulatory control.
- **Hybrid Storage Solutions**: A hybrid solution allows organizations to reap the benefits of scalable cloud storage and store critical data locally on local servers for more control over security and compliance. Using this method, data are available and are duplicated for easy replacement in cases of system failures or network disturbances.

5.4.2 Comparison of the Advantages and Disadvantages of Different Storage Solutions in Terms of Data Accessibility, Scalability, and Security

5.4.2.1 Cloud Storage

Advantages: Provides a great degree of flexibility in terms of ease of use, scalability, and affordability for simple analytics tasks. This makes it possible to be easily compatible with different third-party apps and external service providers.

Disadvantages: Cyber threats and possible breaches of users' confidential data raise concerns over data security and privacy. Second, it requires a good internet connection that might be unavailable in rural and underserved communities.

5.4.2.2 On-Premises Storage

Advantages: Enhances data security, compliance, and management of data in its entirety. First, it guarantees reliable data access regardless of internet connection, with a low chance of data compromise.

Disadvantages: This entails a huge initial investment and running costs, as well as a limited scalable approach when compared to cloud solutions and risky processes such as data backup and disaster management.

5.4.2.3 Hybrid Storage Solutions

Advantages: It has multiple advantages over cloud or premised storage in regard to increased resilience, scalability, and extra security measures. Organizations have the ability to specify the data security and access level they desire.

Disadvantages: The complexity of the data storage infrastructure may arise when it comes to integrated and comprehensive approaches. The system should also possess powerful network connectivity for smooth synchronization of data between on-premises and cloud systems, as shown in Figure 5.4.

5.4.3 Importance of Data Integrity and Compliance with Healthcare Regulations in the Storage of Sensitive Patient Data

- **Data Integrity**: IoMT systems handle healthcare information that must be accurate and consistent; hence data integrity is critical. It entails implementing data validation methods, performing regular data backups, and employing data encryption techniques to maintain data integrity and prevent illegal data manipulation or loss.

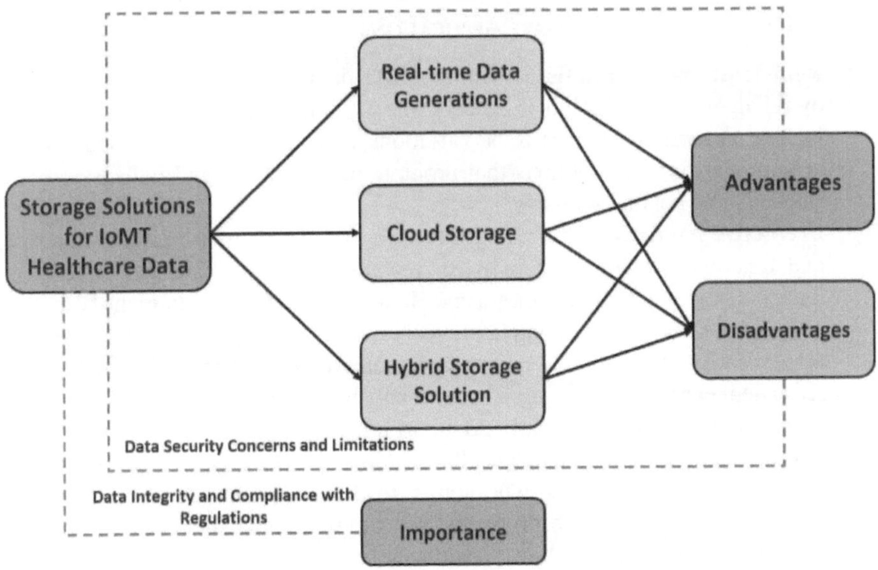

FIGURE 5.4 Storage solutions for IoMT healthcare data.

- **Compliance with Healthcare Regulations**: To maintain patient data privacy, it is critical to comply with healthcare legislation such as HIPAA, GDPR, and industry-specific requirements. To comply with regulatory standards while also respecting patients' privacy and confidentiality, healthcare businesses must have strong data protection mechanisms, access controls, and data retention rules. These policies aid in the development of trust between patients and healthcare practitioners, resulting in a safe and ethical healthcare environment.

5.5 AI-ENABLED PROCESSING IN IOMT HEALTHCARE DATA

5.5.1 Explanation of the Role of Artificial Intelligence (AI) in Processing and Analyzing IoMT Healthcare Data at the Edge

In the healthcare space of IoMT, AI helps to interpret the vast amount of data collected on the edge from which it originates through sophisticated algorithms. By using real-time data interpretation, pattern recognition, and predictive modeling, healthcare professionals can glean important information about patient trends in health, disease progression, and response to treatments through AI. Using edge AI can reduce latency, improve the safety of critical patient data, help healthcare professionals make timely and appropriate decisions based on data, as well as help to monitor patients better, take preventive actions faster, and effectively deliver health services in a cost-effective fashion.

5.5.2 Evaluation of AI Algorithms for Real-Time Data Analysis, Predictive Analytics, and Anomaly Detection in Healthcare Applications

- **Real-Time Data Analysis**: Streaming IoMT data can be quickly processed by AI algorithms, which help detect critically important health events that include abnormal vital signs or variations in patient state. This enables prompt warnings and actions that promote patient safety and reduce possible adverse health outcomes.
- **Predictive Analytics**: Predicting future health risks, disease progression, and treatment outcomes from AI-driven models using historical patient data and real-time health monitoring. Healthcare providers can identify at-risk patients and predict complications before they occur. This is followed by preventive measures and personalized interventions, which result in better patient care and long-term health management.
- **Anomaly Detection**: With such AI algorithms, it is easy for any anomaly or unusual changes in a patient's health data to stand out compared to norms and even predicted trends. The ability to diagnose and adapt treatment plans for emerging health problems in a timely manner helps save lives, improve patient care, and lower healthcare costs.

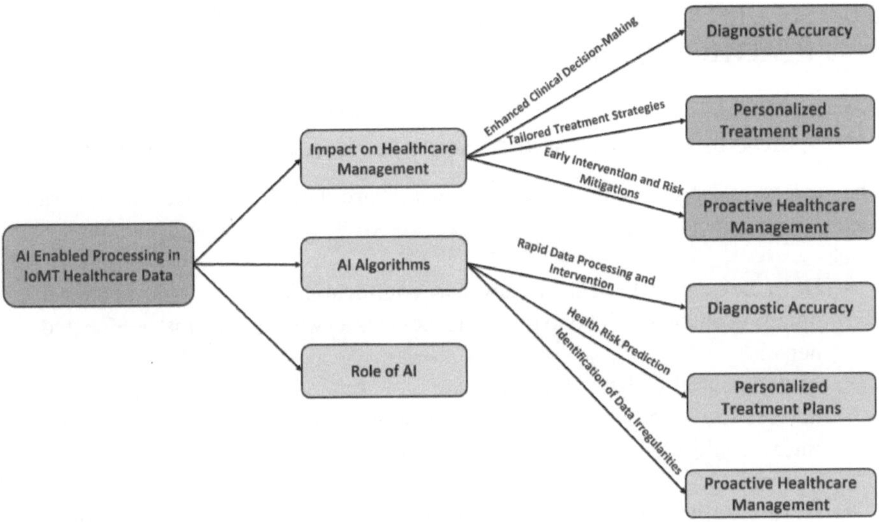

FIGURE 5.5 AI-enabled processing in IoMT healthcare data.

5.5.3 Impact of AI-Enabled Processing on Improving Diagnostic Accuracy, Personalized Treatment Plans, and Proactive Healthcare Management

- **Diagnostic Accuracy**: These AI-enabled diagnostic systems can conduct intricate clinical analyses on such inputs as imaging scans, patient reports, and gene data with great speed and reliability. AI improves the speed and precision of clinical decision-making by automating disease identification, risk assessment, and differential diagnosis, resulting in more dependable diagnosis and an optimal patient outcome.
- **Personalized Treatment Plans**: The use of AI in providing AI-driven insights on patient-specific data helps in the development of customized treatment plans considering health parameters, genes, and lifestyle aspects of the patient. AI is used in the development of patient-centric approaches by tailoring medication regimens, therapy recommendations, and lifestyle interventions to individual needs, leading them to engage with therapy, adhere to treatment protocols, and pursue wellness.
- **Proactive Healthcare Management**: Providing healthcare providers with tools such as AI-enabled proactive monitoring and risk stratification enables them to identify high-risk patients early enough to give them preventative measures as well as timely interventions before health complications set in. Remote monitoring and providing personalized coaching help in creating a more proactive approach to disease management while promoting healthy living and hence better outcomes in health and lower costs related to healthcare, as illustrated in Figure 5.5.

5.6 SECURITY AND PRIVACY CONCERNS IN IOMT HEALTHCARE DATA MANAGEMENT

5.6.1 Assessment of the Potential Security Risks Associated with the Storage and Processing of Sensitive Healthcare Data at the Edge

The storage and processing of sensitive healthcare data at the edge poses various security risks, including:

- **Data Breaches**: Patient privacy and confidentiality are at risk whenever unlawful entry is gained to the IoMT devices as well as their interconnected networks.
- **Malware and Cyber Attacks**: Given how the internet is connected, these devices are vulnerable. Malware, ransomware, or any other type of cyber threat could cause operational delays in health facilities and jeopardize patients' well-being.
- **Data Tampering**: Abuse of patient health information is very dangerous as it has implications for the patient's life because erroneous diagnoses, wrong treatment plans, etc. may be caused by manipulating patient health data, which results in various health risks to the patients concerned.
- **Physical Security Threats**: Healthcare data kept on edge devices and in the data storage infrastructure is susceptible to stealing, damaging, or forced physical entry, which may render it destroyed or corrupted.

5.6.2 Discussion of Privacy Challenges and the Importance of Implementing Robust Encryption, Access Controls, and Data Anonymization Techniques

The storage and processing of sensitive healthcare data at the edge pose various security risks, including:

- **Data Interoperability**: The protection of patients' privacy, while at the same time safeguarding data integrity and security, is maintained by integrating data from multiple sources that utilize standardized data formats and secure data exchange protocols to ensure consistency throughout the system.
- **Identity Protection**: Confidentiality of patients and privacy of information should also prevail for the protection of their identities against theft of identity, fraud, or illegal disclosures. Strong encryption, a multifactor authentication system, and reliable identification control procedures can be used to avoid those vulnerabilities.
- **Consent Management**: Violating patients' autonomy and privacy preferences will arise. Fairness with regard to the consent management framework should be equally considered, and patients will trust the system with their data only when they are sure that s the data are well managed with the utmost professionalism with regard to the data governance strategy set by the hospital or clinic to which they reported.

- **Data Anonymization**: Nonetheless, several data protection measures such as de-identification, aggregation, and pseudonymization are employed to protect individuals' privacy while still facilitating the analyses and research processes. It is possible to strike a balance between the utilization of data in healthcare organizations and privacy protection in relation to confidential data by using the procedure of anonymization, wherein information remains appropriate for ethical use and handling.

5.6.3 Overview of Regulatory Compliance Requirements Such as HIPAA, GDPR, and Other Relevant Standards for Protecting Patient Data in IoMT

The security and privacy of IoMT healthcare data can only be ensured if they comply with healthcare regulations and data breach standards, as illustrated in Figure 5.6. Key regulatory requirements include:

- **Health Insurance Portability and Accountability Act (HIPAA)**: HIPAA stipulates the standards that ought to be followed when dealing with confidential or sensitive patient health information, outlines important security measures, privacy practices, and breach notification protocols in order to protect patients' rights to confidentiality and quality.
- **General Data Protection Regulation (GDPR)**: Data protection requirements under the EU's GDPR include provisions on transparency in data processing, individual data rights, and data breach notification. Data on patients of the members of the European Union is subject to GDPR, which requires healthcare organizations to maintain confidentiality in their handling.
- **Other Relevant Standards**: Besides, other national and international standards like ISO/IEC 27001, the NIST Cybersecurity Framework, and local data protection laws offer further guidance on securing healthcare information and fostering responsible data management processes. Compliance

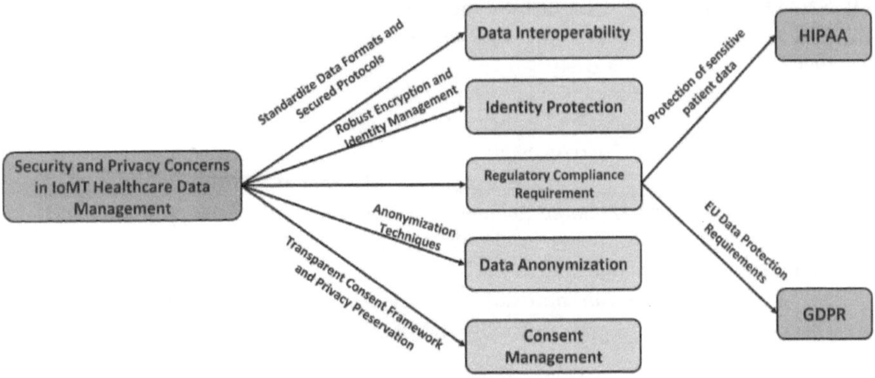

FIGURE 5.6 Security and privacy concerns in IoMT healthcare data management.

with these rules gives rise to an environment that values protection of data privacy, effective risk management, and corporate adherence to ethical rules aimed at building up patients' confidence in their data safety.

5.7 CONCLUSION

This analysis revealed that combining IoMT, edge computing, and AI has opened up unimaginable ways of producing data in real time in the healthcare industry and storing it, as well as making processing easy. It also highlighted the importance of real-time insights in proactive patient care and monitoring, specifically those involving PGD, CRD, and sensor data. An assessment of storage options emphasized an equilibrium approach, taking into account various aspects of data availability, expansion, and security. It also highlights that AI helps with live data analysis, predictive insight, and better health management, leading to increased correctness in diagnoses, better treatment plans based on individual needs, and proactive treatments.

The integration of IoMT, edge computing, and AI opens up a vital window of action for health systems in terms of information-based approaches relating to data safety, confidentiality, and ethics. Healthcare organizations and policymakers must emphasize information privacy and consent for this purpose. Moreover, creating an ethical culture of using data, giving more of a place to a patient-centric health approach, and sticking with regulatory compliance help to build patient trust and apply advanced technologies responsibly. This report proposes that stakeholders take a leading role in developing comprehensive strategies to confront the changing issues as well as the opportunities posed by the ever evolving IoMT environment in relation to edge computing.

REFERENCES

[1] Awad, AI, Fouda, MM, Khashaba, MM, Mohamed, E, Hosny, KM. "Utilization of mobile edge computing on the Internet of Medical Things: A survey", *ICT Express*. 2023, pp. 473–485.

[2] Sun, L, Jiang, X. Ren, H, Guo, Y. "Edge-cloud computing and artificial intelligence in Internet of Medical Things: Architecture, technology and application", *IEEE Access*. 2020, pp. 1–1. https://doi.org/10.1109/ACCESS.2020.2997831.

[3] Kaur, A, Jasuja, A. "Health monitoring based on IoT using raspberry PI", In *Greater Noida: 2017 International Conference on Computing, Communication and Automation (ICCCA)*, 2017, pp. 1335–1340.

[4] Hegde, C. Jiang, Z, Zelko, J, Kamaleswaran, R, Reyna, MA, Clifford, GD. "Autotriage-an open source edge computing raspberry Pi-based clinical screening system", *medRxiv*. https://doi.org/10.1101/2020.04.09.20059840, 2020.

[5] Villarrubia, G, Bajo, J, De Paz, JF, Corchado, JM. "Monitoring and detection platform to prevent anomalous situations in home care", *Sensors*. 14(6), 2014, pp. 9900–9921.

[6] Queralta, JP, Gia, TN, Tenhunen, H, Westerlund, T, "Edge-AI in LoRa-based health monitoring: Fall detection system with fog computing and LSTM recurrent neural networks", In *2019 42nd International Conference on Telecommunications and Signal Processing (TSP)*, IEEE, 2019, pp. 601–604.

[7] Greco, L, Ritrovato, P, Xhafa, F. "An edge-stream computing infrastructure for real-time analysis of wearable sensors data", *Future Gener Comput Syst.* 93, 2019, pp. 515–528.

[8] Pham, M, Mengistu, Y, Do, H, Sheng, W. "Delivering home healthcare through a cloud-based smart home environment (CoSHE)", *Future Gener Comput Syst.* 81, 2018, pp. 129–140.

[9] Dwivedi, R, Mehrotra, D, Chandra, S. "Potential of Internet of Medical Things (IoMT) applications in building a smart healthcare system: A systematic review", *J Oral Biol Craniofac Res.* 12(2), 2022, pp. 302–318.

[10] Dilibal, Ç. "Development of Edge-IoMT computing architecture for smart healthcare monitoring platform", In *Istanbul, Turkey: 2020 4th International Symposium on Multidisciplinary Studies and Innovative Technologies (ISMSIT)*, 2020, pp. 1–4, https://doi.org/10.1109/ISM-SIT50672.2020.9254501.

[11] Thakkar, HK., Chowdhury, SR., Bhoi, AK., Barsocchi, P. "Applications of wearable technologies in healthcare: An analytical study", In *5G IoT and Edge Computing for Smart Healthcare* (pp. 279–299). Academic Press, 2022.

6 Advancements of IoMT and AI for the Advancement of Health Monitoring

Kumar Parmar, Suraj Kothari, Damodharan Palaniappan, and Kirtirajsinh Zala

6.1 INTRODUCTION

Health is necessary for a person to live a comfortable and healthy lifestyle. The WHO describes health as a level of physical and mental fitness free from sickness and disease. Healthcare is the method of keeping or optimizing a person's health via diseases and overall fitness, treatment, and recovery. Most traditional healthcare involves traditional implementation and control of patient statistical details, past cases, lab tests, medicines, payment, and drug asset management, which creates patient failures and has a harmful impact on patients. IoT-based smart healthcare reduces simple mistakes and enables doctors to predict disease more quickly and efficiently by linking all-important element tracking devices than with a software application. The has IoMT focused on health equipment that can transmit files over the internet without requesting person-to-person or person-to-machine learning. Company management consulting projects that, by 2024, the internet will be connected to 20.4 billion items [1]. Furthermore, the IoT sector is expected to be valued at $1.7 trillion before 2024, an increase from $655.8 billion in 2014., at a 16.9% annual growth rate [2]. This huge revenue also includes the creation of IoMT devices. An IoMT system is a main framework that works based on electronic sensors and modules to acquire body parameters from a patient, a machine to process the body parameters, a design to serve as a blueprint to communicate the biological information over the internet, a short-term or long-term storage place, an image processing platform with machine learning schemes to make decisions based on the convenience of the good doctor, and an order to develop this project with machine learning schemes to make choices based on the efficiency of the doctor [3], [4]. Due to the advances in technology and networking technologies, healthcare is currently experiencing an industry transformation. The healthcare system is moving from a responsive healthcare model to something resourceful and customized, from a genetic disorder to a healthcare model. In simple terms, medical systems and basic medical investigations have become way more intelligent.

 DOI: 10.1201/9781003393498-8

6.2 EVOLUTION OF HEALTHCARE TECHNOLOGY

For the past decade, the growth of the healthcare system has given rise to new important rapid progress. The healthcare sector is expanding, and advanced inventions are being created. The growth of the healthcare system assures even more achievements that will enhance healthcare access, reduce prices, and improve health satisfaction. Here are some important positions in the growth of healthcare:

1. **Electronic Health Records (EHRs)**: The massive use of electronic healthcare records has transformed how doctors and hospitals make sure the availability, and distribution of patient data. EHRs enable the more accurate and realistic exchange of information of many suppliers, which would result in positive health outcomes. Even before the initial concepts for EHRs (electronic health records) were stablished in the 1990s, the topics, framework, and advanced technologies of such documents have been commonly modified and updated. The basic concept of promoting and enhancing healthcare has remained accurate [5].
2. **Telemedicine**: Telemedicine was first implemented in 1970 [6]. "Tele" is a Greek word that means "distance," and "mederi" is a Latin word for "to heal." Healthcare is described by the ATA as "the evolution of healthcare system in the virtual world." Telehealth's attraction exists in the use of digital technologies for information and communication to supply and help healthcare services over large places [7]. WHO says that telemedicine is the supply of healthcare services where range is a major element [8]. Sick people can now receive healthcare mostly from the privacy of their own residences thanks to advances in telemedicine. This has improved the availability of care, mainly to those who live in remote or rural locations.
3. **Wearable Devices**: With the massive increase of fitness trackers such as wearable technology and smart glasses, it is now possible to monitor patients' overall health. This information may be utilized to describe possible health problems and levels of popularity. An advanced wearable device is an inner device that serves a particular healthcare role like tracking or advice. The word "wearable" suggests that a gadget is either recognized instantly on the body system or a clothing item and that it has a suitable structure enabling it to operate as a portable device for a longer duration. In general, this involves a device with limited height and shape, responsive and strength independency, and the capacity to be applied and made to wear easily. The data mechanisms handle the creation of isolated from clinical data via physical and other sensor devices, direct input data from customers, and simply other incoming data via wireless data transfer from a server side [9].
4. **Machine Learning and Artificial Intelligence**: Machine learning and artificial intelligence are utilized in the healthcare system to boost symptom efficiency and accuracy, lower the cost, and improve health satisfaction. AI-powered methods can help healthcare organizations study large amounts of information and making smart decisions and provide good

quality outcomes. With the modern lifestyle, danger to human life has increased, and the health sector needs a device that can boost treatment plan to gain maximum accurateness. The merging of ML (machine learning) and specific high technologies improve treatment efficacy in the healthcare field [10]. ML is an important technique for increasing illness prediction scores, ignoring the fact that ML is also successfully mixed with a wide range of other predictive techniques.

6.2.1 IoMT and Its Key Components

IoMT (Internet of Medical Things) refers to a network of connected wearable devices, activity trackers, and many other systems that gather and exchange health-related information. These tools and methods collect information from body sensors and

TABLE 6.1
Summary of Evolution of Healthcare

Technology	Description
X-ray	X-ray infrared energy was used in medical diagnosis to visualize bone fragments and organs of the body in 1895.
Electrocardiogram (ECG)	Electrocardiogram (ECG) is a procedure that records the heart's electrical function to identify heart problems; it was introduced in1901.
Electroencephalogram (EEG	Electroencephalogram (EEG) is a procedure that records the brain's electrical activity to identify psychological issues; it was introduced in 1924.
Ultrasound	Ultrasound is a form of healthcare scan that employs vibrations to examine the inside parts and areas of the body; this innovation was introduced in 1950.
Magnetic resonance imaging (MRI)	Magnetic resonance imaging (MRI) is a form of healthcare examination that utilizes high-frequency sound waves to image inside cells and organs; MRI was introduced in 1977.
Telemedicine	Telemedicine provides remote healthcare and counselling through the use of software such as video calls and monitoring systems.
Electronic health records (EHR)	Electronic health records (EHR) are online documentation of a person's health record, therapies, and prescriptions; EHR was introduced in 1960–1970
Wearable health devices	Wearable medical system gadgets that measure and track health parameters like heartbeat, calories burned, and sleep habits.
Artificial intelligence (AI)	AI is used to assess patient information and help with diseases and therapy suggestions.
Internet of Medical Things (IoMT)	The Internet of Medical Things (IoMT) describes healthcare equipment and networks that are linked and transfer medical information for research and monitoring.

send it to medical professionals for observation, enabling them to discover everything about a person's overall health. This information can be utilized to recognize possible health risks and track trends, enabling healthcare organizations to take better informed choices and reduce medical errors. Biosensors, healthcare products, and smart healthcare systems are different types of IoMT gadgets. These technologies and gadgets communicate to create a more accurate and linked healthcare system, allowing healthcare devices to manage patients more actively and always to provide healthcare and better care.

6.2.1.1 Components of IoMT

The IoMT has major four key components: endpoints, gateway, back end, mobile (Figure 6.1).

6.2.1.2 Endpoints

Endpoints are external hardware components that act like a point of sensing the physical environment, which is one of the phases of a network service, which includes fitness devices, based on GSMA (Global System for Mobile Communication Association) [8]. A medical product is known by the FDA (Food and Drug Administration) as a device, equipment, utility, computer, object, transplant, stem cell reaction, or another comparable or related essay, including a particular element or item of clothing, meant for use in the treatment of illness or other requirements, or in treatment,

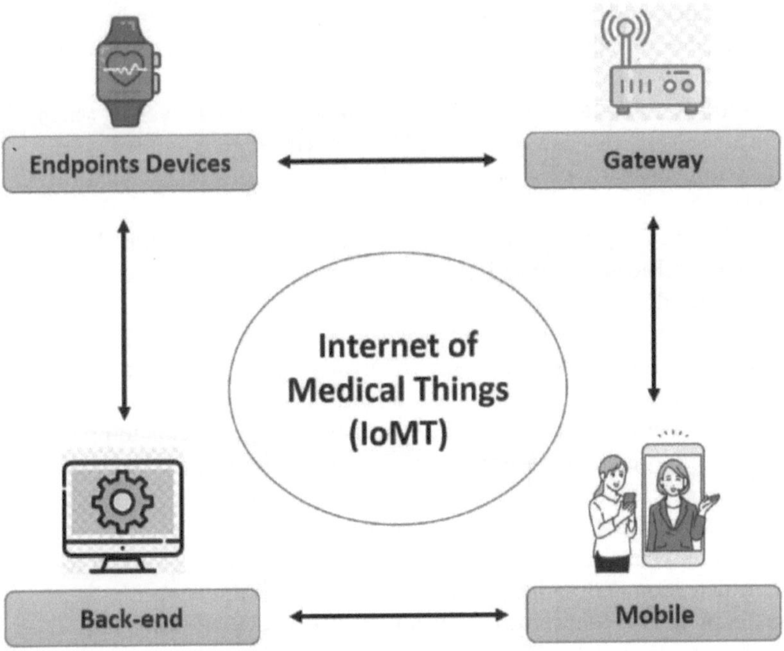

FIGURE 6.1 Classification of IoMT components [11].

management, care, or infection prevention [9]. It also defined as equipment linked to the online platform, healthcare network, or other healthcare product.

6.2.1.3 Gateway

A network gadget collates information and improves communication of limited end points by working as a switching function to the back end.

6.2.1.4 Back End Management

The majority of modern IoT systems use virtualized systems that provide integrated back end functionality such as storage devices, file transfer, environment supervision, reviews and predictive analysis, and internet applications.

6.2.1.5 Mobile

Mobile apps are used in many IoMT frameworks to include back end planning, end point monitoring, and data analysis.

6.2.2 Implementation of IoMT

Effective implementation of the Internet of Medical Things can be a complicated task that needs skillful scheduling and execution. Some common things can be done to implement IoMT:

1. **Describe Your IoMT Task Needs and Objective**: Before you begin, you must accurately describe your IoMT program objectives and the specifications needed to implement them. It could involve improving healthcare quality, improved productivity, or improving efficiency.
2. **Determine Which Gadgets and Sensors Must Be Linked**: Verify which healthcare sensors and gadgets you need to access the server. Smartwatches, medical implants, tracking devices, and other medical instruments are examples.
3. **Select a Technology Platform**: Determine how the gadgets will be linked to the internet. Bluetooth, Wi-Fi, mobile data, and other wireless connectivity may be used.
4. **Choose a Large Data Storage Framework**: Select a framework for keeping data created by connected gadgets. This platform should be capable of securely storing, analyzing, and managing big quantities of information.
5. **Implement Security and Protection Controls**: Set up systems to protect healthcare information data from being stolen or misused. Cryptography, network access, and other safety procedures may be used.
6. **Build Risk Analysis Functionality**: Analyze information recorded from smart objects using data analysis algorithms and software. This can help with the detection of designs, patterns, and possible health dangers.
7. **Transform IoMT Ideas into Current Healthcare Programs**: This is done to guarantee quick information exchange and connectivity.

8. **Create Frameworks for Observing the Information**: Create frameworks for applying information recorded by IoMT devices. Which can include information alert systems, robotic activities, and other reactions.
9. **Guarantee Product Safety**: Make sure that the IoMT execution agrees with legal requirements, such as health insurance portability and accountability or general data protection regulation.
10. **Test the IoMT Method**: Perform a trial of the IoMT system to verify that it functions as designed and achieves the objectives of the project.
11. **Apply the IoMT Approach**: After usability testing, apply the IoMT approach throughout the health sector.

In general, IoMT embellished merging multiple methods and tools into healthcare processes to improve recordkeeping, examination, and selection. During the whole project implementation, it is necessary to work directly with healthcare professionals, IT experts, and other organizations to make sure that the system satisfies the requirements of all parties.

6.2.3 Healthcare Applications Based on Blockchain

Blockchain is reshaping advanced analytics and management in a wide range of healthcare systems. This is mostly due to its flexibility and amazing ability to frame, preserve, and collect medical information and data.

Many existing projects in the healthcare sector are centered on blockchain. Information systems, blockchain, monitoring devices, and organizations are logically categorized into four layers in the growing area of blockchain-based healthcare. Figure 6.2 represents an example of a blockchain-based procedure for smart healthcare. Partially, all records from medicinal products, laboratories, social networks, and other source materials are merged to generate actual data, which is then simplified up to big data. This information is the groundwork of a blockchain in

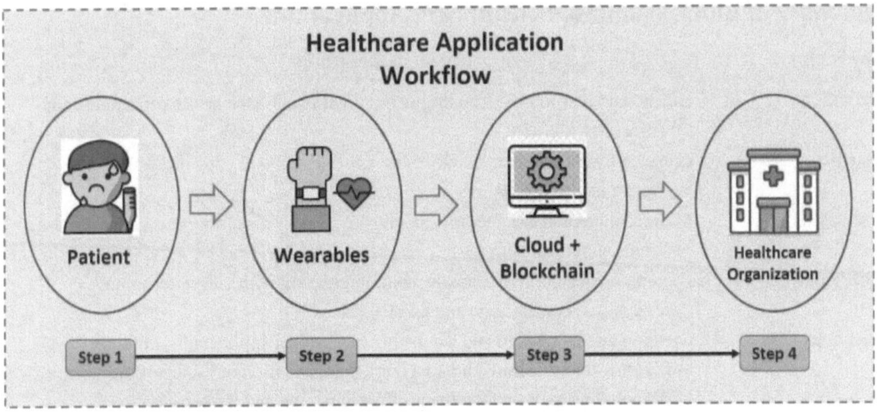

FIGURE 6.2 Workflow of a blockchain-based healthcare application.

the health sector, and it is the major element that generates the first surface of the block. Blockchain is on top of the ground data layer, which is viewed as the base in the view of safe health organizations split into four parts. Each framework has its own characteristics, such as majority view methods and protocols [12]. Blockchain interfaces make it simpler for clients to set up and manage operations. Many other blockchain technologies, including Ripple, Hyperledger Fabric, and Ethereum, have been developed and are in use nowadays. The blockchain's major elements are digital assets, electronic signatures, wallets, activities, subscriptions, and online services. A variety of methods could be used to communicate with other programs and tools between multiple nodes. Figure 6.2 represents blockchain-based applications. The user layer, which includes organizations that profit from blockchain-based applications like corporate users, scientists, and patients, is at the top of the structure.

6.2.4 Challenges and Future Scop of IoMT

6.2.4.1 Challenges of IoMT

IoMT has the ability to give continuous access to a large number of practical digital devices. Users have access to massive amounts of data collected by these gadgets, which heightense privacy concerns that must be solved. The following are some of the problems:

- Even when connected to the internet, most smartwatches cut off to process the data being moved. As regards IoMT, the input signals are mostly blank or much larger, making it difficult for network gadgets to encode such records. There are several choices for encrypting such networks; for example, networks can be encoded on burst-by-burst or per-packet validity.

TABLE 6.2
Summary of BlockchainBased Healthcare Applications

Key Factor	Description
Definition	Blockchain and IoMT technology combined to enhance health procedures and their results
Benefits	Enhanced safety of data, connectivity, cost benefits, privacy protection, and effective health results
Use-cases	Maintenance of health records, handling supply chains, drug testing, monitoring systems, and telehealth
Challenges	Factors to consider: risk management, interaction with current programs, accessibility, consistency, and privacy issues
Best practices	Creating and using safe and extensible blockchain applications, utilizing IoMT platforms for collecting and analyzing data, according to safety requirements, and including all parties in the process of design and implementation
Future perspectives	Growth and use of blockchain and IoMT in healthcare system, increasing stakeholder interaction and the opportunity for fresh companies and profits

- Many gadgets in IoMT depend on simple and defenseless passwords and verifications. Some gadgets will recognize a passcode such as 12345. It is critical to use complicated passwords to secure devices and data from cyber actors. These passcodes must conform to the limits set on the systems' available resources.
- Most gadgets are set to follow the default login and password, facing huge privacy risks to sensitive information. Challenging security elements on these gadgets would be a more efficient and effective solution.
- For a security device, many available methods include a web/mobile layout. Poor access control, bridge scripting risks, and limited default abilities make such a layout defenseless.
- More than one portion of individual data is required by hardware objects in healthcare organizations. These sensors gather information such as age, name, and so on. Because most of these gadgets send information over the internet without authentication, there is a major security threat for the files. When gadgets capture and measure data samples related to their resources, a security risk occurs. A normal buyer of food products, for example, may expose a viewer's beliefs or patient records.
- The information in the majority of IoMT systems is strongly secure and faces different security challenges since it is exchanged. For example, through healthcare organizations, personal data must be protected as a result of private data. Most current methods of data exchange in healthcare systems use a distributed structure that requires central control security mechanisms. As a result, providing reliability against errors and records visibility becomes difficult [13]. To address these issues, blockchain's data center can provide a cost-effective and flexible solution while ensuring security.

6.2.4.2 Future Scope of IoMT

The rise of IoMT comes at a time when the health system is becoming more costly. As a result, for those starting up or growing businesses, healthcare technology institutions must reorganize to compete successfully healthcare sector. They must create better strategies to successfully use big data collected from technically advanced healthcare applications in order to make their separate business model and business strategy more applicable and effective. Thus controls in the healthcare sector, as well as the growth of new methods such as AI, big data, algorithms, 3-D scanners, mobile applications, and sensor technology, will surely present both challenges (such as data security and privacy) and possibilities for the healthcare sector. Even though it is clear that robots and machines will replace some daily tasks, they will also generate new types of tasks that will demand the use of scientific organizational technical skills. Furthermore, some organizations will use IoMT devices to transfer the data, enabling them to provide national healthcare tech support through the use of machine learning algorithms. Thus the expansion of smart healthcare applications and the usage of mobile phones will lead to the fast evolution of IoMT, particularly in the health industry, to provide efficient and high-quality personal healthcare at a less cost.

6.2.5 Security and Privacy

So many methods and rules were created to help in the comfortable construction of a device. The Common CEM [14] and Open Vulnerability Scanning Methodology Manual [15] are two common and widely used security specification methods. The principles of privacy, honesty, and accessibility are the three major computer safety concepts for any kind of security control. Security is the property of not disclosing data to users, procedures, or gadgets unless they are authorized. The feature of confidentiality is the failure of unauthorized modification or destruction of data. The facility of being visible is availability.

As a result of these standards and related research activities [16], each of these protocols involves relevant security methods, which are explained next. The authors of [17] present surveys on safety, design, and frameworks in the IoMT domain, respectively, while [18] proposes a taxonomy of related security threats. The security sectors mentioned in Figure 6.3 are recommended by a large software and hardware supplier as rules for secure IoMT development:

- **Device Security**: Systems and methods for securing the sensor after being installed in the field
- **Connectivity Security**: Structures and tools for ensuring the privacy and trustless transmission of information between IoMT tools and IoMT devices
- **Cloud Security**: Function and mechanisms for protecting data during transmission to and storage in the server

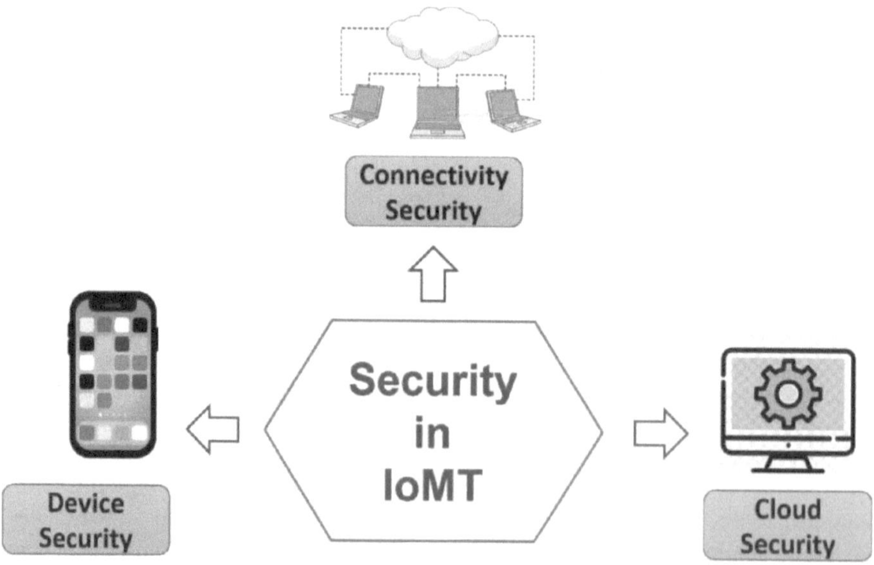

FIGURE 6.3 Security sectors in IoMT.

Popular IoMT platforms, such as the Microsoft Azure IoMT software platform [19] and the IBM Platform [20], address these concerns and offer popular solutions. IoMT security is divided into the three major categories just listed.

In the current world, simply protecting the network isn't enough to ensure its proper functioning. Privacy protection is also critical, particularly for ECG systems. In this portion, we give a brief overview of safety risks and relatively efficient security schemes.

6.2.5.1 Private Data

A large amount of data is transmitted among various systems linked to the network in IoMT-based applications, increasing privacy issues. As a result, various guidelines such as ISO/IEC 27018 [21] and 29100 [22] are created to address these problems to differing levels. Personal identifiable information is the order to get data that is used to display data about a specific person [22]. Based on this, data can be divided into three classifications: general data, statistical data, and personal data.

6.2.5.2 Prevention Mechanisms

Suspicious events that damage PII privacy include interfering with the relationship between smart gadgets or gaining private data access via wearable health devices [23, 24]. As a result, personal data must be secured before it is shared or stored. However, some defenses can be implemented to secure data during its stages, from gathering to storing and processing.

6.2.6 Wearable Healthcare Systems

WBSN (wireless body sensor networks) have been recognized as an important part of IoMT-based healthcare, WBSN is an attractive solution that is used to track a person's routine. It is made up of advanced sensor nodes that do not disrupt common events and help identify long-term illnesses like heart attacks, breathing problems, kidney disease, and so on, as well as warning patients in the event of an emergency. These systems provide attractive services in a variety of sectors. WBSN sensor nodes use very little energy and serve in a variety of fields. We can track tasks, body movement, and important body signals from remote sites using WBSNs and the internet. The demand for these gadgets is increasing by the day, and the creation of reliable small-sized sensors is necessary for the continued development of a system.

6.2.6 Architecture of WBSN

As shown in Figure 6.4, WBSN is made up of small sensor devices that are all different. Several sensors are placed around the human body to perform various functions. One is used to track blood pressure, while the other is used to monitor ECGs, and so on. Body sensor devices (BSDs) is another name for these devices. These BSDs interact with one another and with the rest of the WBSN/tier-1 network. The data from these sensor devices is collected and sent to a central server defined as the

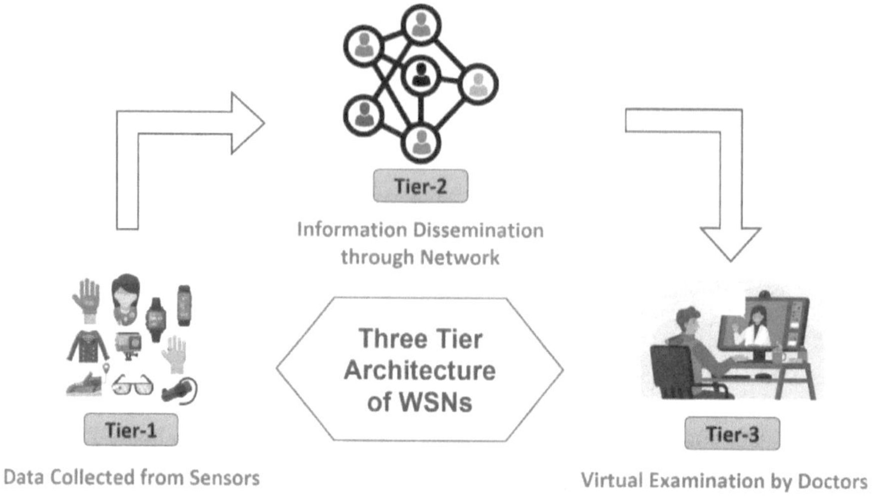

FIGURE 6.4 Architecture of WBSN.

body monitoring system. The data is then sent to other systems or networks, which can be laptops or mobiles, which is known as inter-WBSN/tier-2 interaction. Data is transmitted from these machines to a wireless router via existing communication networks such as Bluetooth, WIFI, and others. The data is then routed to the access point so that it can link to a variety of networks. Once information is sent through the internet, it is easily accessible. The information at these sites can be saved to database servers and used for testing by medical professionals, keeping health records, and other purposes. To prevent misuse, some security protocols can be implemented to access only a few verified individuals. The data can also be saved on our device or smartphone and later uploaded to a PC. While located far away from the patient, the medical professional can examine him or her and manage the necessary medicine. This is referred to as interaction beyond WBSN/tier-3. We can transfer information via the internet using 4G/5G networks.

This part of the research focused on semi- and fewer sensors, except for the monitoring unit. Five basic sensors are recognized: three for tracking vital signs like heart rate, breathing rate, and pulse rate, and two for tracking both heart rate and breathing; both are widely noted in a medical area.

6.2.6.1 Pulse Sensors

Pulse, one of the most noticed important signs, can be utilized to identify a wide range of urgent situations, including heart disease, collapsed lungs, and difficulty breathing. Pulse sensor nodes have been studied, both for device applications and activity trackers. Pulse values can be taken from the body, arm, earlobe, fingers, and other locations. Although scrotum- and finger-measured values are highly accurate, they are not very usable. Although an abdomen system is wearable, arm sensors are generally thought to be the most flexible for long-term use.

6.2.6.2 Breathing Rate Sensors

Another sign is the breathing rate or the percentage of breaths taken per minute by the service user. Observing breathing could help identify situations such as breathing problems, chest tightness due to anxiety disorder, respiratory episodes, lung disease, breathing obstructions, infectious diseases, and others. Many past projects have created sensors that monitor breathing rates of the importance of breathing. Several types of breathing rate sensors have emerged from past projects. One is a thermistor nose sensor. The reason for creating these sensors is that exhaled air is hotter and drier than surrounding air. As a result, the sensor tracks the number of breaths by measuring the increase and decrease in temperature. This has been demonstrated to work pretty well, but exactness may be affected by other causes of seasonal changes, such as a chef trying to work in a kitchen. It's also not very comfortable to wear because it's inflexible and recognizable.

6.2.6.3 Body Temperature Sensors

Body temperature is the third key indicator, and it may be used to identify cold, heat stress, fevers, and other conditions. As a result, body temperature is a useful tool for diagnosis that should be incorporated into a wearable system of healthcare. Recent works involving the monitoring of body temperature have all made use of temperature sensors. The temperature sensor was shown in all studies to monitor an appropriate temperature range for tracking the human body with normal limits of mistakes. As a result, it is highly suggested that future designers continue to use these types of sensors.

6.2.6.4 Blood Pressure

This is not an important indicator in and of itself, pulse rate is usually monitored by the other three vital signs. High blood pressure (hypertension) is a famous risk factor for the heart, including heart disease. It also ranks as one of the greatest common serious illnesses in Australia, directly impacting 32% of adults. Of those impacted, 68% had unchecked or poorly managed high blood pressure [25]. As a result, introducing BP into the WBAN for health services would provide important data to many sick people. Nonetheless, designing a wearable sensor for continuously and noninvasively monitoring blood pressure remains a challenge in the field of healthcare. A lot of research attempted to achieve a precise estimate of blood pressure by calculating pulse travel time (PTT), that is, the time taken between a pulse first at the heart and a pulse at some other spot. Another study attempted to calculate this theory between the throat and the limb. PTT is defined to be comparable to SBP, and it is typically measured with an ECG signal.

6.2.6.5 Pulse Oximetry Sensors

The level of blood oxygen levels is measured using a pulse sensor. Blood oxygen level, like heart rate, is not a key indicator, but it is an indicator of breathing and can help in the diagnosis of illnesses such as oxygen starvation. As such, a sensor is an important part of complete health tracking. Biosensors monitor the amount of oxygen in the blood by receiving PPG waves. Two LEDs are usually targeted through the body. Nearly all of this artificial light is captured by the bloodstream. The receiving detector measures the light that isn't consumed, and the gap between collected lights is utilized to calculate oxygen levels in the blood. LED lights may or may not go through a body part to a photocell on the backside, or they can be driven at an edge in which some light strikes a photodetector located on the side of the part. These sensors are known as PPG sensors.

6.2.6.6 Other Wearable Sensors for Healthcare

Apart from device monitoring, which is an important health criterion, a lot of specialized sensor devices can be useful in tracking a particular diagnosis. ECGs can be utilized to assess overall healthcare, and many wireless sensors nodes have been created to collect these pulses. ECG sensors have also been successfully integrated into helmets and more traditional chest straps. Other sensor devices have been designed for special uses, such a recognizing exhaustion or reducing stress.

TABLE 6.3
Summary of Healthcare Application

Healthcare Application	Description
Remote patient monitoring	Remotely tracking patients through wearable technology, monitors, and smartphone devices to capture and transfer real-time healthcare information to hospitals and doctors for examination and treatment monitoring
Chronic disease management	Utilizing IoMT equipment to manage illnesses including insulin, heart problems, and bronchitis by tracking signs, blood work, and treatment outcomes and alerting clients and medical providers as needed
Telemedicine and telehealth	Remote discussion and treatment, health monitoring, and medical service delivery through the online platform, using teleconference, mail, and other digital equipment
Hospital operations management	Utilizing IoT sensors and gadgets to track operations, such as healthcare system, energy use, and stock management, in order to enhance performance and reduce costs
Medication management	Medicine usage, quantity, and conformance are tracked via smart medicine bottles, medicine distributors, and smartphone apps, with warnings sent to patients as well as doctors when medicines are skipped or missed
Emergency response and disaster management	Monitoring patient's condition, resource usage, and service quality using IoT technology and sensors to identify and react to losses, terrorist attacks, and other crises
Wellness and fitness monitoring	Monitoring physical and mental wellness parameters, including steps, heartbeat, sleep habits, and other health factors via wearable technology and mobile apps, and offering customized exercise and food suggestions
Patient engagement and education	Utilizing online technologies such as mobile applications, sensors, and web-based tools to involve users with their own healthcare, give educational guidance and assistance, and promote serious disease self-management

6.2.7 Conclusion

IoMT is evolving from a research stage to demonstrable forms with brand-new programs growing. By 2025, it is assumed that there may be 41.6 billion smart ways to connect to the internet, generating huge amounts of information. These components' raw data sources must fully satisfy expectations in terms of network capacity, delay, backup, safety configuration, QoS, and QoE, among many other things. In this chapter, we examined IoMT applications. The most recent trends in safety primitives, such as verification, confidentiality, and honesty were discussed, along with security-related challenges, Future scope and the implementation of IoMT's impact on multimedia data were pointed out. The drawbacks of these elements, combined with the demand for storage devices, resulted in the development of blockchain. The blockchain network and its connection with IoMt technology, as well as blockchain's use with multimedia capabilities systems, were discussed. Several research challenges were also mentioned, as well as the key advantages of this merging. With respect to the importance of our work in terms of the future era of multimedia applications, recent works using cloud services for storage devices were introduced to show that cloud computing is the most effective way to store and arrange data in the healthcare system. Some other works have also demonstrated that analysis can be performed more effectively inside the cloud than on wearable gadgets that have limited resources. The major drawback of working with the cloud computing is that it creates security threats. As a conclusion, we offered major works designed to enhance cloud security. Initially it was observed that controls on accessing and encrypting can help to increase security, but no known standard has been prepared to begin execution of a wearable, IoMT-based health service.

REFERENCES

[1] Baker, Stephanie B., Wei Xiang, and Ian Atkinson. "Internet of things for smart healthcare: Technologies, challenges, and opportunities." *IEEE Access* 5 (2017): 26521–26544.

[2] El-Wakeel, Amr S., et al. "Towards a practical crowdsensing system for road surface conditions monitoring." *IEEE Internet of Things Journal* 5.6 (2018): 4672–4685.

[3] Mehmood, Yasir, et al. "Internet-of-things-based smart cities: Recent advances and challenges." *IEEE Communications Magazine* 55.9 (2017): 16–24.

[4] John, Jerrin T., and SR Jino Ramson. "Energy-aware duty cycle scheduling for efficient data collection in wireless sensor networks." *IJARCET* 2 (2013).

[5] Hoerbst, Alexander, and Elske Ammenwerth. "Electronic health records." *Methods of Information in Medicine* 49.4 (2010): 320–336.

[6] Strehle, E. M., and N. Shabde. "One hundred years of telemedicine: Does this new technology have a place in paediatrics?" *Archives of disease in childhood* 91.12 (2006): 956–959.

[7] Allen, Ace, and David Allen. "Telemedicine programs: 2nd annual review reveals doubling of programs in a year." *Telemedicine Today* 3.2 (1995): 10–14.

[8] Sageena, Geetanjali, Munish Sharma, and Ajita Kapur. "Evolution of smart healthcare: Telemedicine during COVID-19 pandemic." *Journal of The Institution of Engineers (India): Series B* (2021): 1–6.

[9] Glaros, Constantine, and Dimitrios I. Fotiadis. "Wearable devices in healthcare." In *Intelligent paradigms for healthcare enterprises*. Berlin, Heidelberg: Springer Berlin Heidelberg, 2005. 237–264.

[10] Saxena, Ankur, and Shivani Chandra. *Artificial intelligence and machine learning in healthcare*. Singapore: Springer, 2021.

[11] Alsubaei, Faisal, Abdullah Abuhussein, and Sajjan Shiva. "Ontology-based security recommendation for the Internet of Medical Things." *IEEE Access* 7 (2019): 48948–48960.

[12] Alsubaei, Faisal, Abdullah Abuhussein, and Sajjan Shiva. "Ontology-based security recommendation for the Internet of Medical Things." *IEEE Access* 7 (2019): 48948–48960.

[13] Dwivedi, Ashutosh Dhar, et al. "A decentralized privacy-preserving healthcare blockchain for IoT." *Sensors* 19.2 (2019): 326.

[14] Hatzivasilis, George, et al. "Review of security and privacy for the Internet of Medical Things (IoMT)." In *2019 15th International Conference on Distributed Computing in Sensor Systems (DCOSS)*. IEEE, 2019.

[15] Herzog, Pete. *Open-source security testing methodology manual*. Institute for Security and Open Methodologies (ISECOM) (2018).

[16] Hatzivasilis, George, Ioannis Papaefstathiou, and Charalampos Manifavas. "Software security, privacy, and dependability: Metrics and measurement." *IEEE Software* 33.4 (2016): 46–54.

[17] Lin, Jie, et al. "A survey on internet of things: Architecture, enabling technologies, security and privacy, and applications." *IEEE Internet of Things Journal* 4.5 (2017): 1125–1142.

[18] Nawir, Mukrimah, et al. "Internet of Things (IoT): Taxonomy of security attacks." In *2016 3rd International Conference on Electronic Design (ICED)*. IEEE, 2016.

[19] Betts, Dominic, C. Street, and Y. Diogenes. *Internet of Things Security Architecture*. Microsoft Azure Documentation (2018).

[20] Chatterjee, Jit, and Tushar Debnath. "Environmental monitoring using sense hat based on IBM Watson IoT platform." *International Research Journal of Engineering and Technology (IRJET)* 5.7 (2018): 392–399.

[21] Rannenberg, Kai. "Enabling identity management and privacy in a global context: ISO/IEC Standardization in JTC 1/SC 27/WG 5 'Identity Management and Privacy Technologies'." *경제규제와 법* 11.2 (2018): 9–24.

[22] Shin, Sanggyu, et al. "Proposal for a Privacy Impact Assessment Manual Conforming to ISO/IEC 29134: 2017." In *Computer Information Systems and Industrial Management: 17th International Conference, CISIM 2018, Olomouc, Czech Republic, September 27–29, 2018, Proceedings 17*. Springer International Publishing, 2018.

[23] Brahma, Joy, and Debanjan Sadhya. "Preserving contextual privacy for smart home IoT devices with dynamic traffic shaping." *IEEE Internet of Things Journal* 9.13 (2021): 11434–11441.

[24] Kerr, Don, Kerryn Butler-Henderson, and Tony Sahama. "Security, privacy, and ownership issues with the use of wearable health technologies." In *Wearable technologies: Concepts, methodologies, tools, and applications*. IGI Global, 2018. 1068–1083.

[25] Banka, Subham, Isha Madan, and S. S. Saranya. "Smart healthcare monitoring using IoT." *International Journal of Applied Engineering Research* 13.15 (2018): 11984–11989.

Part III

IoMT Frameworks and Architectures for Artificial Intelligence (AI) in Augmented Reality

7 AI-Enabled IoMT Frameworks for Automated Health Diagnosis

Suyamoon Pathak, Hiren Kumar Thakkar, and Ketan Sabale

7.1 INTRODUCTION

In the recent past, a revolution has taken place in the field of healthcare and medicine as a result of advancement in AI-supported technologies in several domains. Several avenues are made possible such as in the field of patient care, diagnosis, precision treatment, and customized medication due to the enhanced capacity of AI-based models to analyze the high volume of data, to identify the patterns, and to predict the anomalies using the insightful patterns. Therefore, the integration of AI-based models with the healthcare domain has promised effective healthcare solutions that improve the precision, effectiveness, and customization of the healthcare solutions. In this regard, the Internet of Medical Things (IoMT) is used to enable automated health diagnosis as described in [1].

7.1.1 Background and Significance of AI in Healthcare

A few years back, the application of AI was very limited, and it was not widely adopted by the domain experts. However, in the recent times, the importance of AI in the medical field has become evident, and several medical experts including doctors are recognizing the role of AI in healthcare. The importance of AI in healthcare is unavoidable as traditional techniques of diagnosis and treatment are becoming more and more irrelevant due the ever increasing amount of healthcare data. The traditional models are incapable of processing the voluminous data and unable to find the correlation among various attributes. Although the role of AI is increasing in the healthcare domain, it is still used as a supportive alternative to assist healthcare practitioners, who may make better judgments by augmenting the knowledge obtained using AI algorithms. Such combination of AI-supported decision-making with healthcare practitioners' domain expertise makes the decision process quick and effective. Several practical applications have been noticed in the recent past,

DOI: 10.1201/9781003393498-10

where AI-driven diagnostic systems have successfully tackled the variety of medical problems [2]. It is noticed that AI makes early illness identification, individualized treatment with improved patient outcomes possible. By automating mundane tasks and providing data-driven insights, AI supports healthcare professionals and reduces their overburdened workload without compromising the quality of healthcare services.

7.1.2 Overview of IoMT and Its Role in Healthcare

A key component of this AI-driven healthcare revolution is the Internet of Medical Things (IoMT): an interconnected system of wearables, sensors, and medical equipment. As shown in Figure 7.1, these devices gather and send real-time health data to healthcare systems. This networked ecosystem not only makes remote patient monitoring easier but also makes the data-collecting process more efficient, giving AI systems access to and analysis of a steady supply of crucial health data [3]. The use of IoMT devices, such as intelligent wearable fitness trackers, remote monitoring systems, and implanted sensors, has increased exponentially. These gadgets continuously feed information about many physiological factors, such as heart rate, blood sugar levels, and degree of exercise [4, 5].

7.1.3 Problem Statement and Research Objectives

Several important difficulties and possibilities have arisen in the era of expanding healthcare data and technology breakthroughs. These difficulties mainly concern

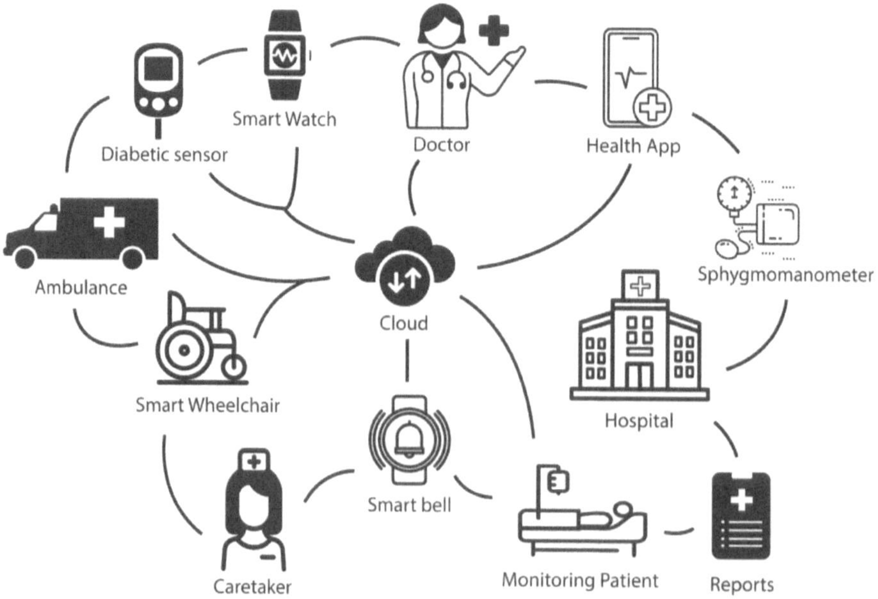

FIGURE 7.1 AI-enabled hospital ecosystem.

improving patient care and healthcare procedures while effectively handling the vast amount of medical data at hand. The following issues are discussed in this chapter, along with particular research goals to solve them.

7.1.3.1 Problem Statement

1. **Data Overload and Diagnosis Complexity**: Massive volumes of patient data, such as electronic health records, medical pictures, and real-time monitoring from IoMT devices, are overwhelming the healthcare sector. Moreover, healthcare diagnostics and decision-making have become much more complicated. Therefore, it is the need of the hour to design an intelligent algorithms that analyzes the data, find crucial insights and trends, and help medical personnel make quick and an accurate diagnoses.
2. **Interoperability and Standardization**: Considering the use of diversified IoMTdevices and systems, the IoMT systems must be equipped with proper standardization and compatibility across the devices. In the absence of standardization, it becomes difficult for any AI-enabled healthcare systems to work efficiently. Comprehensive automated health diagnosis is hampered by the absence of standardized data standards and interfaces.
3. **Ethical and Regulatory Concerns**: The use of AI in healthcare poses ethical questions about the confidentiality, permission, and openness of patient data. To make room for AI in healthcare settings, regulatory frameworks, including data protection laws and healthcare standards, must be modified. To enable the appropriate and secure application of AI in medical diagnostics, ethical and legal issues must be resolved.

7.1.3.2 Research Objectives

The following research goals are meant to address these issues:

1. **Thorough Review**: Give a thorough analysis of AI-enabled IoMT frameworks for automated health diagnosis, covering current practices, advancements in technology, and successful applications.
2. **Technology Exploration**: Learn about the fundamental technologies that support automated health diagnosis, such as computer vision, machine learning, and data collecting.
3. **Interoperability Solutions**: Outline strategies for improving interoperability within the IoMT ecosystem, concentrating on data standards and integration techniques that enable a smooth exchange of health data.
4. **Ethical and Regulatory Analysis**: Examine the ethical ramifications and legal issues related to AI in healthcare, such as data protection, informed consent, and regulatory compliance. Advise on how to utilize AI responsibly.
5. **Impact Assessment**: Assess how patient care, results, and the healthcare ecosystem are affected by AI-enabled health diagnosis. Find examples where the use of AI has improved resource allocation, diagnosis, and treatment.

6. **Challenges and Future Directions**: Examine the shortcomings and difficulties that current frameworks confront, and suggest any areas that might want improvement. Investigate new trends and innovations that show potential for the application of AI in healthcare.

This chapter seeks to give a comprehensive overview of the present status of AI-enabled IoMT frameworks for automated health diagnosis and to offer insights into overcoming obstacles and influencing the future of healthcare with AI by addressing these research objectives.

7.2 LITERATURE REVIEW

7.2.1 History of Healthcare and AI

Artificial intelligence (AI) has been gradually incorporated into the healthcare industry through a complex historical process. Healthcare's potential to be transformed by AI has been understood since the 1960s. The groundwork for AI's use in medical diagnostics was created by innovative efforts like Dendral and MYCIN. These early systems, which emphasized rule-based expert systems, were the beginnings of automated medical diagnosis [6]. The traces of the decision support systems development can be found as early as in the 1970s and 1980s, which later resulted in the advancement of AI in the healthcare industry. By engaging the AI-based models to examine the patients' data, these AI systems attempt to help healthcare personnel to make effective clinical judgments. Although AI systems had a great potential to help healthcare systems, their wider adoption was hampered by the lack of computer power and data availability [7]. Machine learning and data-driven AI started becoming popular around the 1990s and early 2000s with the increase in computation power. AI started to gain momentum with the increasing digitization of electronic health records (EHRs) and the accessibility of huge healthcare datasets. For applications such as medical image analysis and predictive modeling, machine learning techniques have become very popular such as neural networks, deep neural networks, etc. [8].

7.2.2 AI's Current State in Healthcare

AI in healthcare is currently a booming field with applications in many different medical disciplines. In the recent past, the AI-driven diagnostic systems have shown remarkable results in spotting diseases such as cancer, diabetes, and heart-related anomalies. For instance, in medical image-based diagnosis, the state-of-the-art deep learning models are now outperforming human experts in detecting anomalies in images such as in X-rays, MRIs, and CT scans, which are all types of medical pictures. In addition to the diagnosis, AI is equally becoming robust in assisting experts in drug development, genomics, remote patient monitoring, and health treatment planning. For instance, the robust design of the natural language processing (NLP) model helps to extract meaningful insights from written clinical notes and from verbal patient–doctor narratives. To conclude the AI's current state in healthcare,

AI-based predictive analytics help healthcare professionals and institutions to estimate the overall patient outcome and also optimize the allocation of resources.

7.2.3 IoMT Applications in Healthcare

In the era of internet technology and wearable devices, an essential component for contemporary healthcare is emerging in the form of the Internet of Medical Things (IoMT). The IoMT is considered as a subset of the Internet of Things (IoT), and it refers to a variety of wearable devices, low-cost sensors, and any tiny wireless devices with limited computation power that collect the real-time health information. Such tiny low-powered wearable devices help to remotely monitor a patient's condition and provide continuous feeds of information such as heart rate, blood pressure, body temperature, and glucose levels. These wearable devices have revolutionized the way patient data is collected followed up by support to healthcare service delivery. The emergence of IoMT devices has made it possible to effectively manage chronic illnesses and provide telemedicine services. Moreover, the IoMT devices have made the individuals to actively participate in the healthcare system with the help of wearable fitness trackers, implanted sensors leading to early disease detection [9].

7.2.4 Automated Health Diagnosis Frameworks

The use of AI coupled with IoMT for health diagnosis has given a birth to several paradigms recently. These proposed AI-supported IoMT frameworks offer alternative mechanisms to gather, process, and analyze data to produce meaningful diagnostic insights. A few notable frameworks are IBM's Medical Sieve, Google Health's DeepMind, and Watson for Health. These systems offer automated health diagnosis by effectively using IoMT data with AI-based approaches such as deep learning, NLP, and computer vision [10]. The careful adoption and application of these frameworks may reduce the misdiagnosis of the disease, with a quick diagnosis and overall improvement of diagnosis standards. In this regard, several healthcare environments, such as radiology departments and primary care clinics, have shown their effectiveness [11].

7.2.5 Related Technologies and Trends

The future of healthcare delivery will be shaped by several connected technologies and trends, including AI. A few of these are:

1. **Blockchain for Health Data Security**: Blockchain technology is gaining popularity for protecting privacy, safeguarding healthcare data, and facilitating secure record sharing.
2. **Telemedicine and Remote Monitoring**: Patients may consult with medical professionals and get care from the convenience of their homes thanks to telemedicine platforms and remote monitoring technologies, which are gaining popularity.

3. **Personalized Medicine**: By customizing treatment strategies for specific patients based on their genetic and clinical data, AI is enabling the age of personalized medicine.
4. **Explainable AI**: To increase openness and trust, explainable AI models are becoming more and more important as AI is incorporated into healthcare decision-making.
5. **AI in Drug Discovery**: AI-driven drug discovery streamlines the identification of promising drug candidates, reducing the amount of time and money needed to create novel treatments.

AI and IoMT interact with these linked technologies and trends, advancing patient care and healthcare services as a whole [12].

7.3 AI TECHNOLOGIES IN HEALTH DIAGNOSIS

7.3.1 Machine Learning, Deep Learning, and Their Relevance

The foundation of AI technologies used in medical diagnostics is machine learning (ML) and deep learning (DL). As shown in Figure 7.2, ML is a subset of DL and employs artificial neural networks to model complicated relationships, whereas DL is a subset of ML and includes training algorithms to learn patterns and generate predictions from data. These technologies' usefulness in diagnosing medical conditions stems from their capacity to analyze massive healthcare databases, spot tiny trends, and make precise predictions. For a variety of tasks in healthcare, including illness diagnosis, risk assessment, and therapy suggestion, ML and DL models are utilized. For instance, by automating the identification of anomalies in X-rays, MRIs, and CT scans, convolutional neural networks (CNNs) have transformed medical imaging. For tracking patient vitals and foretelling unfavorable outcomes, time-series analysis is used with recurrent neural networks (RNNs) [13].

7.3.2 Natural Language Processing (NLP) for Clinical Data

As shown in Figure 7.3, first the raw data is fed into the system. The system extracts the raw data and removes all the placebo text present in the data. When the data contains only the keyword, NLP algorithms are applied to formulate the results required. NLP is an area of AI that focuses on how computers and human language interact. NLP is essential in the healthcare industry for obtaining important information from patient narratives, medical data, and clinical notes. Unstructured text data may be analyzed using NLP algorithms, yielding information that aids in clinical research and decision-making. Applications of NLP in medical diagnosis include sentiment analysis of patient records, clinical fact extraction, and the creation of structured data from unstructured notes. Understanding patient experiences and sentiments through sentiment analysis contributes to better patient care. To facilitate diagnostic procedures, NLP can also help in detecting important clinical terminology, illnesses, and patient demographics.

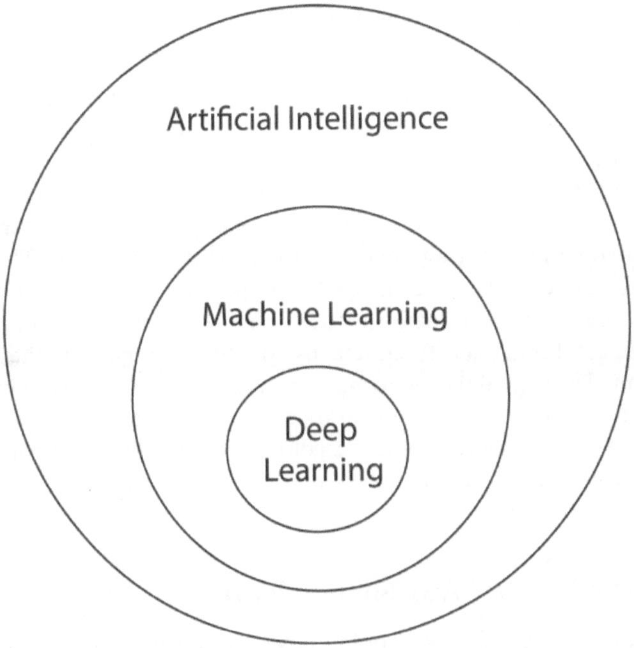

FIGURE 7.2 Relationships among artificial intelligence, machine learning, and deep learning.

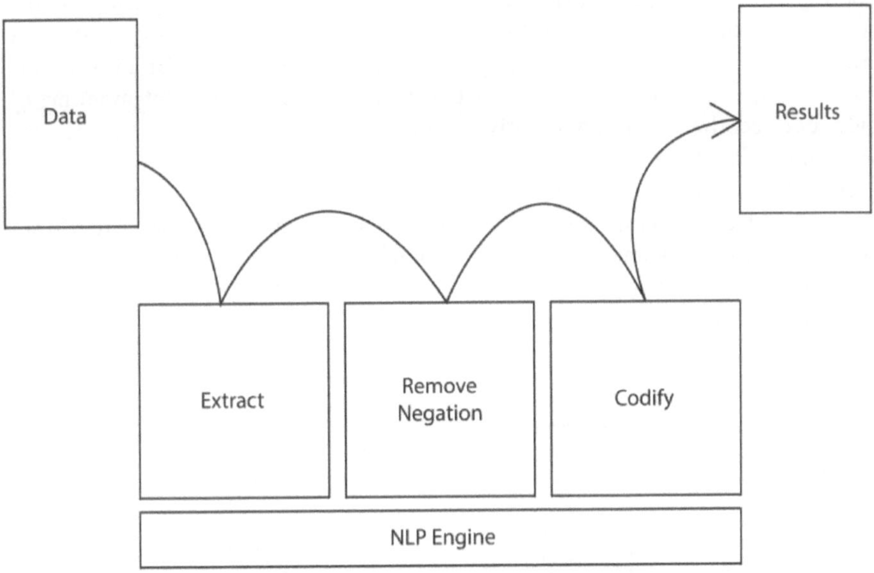

FIGURE 7.3 How natural language processing works.

7.3.3 Computer Vision in Medical Imaging

Another AI innovation that is essential for diagnosing illnesses is computer vision, especially when it comes to the evaluation of medical photographs. X-ray, MRI, and CT scan pictures may be used to diagnose abnormalities, cancers, and other medical issues thanks to computer vision algorithms' ability to process and interpret visual data. As shown in Figure 7.4, computer vision systems take image inputs from a sensory device, primarily a camera, and it is processed in some interpreting device that is loaded with CNNs. These help us interpret what the object in the image looks like and make inferences accordingly. CNN and other deep learning-based computer vision models have been incredibly successful in classifying images, identifying objects in them, and segmenting them. These models can identify even minute anomalies, increasing the precision and effectiveness of medical diagnostics. The extension of healthcare access to rural or underserved areas is made possible by the combination of computer vision with IoMT, which enables real-time picture processing and remote diagnosis [14].

7.3.4 Sensors and Data Acquisition in IoMT

The Internet of Medical Things (IoMT) combines a variety of sensors and data collection systems to collect and send real-time health data. These sensors include those found in smartwatches, implanted medical devices, wearable fitness trackers, and remote monitoring systems. Data collection is the foundation for IoMT's ability to continuously monitor patient health. As shown in Figure 7.5, IoMT sensors capture a wide range of physiological data, including temperature, heart rate, blood pressure, blood glucose levels, intensity of activity, and many other metrics. The obtained data is given to healthcare systems for analysis and interpretation. The use of sensors in IoMT enables remote patient monitoring, individualized healthcare, and early sickness detection. It gives a complete and up-to-date picture of a patient's health status, enabling medical professionals to make informed decisions. Naturally, this section of your report will concentrate on the IoMT architecture and components, including an overview of the IoMT architecture, sensors and wearable technologies, connection and data transmission protocols, cloud computing, edge computing, and security and privacy concerns in IoMT [15].

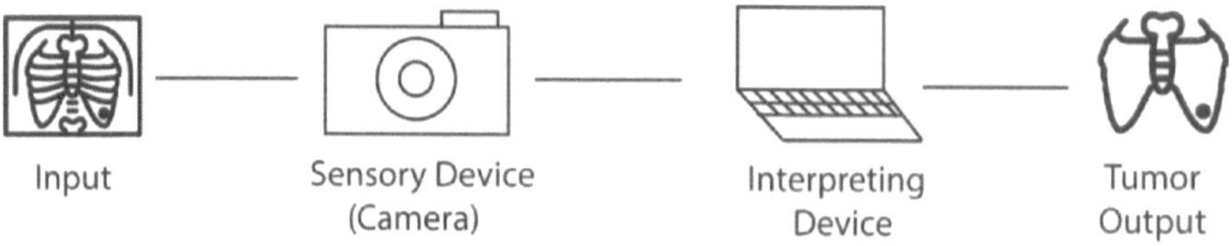

FIGURE 7.4 How computer vision works.

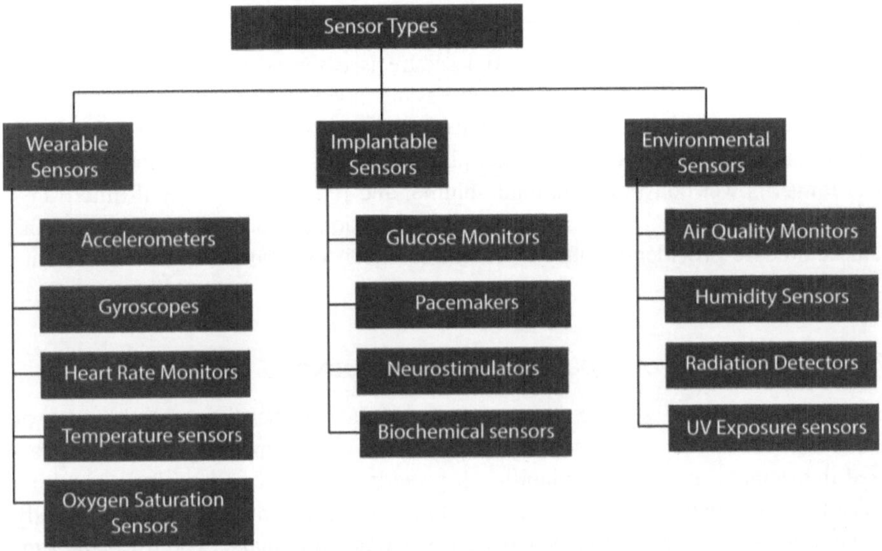

FIGURE 7.5 Types of sensors in IoMT.

7.4 IOMT COMPONENTS AND ARCHITECTURE

7.4.1 Overview

The purpose of the Internet of Medical Things (IoMT), a complex ecosystem that is continually growing, is to transform healthcare by connecting a wide range of devices, sensors, and medical equipment. Its structure is made up of many essential components that work together to collect, transmit, and analyze health data. The core elements of IoMT architecture are sensors and wearables for data collection, secure connection and data transmission protocols, and data storage and processing systems, either in the cloud or at the edge, for data management and analysis. The design ensures real-time monitoring, quick reactions, and the seamless integration of data into healthcare systems.

7.4.2 Sensors and Wearable Devices

IoMT's frontline sensors and wearable tech are in charge of gathering patient physiological data. Several sensors, including accelerometers, heart rate monitors, and GPS receivers, are included in wearable technology, such as fitness trackers, smartwatches, and smart clothing. The IoMT ecosystem includes implantable devices like pacemakers and continuous glucose monitoring. These gadgets record information on a range of variables, including heart rate, blood pressure, body temperature, physical activity, and more. The information gathered is crucial for tracking medical problems, managing chronic diseases, and giving ongoing insights into a person's well-being [16].

7.4.3 Protocols for Data Transmission and Connectivity

Data transmission that is effective and secure is essential to IoMT. By allowing data to be sent from sensors to healthcare systems via connectivity protocols, real-time access to health information is made possible. Zigbee, LoRaWAN, Bluetooth, Wi-Fi, and cellular networks are examples of common communication protocols. The range, power consumption, data volume, and requirement for real-time transmission all play a role in the choice of communication protocol. To educate patients and healthcare providers about key health occurrences, seamless and reliable data transfer is necessary.

7.4.4 IoMT's Use of Cloud and Edge Computing

IoMT depends on the storage and processing of data. Either the network's edge or the cloud can be used to process and store data. Cloud computing enables centralized data management and scalability. It provides sophisticated analysis, machine learning, and global access to healthcare data. No matter where they are physically located, healthcare professionals may access patient data, make diagnoses, and suggest treatments in real time. While lowering latency and improving real-time capabilities, edge computing processes data locally on the device or at the edge of the network. The local processing and analyses of the healthcare data produces quick results, which are highly beneficial in emergency situations such as irregular heartbeat and glucose level increase in blood by wearable sensors [17]. The choice between the cloud infrastructure and edge computing is entirely dependent on the constraints of the healthcare systems. For instance, if the quick processing and analysis of a low volume of the data is needed, then one can choose edge computing. However, if the latency is not the constraint but processing of huge amount of the data is the need, then cloud infrastructure is preferable. To conclude, cloud and edge computing provide benefits that support the demands of many healthcare applications.

7.4.5 Security and Privacy Considerations in IoMT

In the domain of IoMT-enabled healthcare service delivery, the secured methods for data collection, data transmission, and data storage of patients' sensitive healthcare data are highly essential for the overall of success of IoMT systems [18]. In IoMT-enabled healthcare environment, the security and privacy of data are very important as follows:

1. **Data Encryption**: The suitable data encryption likely prevents unwanted access, and therefore data encryption should be done during data transmission and storage as well.
2. **Access Control**: The stringent data access protocols ensure that the authorized data access and manipulation, and therefore it is desirable to have robust access control protocols in place.
3. **Device Authentication**: Several IoMT devices in a system work in parallel, and therefore, to stop any hostile remote device from penetrating the IoMT system, each IoMT device must be authenticated.

4. **Regulation Compliance**: Each country establishes the legal compliances to be followed while dealing with healthcare data. In order to ensure the protection of the sensitive healthcare data of the patient, the IoMT system must follow the healthcare standards established by the country such as HIPAA and DGPR proposed by the United States of America and European Union, respectively.
5. **Security Updates**: Routine security updates need to be provided to reduce vulnerabilities in IoMT networks and devices [19].

7.5 DATA COLLECTION AND PREPROCESSING

7.5.1 Data Collection and Aggregation Techniques

As AI-enabled health diagnosis frameworks significantly rely on a variety of data sources, data gathering is the cornerstone of these systems. In IoMT ecosystems, a variety of techniques are used for data collecting and aggregation.

1 **Wearable Technology and Sensors**: Wearable technology with sensors, such as accelerometers and heart rate monitors, continually gathers patient information. For additional analysis, these devices provide data to centralized databases.
2. **Electronic Health Records (EHRs)**: EHRs store detailed information about patients, such as medical histories, test findings, and prescription histories. EHRs are a great resource for organized data that may be used for prognosis and diagnosis.
3. **Mobile Applications and Telemedicine Platforms**: These tools allow for data collecting and remote patient monitoring. They make it easier for healthcare systems to incorporate patient-generated health data.
4. **IoMT Gateways**: IoMT gateways act as go-betweens, transferring data gathered from various sensors and gadgets to the cloud or data storage systems. They aid in managing and regulating the data flow.
5. **IoMT Data Hubs**: By combining data from many sources, data hubs guarantee smooth data flow and storage. These hubs are essential for effectively handling massive amounts of health data.

7.5.2 Data Cleaning and Preprocessing

Data gathered from several sources may be erroneous, lacking, or conflicting. To guarantee that the data is prepared for analysis, preprocessing and cleaning the data are crucial processes. This entails numerous critical procedures:

1. **Cleansing the Data**: Find and fix any incorrect or missing data points. Problematic data may need to be interpolated, imputed, or removed to achieve this.
2. **Data Transformation**: Put data into a consistent format for analysis. For instance, resampling time-series data to regular intervals may be necessary.

3. **Feature Engineering**: From unprocessed data, produce useful features. For creating pertinent input variables for AI models, feature engineering is essential.
4. **Outlier Detection**: Find outliers that might bias analysis and diagnostics and deal with them. For this, a variety of statistical and machine-learning approaches can be applied.
5. **Normalization and Standardization**: To make it easier to train machine learning models, make sure data is distributed and scaled consistently.

7.5.3 Assurance of Data Integrity and Quality

In the healthcare industry, where mistakes can have serious repercussions, data integrity and quality are of utmost importance. Several procedures are involved in quality assurance:

1. **Data Validation**: Validate data often against established guidelines and benchmarks to guarantee correctness and consistency.
2. **Data Security**: Put in place strong security measures to safeguard health information from unauthorized access, breaches, and online dangers.
3. **Data Redundancy Management**: Take steps to manage redundant data to avoid record duplication and to preserve a single source of truth.
4. **Data Backup and Recovery**: Set up mechanisms for data backup and recovery to protect information in the event of hardware failure or data loss.
5. **Data Governance**: Establish rules and guidelines to make sure data is handled responsibly and in compliance with all applicable laws.
6. **Data Audit and Monitoring**: Constantly keep an eye on the usage, access, and integrity of data to spot and correct irregularities.

7.6 MACHINE LEARNING MODELS

7.6.1 Supervised, Unsupervised, and Reinforcement Learning

AI-enabled health diagnostic frameworks that use machine learning for data analysis use a variety of methods, including:

1. **Supervised Learning**: Using labeled data and known input and target, supervised learning includes training machine learning models. Supervisory learning is employed in the field of medical diagnostics for tasks including illness categorization, risk assessment, and therapy prescription. Deep neural networks, decision trees, and support vector machines are examples of common algorithms.
2. **Unsupervised Learning**: When the target variable is unknown, unsupervised learning is performed. It entails looking for trends, connections, and structures in the data. In healthcare, clustering is frequently used to categorize individuals that have similar traits.

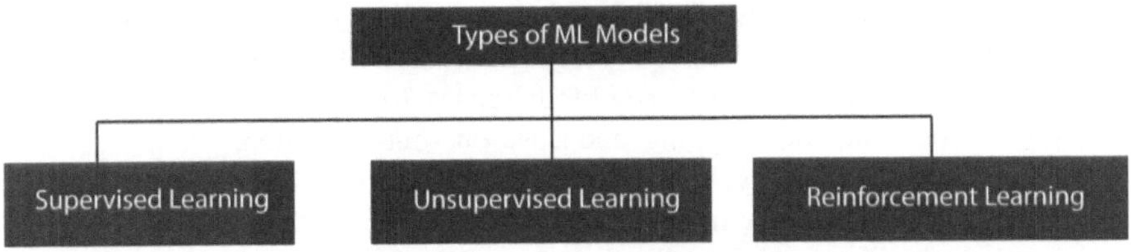

FIGURE 7.6. Different types of models in machine learning.

3. **Reinforcement Learning**: The reinforcement learning is rarely used in medical diagnosis. However, it may help in designing customized treatment plans to enhance therapy.

7.6.2 Feature Selection and Engineering

The feature selection and engineering are the fundamental steps required to prepare the data for the machine learning models.

1. **Feature Selection**: The feature selection is the process of selecting the relevant attributes from the pool of all the attributes to reduce the dimensionality and increase model effectiveness. The selection of the subset of the most relevant and useful features for the given healthcare problem is carried out using variety of methods such as correlation analysis, mutual information, and recursive feature removal.
2. **Feature Engineering**: On the contrary, the feature engineering is the process of generating new features from the existing set of attributes or of altering the existing attributes in a way to improvise the performance of the machine learning model. For instance, in the healthcare domain, feature engineering can be done through aggregated statistics, derived variables, and time-series modifications. For example, one can derive the average heart rate over a period of time as a new feature to identify arrhythmias.

7.6.3 Model Selection and Evaluation Techniques

Critical components of AI-enabled health diagnostics include choosing a suitable machine learning model and assessing its performance:

1. **Model Selection**: Depending on the nature of the diagnostic work, a model may be chosen. Convolutional neural networks for medical image analysis, random forests for decision support, and logistic regression for binary classification are common models in healthcare. Understanding the dataset and the desired result is necessary for choosing the appropriate model.
2. **Assessment Techniques**: The approach that is used for an assessment relies on the issue type (such as classification or regression) and the type of data

being used (such as unbalanced data). Accuracy, precision, recall, F_1-score, and the area under the receiver operating characteristic curve (AUC-ROC) are common assessment criteria. Model generalization is evaluated using cross-validation, bootstrapping, and leave-one-out validation.

3. **Model Interpretability**: To comprehend and believe AI-driven diagnostic results in the healthcare industry, model interpretability is essential, which can be carried out using methods such as SHapley Additive exPlanations (SHAP), local interpretable model-agnostic explanations (LIME), and feature significance scores.

7.7 NATURAL LANGUAGE PROCESSING IN HEALTH DIAGNOSIS

7.7.1 Unlocking the Power of NLP in Healthcare

Natural language processing (NLP) deals with extracting the meaningful insights from the unstructured text data and provide the knowledge such as sentiment analysis, summarization, language translation, etc. In the field of healthcare, NLP would be useful to extract insight from massive amounts of unstructured clinical text data. It can efficiently extract information from clinical notes, medical data, and perform a variety of tasks such as summarization, translation, sentiment analysis, etc.

7.7.2 NLP Techniques for Medical Records

NLP has revolutionized the way healthcare professionals interact with clinical records. Several NLP approaches exist to handle and analyze unstructured medical text data, as shown in Figure 7.7.

1. **Named Entity Recognition (NER)**: The automatic extraction of entities from the messy and unstructured clinical data can be accomplished using NER. For example, NER can extract entities such as the patient names, healthcare providers, type of illnesses, drug names, and procedures followed from the clinical records. To conclude, NER would help processing unstructured data for quick data accessibility.
2. **Text Classification**: The text classification of healthcare records can help patient classification, disease classification, drug classification, and treatment classification. The text classification of the healthcare data can be done in a supervised as well as an unsupervised manner depending on the information about the predetermined classes.
3. **Information Retrieval (IR)**: IR is an important subdomain of NLP, which helps to access relevant healthcare data quickly and efficiently. IR performs focused searches and provides relevant information quickly.
4. **Topic Modeling**: Topic modeling methods such as Latent Dirichlet Allocation (LDA) is useful in mining the obscure topics from the huge collection of clinical papers, and it makes it easier to identify health patterns, study direction, and open questions for the research.

5. **Text Summarization**: Usually, the clinical record and other healthcare documents are lengthy in nature and do not provide a quick summary. The text summarization methods have the ability to compress these documents and extract the meaningful summaries for further processing.

7.7.3 Clinical Note Extraction and Sentiment Analysis

Clinical notes, which may be found in electronic health records, discharge summaries, and doctor's notes, include a wealth of crucial data. These insights can be unlocked by healthcare experts using NLP techniques:

1. **Clinical Note Extraction**: To discover critical clinical information, such as diagnoses, treatments, and patient histories, clinical note extraction entails a thorough study and parsing of electronic health data. This automated procedure makes it possible to convert unstructured clinical writing into structured data, which improves the effectiveness of managing medical records and decision assistance.

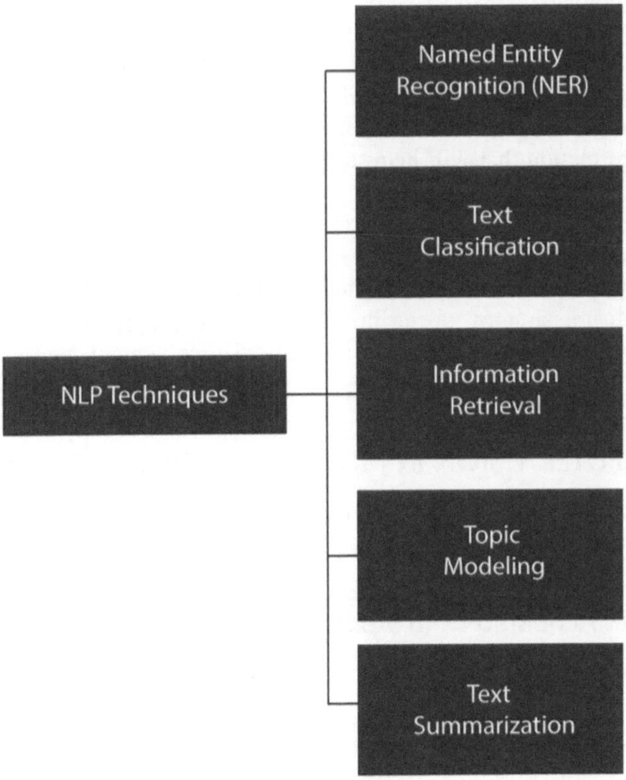

FIGURE 7.7 NLP techniques that can be applied in IoMT.

2. **Sentiment Analysis**: Sentiment analysis in healthcare is a fascinating application that is also really helpful. The emotional content of clinical notes and narratives is assessed using this technique. Sentiment analysis may be a driving force in improving patient care by comprehending patient experiences, evaluating the caliber of doctor–patient interactions, and detecting possible problems or opportunities for change in healthcare delivery [20].

7.7.4 Language Models and Their Applications

Language models have become game-changers in NLP, especially transformer-based models like BERT (bidirectional encoder representations from transformers) and GPT (generative pretrained transformer). They have a wide range of uses in healthcare:

1. **Clinical Data Processing**: Language models are an excellent option for fine-tuning clinical entity recognition and the identification of complicated connections in medical records because they can absorb, understand, and extract structured information from clinical literature. Healthcare workers may automate the extraction of clinical entities and connections from the vast amount of clinical data by utilizing models like BERT.
2. **Clinical Question Answering**: Language models, especially GPT-3, show incredible promise in this domain. These models can quickly respond to medical inquiries, assisting healthcare professionals in quickly obtaining information that will help them make decisions and improve clinical practice.
3. **Clinical Chatbots**: Conversational exchanges between patients and healthcare providers have entered a new era thanks to chatbots with language models like GPT. These chatbots are crucial in simplifying the transmission of prescription information, appointment booking, and symptom analysis, increasing patient involvement, and expanding access to healthcare.

7.8 COMPUTER VISION IN MEDICAL IMAGING

In this section, we discuss about the visual data acquisition cum storage, data processing, and data analysis components.

7.8.1 Image Acquisition and Storage

The first step in medical imaging is data gathering followed by processing using a variety of modalities.

1. **X-Ray Imaging**: X-ray machines are widely used to capture the view of the inside organs and bones of the body. X-ray images are preferably stored in a digital format for their quick retrieval and subsequent processing.

2. **Magnetic Resonance Imaging (MRI)**: MRI devices produce precise cross-sectional pictures of the body using strong magnets and radio waves. An MRI scan produces digital files that are used to store the pictures.
3. **Computed Tomography (CT)**: CT scanners take several cross-sectional pictures using X-rays. These digitally recorded and rebuilt pictures provide an in-depth understanding of anatomical components.
4. **Ultrasound Imaging**: To create pictures of interior organs, ultrasound equipment uses high-frequency sound waves. Health information systems frequently record and preserve these pictures digitally.
5. **Endoscopic and Microscopy**: Visual information obtained during endoscopic operations and microscopy is needed for microscopic inspections and is digitally saved, frequently in specialized systems.

Digital storage systems, such as picture archiving and communication systems (PACS), electronic health records (EHRs), and cloud-based solutions, ensure that these visual records are readily accessible to healthcare providers [21].

7.8.2 Image Enhancement and Preprocessing

Medical pictures are frequently enhanced and preprocessed before being analyzed to guarantee the best quality and clinically relevant extraction of data:

1. **Noise Reduction**: To improve picture quality, noise, which is frequently present in medical images owing to a variety of circumstances, is reduced or removed.
2. **Picture Contrast Adjustment**: Increasing picture contrast makes it easier to distinguish between distinct structures and abnormalities, which increases the accuracy of diagnostics.
3. **Registration And Alignment**: For comparison analysis, numerous pictures from various modalities or periods are aligned using registration techniques.
4. **Picture Segmentation**: To isolate certain areas of interest within a picture, image segmentation is essential. It enables focused examination of certain anatomical or pathological locations.
5. **Resolution Enhancement**: Techniques for enhancing resolution make images sharper and more detailed, especially when it's necessary to see minute structures.
6. **Artifacts Removal**: To maintain the quality of the data, artifacts created during picture capture, such as motion artifacts, are either rectified or deleted.

7.8.3 Deep Learning Models for Medical Image Analysis

Deep learning models' outstanding performance in tasks like image classification, object recognition, and segmentation has made them vital tools for medical image analysis:

1. **Convolutional Neural Networks (CNNs)**: CNNs are now the standard for analyzing medical imaging data. They have been designed to pick up on hierarchical characteristics and patterns in photos. CNNs are particularly adept at jobs like spotting anomalies in X-rays, CT scans, and MRIs. As shown in Figure 7.8, first the CNN starts from taking X-ray input, and then it undergoes different rounds of convolutions—realigning the image, cropping/resizing the image, rotations—to get the final output of the tumor.
2. **Segmentation Networks**: For accurate segmentation of anatomical features, tumors, or lesions inside medical pictures, models like U-Net and Mask R-CNN are used.
3. **Transfer Learning**: Using medical datasets, transfer learning optimizes previously learned deep learning models. Performance is enhanced, and model creation is sped up using this method.
4. **Generative Adversarial Networks (GANs)**: GANs improve the clarity and interpretability of medical pictures through super-resolution, artifact removal, and image-to-image translation.
5. **3-D Deep Learning**: Three-dimensional deep learning models are used to assess spatial connections and detect problems in volumetric medical data, such as CT and MRI images [22].

7.9 ETHICAL AND LEGAL CONSIDERATIONS

7.9.1 Ethical and Legal Imperatives

In this section, we discuss the ethical and moral implications on AI models and IoMT systems including patient data security, privacy, regulatory compliance, etc.

7.9.2 Patient Data Privacy and Security

1. **Data Encryption**: The AI-enabled IoMT systems are bound to transmit the health data continuously, and therefore it is necessary to preserve this data during transmission and storage by applying the appropriate encryption technique.
2. **Access Control**: The IoMT systems must be equipped with strict access control procedures such as role-based access restrictions and multifactor authentications to guarantee the authorized access.
3. **Data Anonymization**: The data anonymization methods help in hiding the identity of the patient and thereby preserve privacy while reducing the risk of data exposure.
4. **Data Minimization**: Data minimization deals with the collection of only the relevant data of the patient and thereby reduces the chances of exposure of the sensitive health related data.
5. **Consent Management**: Patients must be informed about data usage and options. Procedures for obtaining patients' informed permission should be transparent and explain how their data will be used.

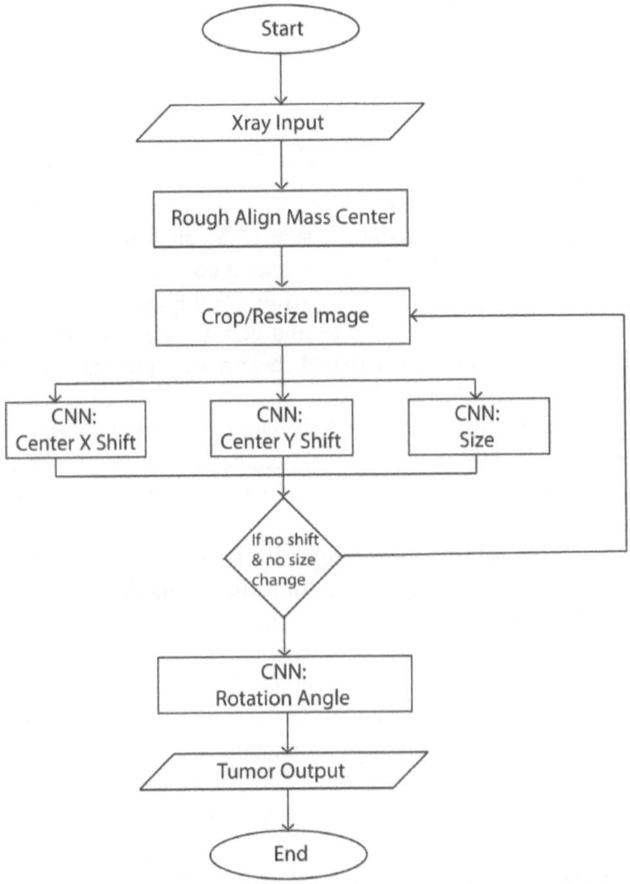

FIGURE 7.8 How CNN works in medical image analysis.

7.9.3 Regulatory Compliance and Standards

1. **HIPAA Compliance**: The Health Insurance Portability and Accountability Act(HIPAA) in the United States establishes guidelines for the privacy protection of patient data. HIPAA guidelines must be followed by AI-enabled IoMT systems to guarantee patient confidentiality and data protection.
2. **GDPR Compliance**: The General Data Protection Regulation (GDPR) of the European Union enforces stringent data protection guidelines. Healthcare organizations employing AI and IoMT must abide by GDPR, particularly when working with patient data from other countries.
3. **Healthcare Standards**: The interoperability and safe sharing of patient data between IoMT devices and healthcare systems depends on compliance with healthcare data exchange standards (such as HL7 and DICOM).

4. **FDA Regulations**: In the US, the Food and Drug Administration (FDA) is in charge of enforcing laws governing medical devices, including those utilizing AI.

7.9.4 Ethical Dilemmas in AI-Based Diagnosis

1. **Transparency and Accountability**: Transparency is an essential component in any healthcare system. Usually, AI algorithms work as "black boxes," which make it difficult to understand how they make decisions.
2. **Fairness and Bias**: AI models learn from training data. With biased training data, AI models inherit the bias and may treat a few patients unfairly. Therefore, ensuring the fairness and minimizing the bias are important ethical issues in AI-based diagnosis.
3. **Patient Autonomy and Informed Consent**: The patient's informed consent is necessary before using critical healthcare data. However, the use of AI in medical decision-making may violate the patient's autonomy and can affect medical decisions.
4. **Data Ownership and Authorization**: There is a chance that the patients' healthcare data may be utilized to train the AI models without consent. Therefore, data ownership and patient rights over their health information raise serious ethical concerns.
5. **Accountability for Errors**: It is very hard to pinpoint accountability in the cases when AI systems produce erroneous results such as mistakes in diagnosis or wrong treatment recommendations.
6. **Job Displacement**: The automation of tasks by AI models is likely to cause job displacement among healthcare professionals and may create moral concerns.
7. **Resource Allocation**: The AI-based diagnosis may affect the distribution of healthcare resources among the doctors, patients, and other service providers such as treatment priority, leading to ethical issues.

7.10 CHALLENGES AND FUTURE DIRECTIONS

7.10.1 Navigating Complexities and Forging Ahead

The use of AI coupled with IoMT in the domain of healthcare service delivery offers exciting prospects. However, there are several challenges for its successful deployment. The following are the selected challenges and future directions for the further improvement.

7.10.2 Limitations of Current Frameworks

The following are the major limitations of current frameworks such as data privacy, data security, compatibility, bias and fairness, data quality, and regulatory compliance.

1. **Patient Data Privacy and Security**: This limitation restricts the current frameworks' wider acceptability. In spite of the progress in data encryption front, this is still considered a major concern.
2. **Compatibility Problems**: Since wearable IoMT devices are designed by different companies, they lack the common standard protocols, and therefore there exists a lack of compatibility among the various IoMT devices in healthcare systems. Despite making efforts to standardize the protocols in the recent years, the integration of the various technologies and data formats poses a challenge.
3. **Bias and Fairness**: The lack of balanced training data may lead to AI systems picking up biases. Later, the biased AI system may cause problems in accurate medical diagnosis.
4. **Data Quality and Consistency**: The accuracy of any AI-driven diagnostic system heavily relies on the consistency and quality of the data gathered by the IoMT devices. However, it is very challenging to maintain the data quality and integrity under different environmental conditions.
5. **Regulatory Obstacles**: Since IoMT systems are supposed to be deployed for healthcare quality service delivery, they have to comply with the regulations such as obtaining FDA clearance for medical devices. Sometimes, regulatory compliance creates a financial burden and is time-consuming.

7.10.3 Potential Areas for Improvement

To counter these challenges, the following are the areas for the potential improvements.

1. **Improved Data Privacy**: The designing of robust access controls methods in a decentralized data storage mechanism and applying cutting-edge encryption methods help protect the healthcare data. For example, homomorphic encryption is one privacy-preserving method popular for data privacy.
2. **Interoperability Solutions**: The IoMT systems can be made interoperable by designing open standards and application programming interfaces (APIs). Diverse technologies can communicate seamlessly using open standards and APIs.
3. **Bias Mitigation**: The bias mitigation can be done by methods such as the resampling of training data, bias-aware model training, and fairness-aware machine learning model designing. Moreover, transparent AI models can be used to detect and reduce bias and variance.

7.10.4 Emerging Trends in AI and IoMT

1. **Edge Computing**: The deployment of edge computing in IoMT-supported healthcare service delivery is gaining popularity as a result of its ability to analyze data close to the data generation point, resulting in lower latency for quick decision-making.

2. **Federated Learning**: The federated learning in IoMT healthcare facilitates the training of AI models across several decentralized IoMT devices and therefore helps protect data privacy.
3. **Explainable AI**: The deployment of explainable AI models is essential to make the IoMT systems transparent and to build trust in the healthcare services. The XAI models are preferable as they make the predictive choice more transparent for openness.
4. **AI-Driven Drug Discovery**: The AI models are used in healthcare services to expedite the identification of alternate treatment plans and therapies. The AI models are also helpful for new drug production and discovery.
5. **Blockchain for Data Security**: The use of blockchain technology in the healthcare industry is being investigated to improve data security, auditability, and consent management.

7.11 CONCLUSION

The integration of AI with the IoMT is transforming healthcare into a realm of continuous monitoring and personalized care. This report has highlighted the significance of AI in enhancing diagnostic accuracy and operational efficiency within healthcare systems. By examining the historical context, current applications, and technical frameworks, it has become clear that AI-enabled IoMT can revolutionize patient management and treatment strategies. The detailed analysis of AI technologies, including machine learning, natural language processing, and computer vision, illustrates their crucial roles in improving health outcomes. Moreover, the exploration of ethical and regulatory considerations underscores the importance of safeguarding patient data and ensuring compliance within these innovative frameworks. As the healthcare landscape continues to evolve, the recommendations presented advocate for ongoing collaboration, patient-centric approaches, and a steadfast commitment to ethical practices. The findings affirm that while challenges exist, the potential benefits of AI-enabled IoMT frameworks are substantial, promising to enhance not only the quality of patient care but also the overall efficiency of healthcare delivery systems. As we look to the future, embracing these advancements with a focus on ethical implementation and regulatory alignment will be essential in realizing a dynamic, patient-focused healthcare environment. The journey toward this transformative future is not just a technological evolution but a pivotal shift toward more responsive and responsible healthcare.

REFERENCES

[1] Singh P, Devi KJ, Thakkar HK, et al. Robust and secure medical image water-marking for edge-enabled e-healthcare. *IEEE Access*. 2023;11:135831–135845.

[2] IBM. The benefits of AI in healthcare [http://www.ibm.com/blog/the-benefits-of-ai-in-healthcare/], 2023. [Online; accessed 28-Feb-2024].

[3] Lutkevich B, DelVecchio A. Internet of Medical Things (IoMT) or healthcare IoT [https://www.techtarget.com/iotagenda/definition/IoMT-Internet-of-Medical-Things#:~:text=IoMT%20devices%20are%20used%20to,fewer%20mix%2Dups%20and%20mistakes.%20a%20History%20of%20artificial%20intelligence%20in%20healthcare:%20the%20first.%20.%20.%20(n.d.-b)]; 2024. [Online; accessed 28-Feb-2024].

[4] Thakkar HK, Dehury CK, Sahoo PK, et al. *Predictive analytics in cloud, fog, and edge computing: Perspectives and practices of blockchain, IoT, and 5G*. Springer; 2023.

[5] Thakkar HK, Chowdhury SR, Bhoi AK, et al. Applications of wearable technologies in healthcare: An analytical study. In: *5G IoT and edge computing for smart healthcare*. Elsevier; 2022. pp. 279–299.

[6] Bohr A, Memarzadeh K. The rise of artificial intelligence in healthcare applications. In: *Artificial intelligence in healthcare*. Elsevier; 2020. pp. 25–60.

[7] Jiang F, Jiang Y, Zhi H, et al. Artificial intelligence in healthcare: Past, present and future. *Stroke and Vascular Neurology*. 2017;2(4).

[8] Gupta R, Srivastava D, Sahu M, et al. Artificial intelligence to deep learning: Machine intelligence approach for drug discovery. *Molecular Diversity*. 2021;25:1315–1360.

[9] Dwivedi R, Mehrotra D, Chandra S. Potential of Internet of Medical Things (IoMT) applications in building a smart healthcare system: A systematic review. *Journal of Oral Biology and Craniofacial Research*. 2022;12(2):302–318.

[10] Jiang R. *Recent advances in AI-enabled automated medical diagnosis*, edited by Crookes D, Wei H-L, Zhang L, Chazot P. CRC Press; 2022.

[11] Nguyen DC, Nguyen KD, Pathirana PN. A mobile cloud based IoMT framework for automated health assessment and management. In: *2019 41st annual international conference of the IEEE Engineering in Medicine and Biology Society (EMBC)*; IEEE; 2019. pp. 6517–6520.

[12] Haleem A, Javaid M, Singh RP, et al. Medical 4.0 technologies for healthcare: Features, capabilities, and applications. *Internet of Things and Cyber-Physical Systems*. 2022;2:12–30.

[13] Wolfewicz A. Deep learning vs. machine learning—what's the difference? [http://levity.ai/blog/difference-machine-learning-deep-learning]; 2023. [Online; accessed 28-Feb-2024].

[14] Esteva A, Chou K, Yeung S, et al. Deep learning-enabled medical computer vision. *NPJ Digital Medicine*. 2021;4(1):5.

[15] Vishnu S, Ramson SJ, Jegan R. Internet of Medical Things (IoMT)-An overview. In: *2020 5th international conference on devices, circuits and systems (ICDCS)*; IEEE; 2020. pp. 101–104.

[16] Ates HC, Nguyen PQ, Gonzalez-Macia L, et al. End-to-end design of wearable sensors. *Nature Reviews Materials*. 2022;7(11):887–907.

[17] Awad AI, Fouda MM, Khashaba MM, et al. Utilization of mobile edge computing on the Internet of Medical Things: A survey. *ICT Express*. 2023;9(3):473–485.

[18] Devi KJ, Singh P, Dash JK, et al. Secure transmission of medical images in multicloud e-healthcare applications using data hiding scheme. *Journal of Information Security and Applications*. 2023;79:103655.

[19] Saxena A, Mittal S. Internet of Medical Things (IoMT) security and privacy: A survey of recent advances and enabling technologies. In: *Proceedings of the 2022 fourteenth international conference on contemporary computing*. 2022. pp. 550–559.

[20] Denecke K, Reichenpfader D. Sentiment analysis of clinical narratives: A scoping review. *Journal of Biomedical Informatics*. 2023:104336.

[21] Selvakanmani S, Ashreetha B, Devi GNR, et al. Deep learning approach to solve image retrieval issues associated with IoT sensors. *Measurement: Sensors*. 2022;24:100458.

[22] Sistaninejhad B, Rasi H, Nayeri P. A review paper about deep learning for medical image analysis. *Computational and Mathematical Methods in Medicine*. 2023;1(2023):7091301.

8 AI-Enabled Mobile Cloud-Based Federated IoMT Architecture for Ambient-Assisted Healthy Living

Abhijeetsingh Meena, Hiren Kumar Thakkar, and Apriandy Angdresey

8.1 INTRODUCTION

The rapid evolution of artificial intelligence (AI), the Internet of Things (IoT), and cloud computing has ushered in a transformative era for healthcare. This report delves into the development of an innovative AI-Enabled Mobile Cloud-Based Federated IoMT Architecture dedicated to ambient-assisted healthy living. The primary objective is to harness the synergies of AI, IoT, and cloud computing to craft intelligent and context-aware healthcare solutions, fostering personalized and efficient approaches to promoting well-being.

By integrating AI with the Internet of Medical Things (IoMT), this architecture gives rise to ambient-assisted living (AAL) environments. These environments leverage IoT devices and sensors to offer support that is tailored to individuals' daily routines, collecting real-time data to enable personalized healthcare services. The emphasis is on empowering individuals to lead independent and secure lives.

Security and efficiency are paramount considerations in the operation of this architecture. The report investigates lightweight two-factor authentication frameworks, emphasizing privacy preservation for mobile sinks within the social IoMT, with a focus on safeguarding sensitive healthcare data transmitted through the IoMT ecosystem.

Exploration extends to IoT architectures based on microservices tailored for AAL environments, striving to provide personalized assistance and healthcare support, especially for seniors. The integration of these architectures into smart cities aims to promote aging in place, facilitating seamless interconnection of AAL systems within the urban environment. Additionally, the application of federated learning techniques enhances network intrusion detection in AAL environments, ensuring collaborative and privacy-preserving model training using distributed datasets from multiple AAL systems.

 DOI: 10.1201/9781003393498-11

The successful implementation of this architecture faces challenges such as privacy concerns, data security, interoperability, and scalability. Overcoming these challenges holds the key to realizing the full potential of the AI-Enabled Mobile Cloud-Based Federated IoMT architecture for ambient-assisted healthy living. The anticipated outcomes include continuous monitoring, personalized healthcare services, and timely interventions based on real-time data analysis, shaping the future landscape of healthcare technology. With the use of these gadgets, people may now manage their own health directly because they serve as hubs for data collecting, communication, and control. No matter where people are, they can interact with their health and well-being caregivers because of the portability and accessibility of mobile technology. This architecture introduces the idea of remote data processing and storage through its cloud-based features. It allows for easy access to health information from any location with an internet connection by shifting the labor-intensive data maintenance and analysis to remote servers. Collaboration between healthcare professionals and caregivers is made easier as a result, ensuring that patients get proper care at the appropriate time. Federated IoMT refers to the interconnection and cooperative operation of a variety of medical devices and sensors. These interconnected gadgets—from wearable fitness trackers to home health monitors—share information and insights to build a thoroughgoing picture of one's health. The accuracy of health assessments is improved, and potential problems can be identified early thanks to this collaborative method. The emphasis on ambient-assisted healthy living further emphasizes the need to incorporate these technologies into the very foundation of our daily life. This strategy encourages continuous medical monitoring and support within our living environments instead of separate, episodic healthcare. Smart sensors in offices, residences, and public locations collect information on how we live and the environment, promoting a proactive and healthy way of life.

8.1.1 Introduction of Medical Things or IoT in Healthcare

The network of hardware platforms, software applications (protocols), and connected medical equipment that is connected to the internet is known as the Internet of Medical Things (IoMT). IoMT, also known as IoT in healthcare, enables wireless and remote devices to safely connect via the internet to enable quick and adaptable analysis of medical data. The market for healthcare will unquestionably and permanently be affected by IoMT. By 2030, the IoMT industry, according to certain analysts of the healthcare technology sector, is anticipated to reach $861.3 billion. IoMT has numerous effects on the healthcare sector. The following changes are most noticeable when IoMT is used in the home, on the body, in the community, and in hospitals:

- In-hospital IoMT
- In-home IoMT
- On-body IoMT
- Community IoMT

Hospitals must keep track of their medical supplies, equipment, and staff members' and patients' movements within the facility. They do this by using specialized sensors and online-connected tracking devices. These systems aid hospital administrators in having a clearer understanding of what is happening in the hospital. They are able to observe where everything is as well as how individuals are moving.

8.2 OVERVIEW OF THE INTERNET OF MEDICAL THINGS (IOMT)

8.2.1 What Is the Internet of Medical Things?

The Internet of Things (IoT) refers to a concept wherein an object or device is imbued with technologies like sensors and software, enabling it to communicate, control, connect, and exchange data with other devices as long as they remain connected to the internet [1]. IoT shares a close association with the term "machine-to-machine," and devices equipped with machine-to-machine communication capabilities are commonly referred to as smart devices. These intelligent devices are anticipated to assist humans in accomplishing various tasks and responsibilities [2,3]. The Internet of Things offers numerous advantages in enhancing human life, with one notable application being the realm of the Internet of Medical Things.

The Internet of Medical Things (IoMT) refers to the application of IoT technologies and intelligent devices in healthcare [4,5]. IoMT utilizes interconnected sensors and devices to collect medical and health data, which is then analyzed by artificial intelligence//machine learning algorithms to derive insights [6,7]. Key IoMT applications include remote health monitoring, chronic disease management, fitness tracking, smart hospitals, etc. [8,9]. However, centralized IoMT systems can face challenges related to privacy, scalability, latency, and network throughput [10]. The IoMT comprises a network of interconnected medical devices, sensors, and healthcare systems that leverage IoT technologies to gather, track, and analyze health data [6,8]. This interconnectivity facilitates seamless communication and collaboration among various healthcare stakeholders, transforming traditional healthcare into a more proactive, personalized, and efficient ecosystem [7].

The IoMT ecosystem includes a multitude of devices like wearable trackers, smart implants, remote monitoring systems, hospital equipment, and telemedicine platforms [8,9]. These devices collect real-time data such as vital signs, biometrics, medication adherence, and environmental factors. This data is transmitted to the cloud for storage, analysis, and decision-making [9,11]. The key benefit of IoMT is its ability to empower healthcare providers, patients, and caregivers by enabling continuous monitoring, early anomaly detection, and timely interventions [11,12]. By utilizing AI, cloud computing, and advanced analytics, IoMT allows deriving valuable insights.

Furthermore, IoMT plays a vital role in ambient-assisted healthy living by integrating AI-enabled mobile and cloud technologies into daily environments [6,13]. For instance, IoMT-enabled smart homes can detect fall risks, monitor adherence, and adjust conditions to optimize comfort and safety for the elderly or disabled [6]. Figure 8.1 shows the flow of data in a cloud-based federated IoMT architecture. The data is being generated by patients with sensors at home; the user end device is connected to fog servers, which help to decentralize the processing and data storing. We can view Fog servers as helpers in the overall process. This data is connected to

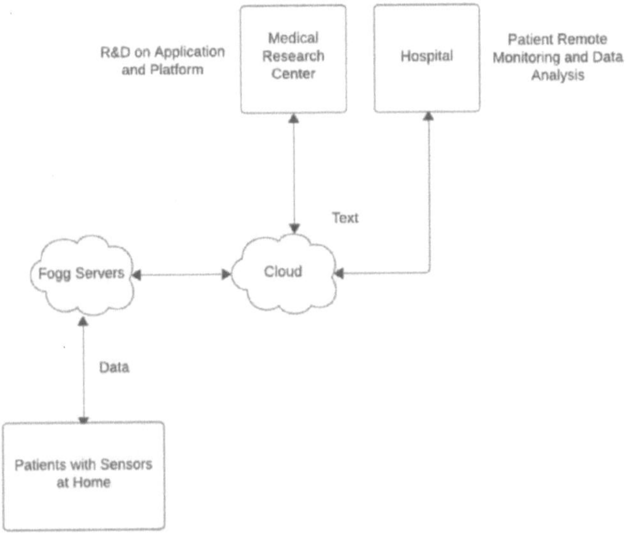

FIGURE 8.1 Flow of data in a cloud-based federated IoMT architecture.

cloud infrastructure, which enables access to research and development departments and hospitals where doctors can track their patients' health and metrics.

8.2.2 Importance of IoMT

IoMT is of paramount importance due to its potential to improve healthcare outcomes and the patient experience. Figure 8.2 portrays some of the key aspects of the importance of IoMT with a flow diagram.

IoMT plays a significant role in five ways:

- **Continuous Health Monitoring**: IoMT devices permit real-time tracking of patients' vital health metrics. For example, wearable devices including smartwatches and fitness bands can continuously monitor parameters like heart rate, activity levels, and sleep patterns. This constant monitoring generates valuable data to enable early disease detection and preventative healthcare [6,11].
- **Chronic Disease Management**: IoMT is transformative for people with chronic illnesses. Patients with diabetes, for instance, can benefit from connected glucose monitors that transmit data to healthcare providers. This allows healthcare professionals to make timely interventions, adjust treatment regimens, and improve patient outcomes [8,12].
- **Remote Patient Care**: For remote patient care, IoMT enables virtual consultations and monitoring from afar. Patients in rural or underserved regions can access healthcare services without frequent travel. This is especially relevant in situations like the COVID-19 pandemic, when telehealth and remote monitoring gained widespread acceptance [4,9].

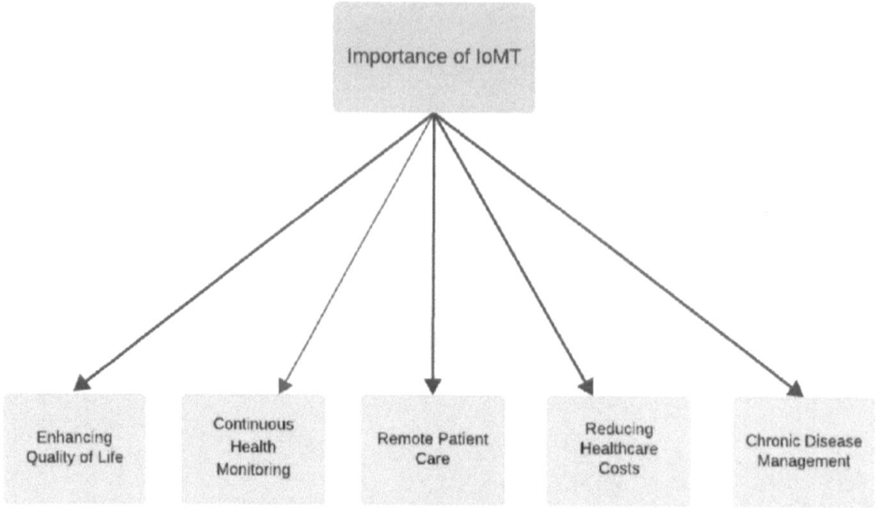

FIGURE 8.2 Flow diagram of importance of IoMT.

TABLE 8.1
IoT Protocols

Protocol	Bandwidth	Range	Use-Cases
Infrared	Not applicable (NA)	Short (few meters)	Short-range data transmission
Bluetooth	2.4 GHz	Short (10–100 meters)	Wireless gadgets communication
Cellular	800 MHz–2.5 GHz	Long (kilometers)	Mobile communications
CoAP	Not applicable (NA)	Short to moderate	IoT applications
WiFi	2.4 GHz, 5 GHz	Moderate to long	Wireless internet access
Zigbee	2.4 GHz	Short to moderate	Home automation

- **Reducing Healthcare Costs**: By providing more data-driven insights and early interventions, IoMT can potentially reduce the overall cost of healthcare. It helps in preventing hospital readmission, reducing emergency room visits, and improving medication adherence.
- **Enhancing Quality of Life**: IoMT is not limited to patient care; it also addresses the overall well-being of individuals. For seniors, IoMT can provide safety and independence through fall detection systems and smart home automation.

8.2.3 Protocol Used in IoMT

- **Infrared**: An infrared protocol is a set of rules for sending information using invisible light; it's often used in remote controls, where you press a button, and the remote sends secret light signals that make your TV or other devices do things.

- **Bluetooth**: The Bluetooth protocol acts as a wireless language that enables wireless communication between gadgets like speakers, headphones, and phones. It makes it simpler for us to use our devices without having to plug in wires because it enables them to share music, calls, and data across short distances.
- **Cellular**: Our mobile phones connect to a network of towers using the cellular protocol, which is comparable to the HTTP or HTTPS protocols used on the internet, to make calls, send messages, and access the internet. Our phones interact with the network and other devices using what seems to be a secret code, allowing us to stay connected and carry out chores like web browsing or texting friends while on the go.
- **CoAP**: Constrained application protocol (CoAP), also known as the Internet of Things (IoT) and limited devices, such as sensors and small embedded systems, is a lightweight communication protocol. Similar to a condensed form of HTTP, which is the standard protocol for internet connection, it is designed to function effectively on hardware with poor processing and memory capabilities. These devices can communicate with one another over the internet or a local network using CoAP, which uses less bandwidth and energy. It is especially helpful for Internet of Things (IoT) applications where a large number of small devices must communicate and share data without consuming excessive power or congesting the network.
- **WI-FI**: The term "wireless fidelity" or "Wi-Fi," refers to a technology that enables smart home appliances, laptops, and smartphones to connect to the internet wirelessly. Devices can communicate with a wireless router or access point by transmitting data using radio waves. Wi-Fi is widely used, making it an easy and flexible means to access the internet in such places as homes, workplaces, and public areas. It now supports numerous daily activities, including web surfing, streaming videos, online gaming, and more. In order to prevent unauthorized access, Wi-Fi networks are often password-protected. This ensures the privacy and security of data sent over the wireless connection. The description of bandwidth, range, and use-cases of each protocol is described in Table 8.1.

8.2.4 AI-ML Algorithms in Healthcare

Various machine learning algorithms have been developed in the recent past for several healthcare domains such as cancer diagnosis, disease predictions, glucose monitoring, etc. Table 8.2 describes the popular ML algorithms with corresponding applications in the healthcare domain.

8.3 EVOLUTION OF FEDERATED LEARNING FOR DISTRIBUTED IOT SYSTEMS

Federated learning is a decentralized machine learning technique that addresses many limitations of centralized systems. It enables distributed training of a shared machine learning model without exchanging raw data. This was pioneered by

TABLE 8.2
ML Algorithms and Applications in the Healthcare Domain

AI Algorithms	Applications in Healthcare Domain
SVM	1. Biomarker imaging 2. Human–machine interface 3. Cancer diagnosis
Neural network	1. Cancer diagnosis 2. Identifying 3. Parkinson's disease 4. Image-based cardiac monitoring
Naïve bayes	1. Disease prediction 2. Medical diagnosis
KNN	1. Glucose monitoring for diabetes 2. Pandemic resource management 3. Disease prediction
Decision tree	1. Glucose monitoring for diabetes 2. Surgery 3. Medical diagnosis
Random forest	1. Disease prediction 2. Healthcare monitoring system 3. Heart disease prediction
Logistic regression	1. Image-based cardiac monitoring 2. Glucose monitoring for diabetes 3. Pandemic resource management 4. Healthcare monitoring system

Google for keyboard prediction and has since evolved for various IoT applications. Compared to traditional distributed learning approaches like parallelization, federated learning better preserves data privacy and reduces communication costs in large-scale distributed IoT systems.

Some key works on improving federated learning techniques include McMahan, who proposed federated averaging to address the client–server communication bottleneck. This introduced the methodology of local model training that clients followed by parameter aggregation at the server. To handle imbalanced and non-IID data, this chapter [4] developed FedProx, which adds a proximal term to the objective function. This prevents client models from diverging too much, so this research [7] designed MoDL, which adaptively tunes client sampling frequencies based on their relative data heterogeneity.

For enhanced communication efficiency, techniques like quantization, sparsification, and gradient coding were explored. Wang studied the effects of gradient quantization and demonstrated that 1-bit quantization works well for distributed training of CNNs. This study [7] proposed top-k sparsification as a way to compress full gradients into sparse vectors and studied their convergence properties. Coded distributed computing was used by [11], where redundant gradients are calculated at client side, and gradient-coded aggregation is provided for robustness against the stragglers of failures.

For heterogeneity in this study, SCAFFOLD [12] used control varieties for reducing variance and adopted per-client learning rates. This worked on partial client participation through conditional gradients that outperform random sampling when clients have limited resources [8]. Furthermore, the study [10] paved the way for cross-silo federated learning through secure aggregation where individual encryptions can be summed without decrypting. Federated learning has emerged as a promising approach to address privacy and data security concerns in distributed IoT systems. It allows multiple edge devices, such as smartphones, wearables, and sensors, to collaboratively learn a shared model without the need to share raw data. This decentralized learning paradigm has experienced notable evolution, driven by advancements in AI, IoT, and cloud computing technologies.

Federated learning began with a focus on mobile devices while taking advantage of their computational capabilities to train models locally [6]. In fact, the year 2017 brought an important breakthrough opportunity after Google had proposed federated averaging. This work highlights the benefits of collaborative learning that implies performing local device-level updates and sharing only aggregate updates with the central server, thus preserving data privacy and diminishing transmission needs. As a result, it is particularly popular among IoT devices, which often lack resources.

With the widespread adoption of IoT, an extension of federated learning to various distributed IoT systems is obvious [14]. Many researchers began to further explore the federated approaches in different fields: health monitoring, smart grid networks, and various transportation systems [4,8]. An example is a federated learning system with healthcare IoT devices, which can facilitate collective model training while keeping all the data private and secure as in the previous example [8]. Another example is a traffic prediction system for intelligent transportation, based on the federated learning approach and distributed sensors that can also improve the quality of prognosis with more data [4].

In order to improve federated learning for distributed IoT, researchers have started to introduce cloud-based architectures. Specifically, cloud-assisted federated learning allows for cloud systems to help edge devices execute the most computationally intensive tasks, while keeping their data secure. Such an approach is beneficial as it makes the best use of both edge computing and cloud. For instance, a cloud-assisted federated learning scheme for IoT devices was introduced, which allows the devices to efficiently train their models and run an inference, while limiting communication overhead [13].

8.4 MOBILE CLOUD ARCHITECTURE FOR FEDERATED IOMT SYSTEMS

To enable federated learning for distributed IoMT devices, a mobile cloud architecture is proposed. IoMT sensors/devices located at the network edge collect and preprocess data locally. Mobile devices like smartphones act as edge processors to train local models using federated averaging. The cloud serves as a centralized coordinating entity to manage the federated training process without accessing raw data. This distributed architecture leverages edge/fog computing benefits for reduced latency, extended coverage, and improved efficiency.

The mobile cloud architecture for a federated IoMT system typically includes four layers as described by [6]:

- **Perception Layer**: This consists of IoMT devices like smartwatches, fitness bands, and medical equipment that collect health data like heart rate, glucose levels, activity records, etc., as mentioned earlier [15].
- **Network Layer**: Network technologies like WiFi, Bluetooth, and 4G/5G cellular networks are used to transmit this data from perception devices to edge nodes as studied in [4]. Edge positions track resource usage to optimize network transmissions effectively.
- **Edge Computing Layer**: Edge nodes located near end devices perform data preprocessing, integration, and contextualization as proposed in [8]. This includes tasks like data cleaning, feature extraction, and encryption.
- **Cloud Computing Layer**: Large cloud platforms pool resources for tasks like distributed training of federated models, longitudinal record storage, and advanced analysis on enormous multimedia and time-series data pools according to [12]. Interfaces and APIs give access to health applications, physicians, and other consumers.

This distributed architecture leverages both edge and cloud advantages effectively for privacy-preserving federated learning with real-time and personalized healthcare assistance as explored by [8]. The mobile cloud architecture for federated IoMT systems combines the power of mobile devices with the scalability and resources offered by cloud computing. This architecture enables seamless integration of AI-enabled analytics, secure data sharing, and real-time decision-making, fostering ambient-assisted healthy living environments.

Mobile devices such as wearable devices and smartphones are the central components of the architecture. These mobile devices act as a gateway for collecting and analyzing health-related data from various IoMT devices. In order to reduce the load on the cloud infrastructure, the mobile device acts as an edge node, performing basic tasks such as data preprocessing and feature extraction. It is noticed that time-sensitive healthcare applications require real-time data analysis and responsiveness. Therefore, a mobile cloud infrastructure is required for sufficient computational power and scalability in federated IoMT systems to work in the real-time manner [4,6,8]. In such cases, the cloud acts as a centralized server to store the processed data, to train the models, and to perform intensive complex calculations [2,3]. The real-time and responsive applications can be further enhanced by making them scalable and secured, making them deployable.

A federated learning framework in a mobile cloud infrastructure is comprised of a central server, local devices, and communication protocols [4,6]. The global model is made consistent when the central server supervises the learning process of all the local devices and combines the updates [4,8]. On the contrary, the local devices guarantee privacy during data generation and contribute to the training process [13].

Moreover, the mobile cloud architecture integrates AI-powered analytics modules that utilize machine learning algorithms to extract insights, from the gathered data. These modules can detect patterns, anomalies, and trends in health-related information, allowing for early detection of potential health risks and personalized interventions. For example, AI algorithms can analyze vital signs, activity levels, and environmental data to provide context-aware recommendations for medication adherence, exercise routines, and lifestyle modifications [16,17].

8.5 AI/ML MODELS FOR AMBIENT-ASSISTED HEALTHY LIVING

Important ML models for ambient-assisted living applications include activity recognition using CNNs/RNNs, health assessment using ML classifiers, predictive models for disease management, etc. Federated learning enables distributed training of these complex models across IoMT devices in a privacy-preserving manner for a large population. Regular model updates help develop personalized and contextualized ML models for each individual. Key ML techniques used include computer-vision-based activity recognition CNNs from camera streams. For example, a ResNet architecture was used by [12] to classify six behaviors with 98.4% accuracy on ADL datasets. NLP models like LSTMs and transformers are gaining traction for conversational agents. Li developed a transformer-based chatbot that answers clinical questions with a mean reciprocal rank of 0.89.

In the realm of healthcare analytics, the study employs advanced techniques to analyze time-series data derived from vital signs. Long short-term memory (LSTM) networks, and gated recurrent units (GRUs) are utilized to model health trends. The comparative analysis conducted by the authors reveals that LSTMs outperform GRUs, particularly in accurately forecasting blood pressure and heart rate 14 days in advance [12]. To gain deeper insights into the data, multivariate clustering is facilitated by uniform manifold approximation and projection (UMAP) and *t*-distributed stochastic neighbor embedding (t-SNE), as demonstrated by a previous study [11]. This approach aids in uncovering novel patterns and relationships within the dataset. Moreover, the proposed study analyzes the optimization of autoencoder models through attention mechanisms and generative adversarial networks (GANs). This optimization of autoencoder models is targeted to enhance the representation learning of Internet of Medical Things (IoMT) data [13].

Healthcare-recommended systems are essential for ambient-assisted living, for which the techniques such as matrix factorization (MF) and collaborative filtering (CF) are essential. In [4], a personalized health risk prediction and preventive advice method using the electronic medical records (EMRs) is proposed using the CF. The healthcare-recommended system based on MF and CF is considered an advanced analytics-based approach that analyzes the individual medical records to predict health and prevent illnesses. Federated model development is leading the way, prioritizing the protection of privacy and providing proactive healthcare support to citizens. This collective advancement shows a dedication to developing technology that supports proactive and individualized healthcare treatments in addition to analyzing health trends.

The goal of ambient-assisted healthy living is to deliver individualized healthcare services by analyzing data gathered from IoMT devices using AI and machine learning models. These models are necessary to identify irregularities, to forecast health hazards, and to produce useful information that helps people lead healthy lives. A flow diagram as shown in Figure 8.3 shows various AI/ML models that can be used to build AAL. Moreover, the summary of types of models is described in Table 8.3.

- **Predictive Analytics Models**: Predictive analytics models detect potential health hazards and take preemptive measures by combining previous IoMT data with AI algorithms. For instance, depending on a variety of variables such as age, lifestyle, and biometric data [18], machine learning techniques such as decision trees, random forests, and support vector machines forecast the probability of finding chronic illnesses.
- **Activity Recognition Models**: To infer a user's behaviors and activities, such as eating, sleeping, or walking, activity recognition algorithms examine sensor data from environmental sensors or wearables. For activity tracking and classification, methods such as recurrent neural networks, hidden Markov models, and supervised learning are used. Through the comprehension of activity patterns, these models are able to recognize potential health risks or falls and identify departures from regular routines, therefore initiating the necessary alarms [6,8].
- **Decision Support Systems**: Healthcare workers can make better decisions with the help of machine learning algorithms and decision support systems. They combine AI, medical knowledge, and patient data to diagnose

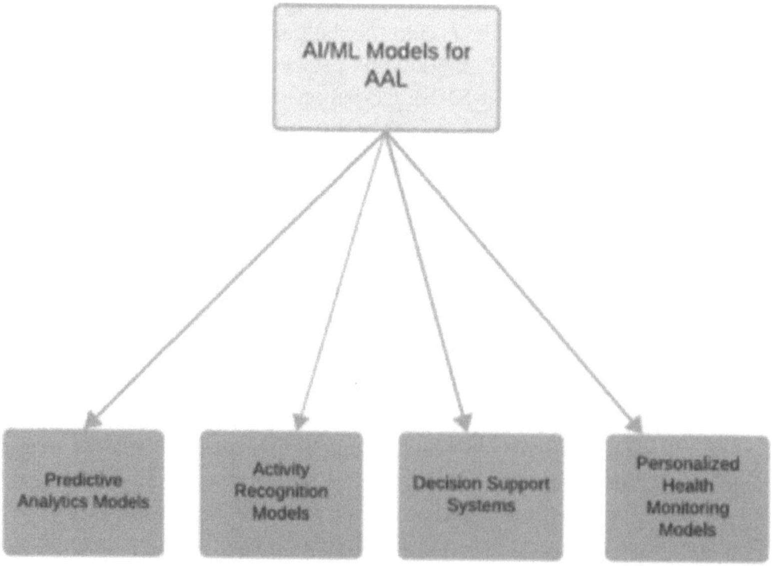

FIGURE 8.3 Flow diagram of types of AI/ML models for ambient-assisted healthy living.

TABLE 8.3
Summary of Types of Models [4,6–9,11].

Types of Model	Summary about Model
Predictive analytics models	Predictive analytics models use historical healthcare data and AI algorithms to anticipate potential health risks and proactively intervene.
Activity recognition models [6,8].	Activity recognition models analyze sensor data from wearable or environmental sensors to identify and track a person's daily activities, aiding in identifying deviations and potential health issues.
Decision support systems [4,11].	Decision support systems employ machine learning algorithms to assist healthcare professionals in diagnosing diseases, recommending treatment plans, and improving healthcare accuracy and delivery.
Personalized health monitoring models [7,9].	Personalized health monitoring models use AI to analyze real-time health data from IoT devices, providing personalized feedback and recommendations to optimize an individual's well-being.

conditions, suggest courses of therapy, and offer customized guidance. CNNs and other deep learning models can help with medical picture analysis, helping to identify diseases such as cancer or retinal disorders. This improves healthcare delivery [4,11] and increases accuracy while reducing human error.

- **Personalized Health Monitoring Models**: AI-powered health tracking systems use data from wearable devices to give feedback on a person's health in real time. For instance, recurrent neural networks (RNNs) or long short-term memory (LSTM) can be used to analyze data that changes over time, such as heart rate, to identify unusual patterns or trends. These models can provide customized suggestions to enhance the person's health and well-being [7,9].

8.6 CONCLUSION

In this chapter, we described the significant influence of AI, the IoT, and cloud computing on healthcare, particularly through the development of an AI-enabled Mobile Cloud-based Federated IoMT Architecture aimed at enhancing AAL. The integration of AI with IoMT facilitates real-time data collection via IoT devices, supporting personalized healthcare solutions and promoting independent living for seniors. The report delves into lightweight two-factor authentication frameworks to ensure secure operations within IoMT environments. Additionally, microservices-based IoT architectures are explored as means to deliver tailored assistance and are adaptable for integration within smart cities to foster aging in place. Federated learning techniques are highlighted as crucial for improving network intrusion detection while maintaining privacy during collaborative model training. Addressing challenges such as privacy concerns, data security, interoperability, and scalability is vital for effective implementation. The promise of this integrated approach lies in its ability to enable continuous monitoring and personalized healthcare, ultimately leading to timely interventions that enhance overall well-being. The report underscores the potential of these technologies to revolutionize healthcare delivery and create supportive environments for aging populations, paving the way for more efficient and responsive health solutions in modern society.

REFERENCES

[1] F.Meneghello, M. Calore, D. Zucchetto, M. Polese, and A. Zanella. IoT: Internet of threats? a survey of practical security vulnerabilities in real IoT devices. *IEEE Internet of Things Journal*, 6(5):8182–8201, 2019.

[2] L.Sitanayah, A.Angdresey, and E.Kristalino. A real-time application for road conditions detection based on the internet of things. *JOIV: International Journal on Informatics Visualization*, 6(3):629–635, 2022.

[3] Y.Yang, X.Luo, X.Chu, M.-T.Zhou, Y.Yang, X.Luo, X.Chu, and M.-T.Zhou. IoT technologies and applications. *Fog-Enabled Intelligent IoT Systems*, 1–37, 2020.

[4] D.J.Cook, J.C.Augusto, and V.R.Jakkula. Review: Ambient intelligence: Technologies, applications, and opportunities. *Pervasive and Mobile Computing*, 5(4):277–298, 2009.

[5] F.Wu, T.Wu, and M.R.Yuce. Design and implementation of a wearable sensor network system for IoT-connected safety and health applications. In *2019 IEEE 5th World Forum on Internet of Things (WF-IoT)*, 87–90. IEEE, 2019.

[6] M.-L.M.-Llacuna, J.C.-Llin'as, and J.M.-Frigola. Lessons in urban monitoring taken from sustainable and livable cities to better address the smart cities initiative. *Technological Forecasting and Social Change*, 90:611–622, 2015.

[7] S.Blackman, C.Matlo, C.Bobrovitskiy, A.Waldoch, M.Fang, P.Jackson, A.Mihailidis, L.Nygård, A.Astell, and A.Sixsmith. Ambient assisted living technologies for aging well: A scoping review. *Journal of Intelligent Systems*, 25(1):55–69, 2016.

[8] R.Giffinger and H.Gudrun. Smart cities ranking: An effective instrument for the positioning of the cities? *ACE: Architecture, City and Environment*, 4:7–26, 2010.

[9] P.Rashidi and A.Mihailidis. A survey on ambient-assisted living tools for older adults. *IEEE Journal of Biomedical and Health Informatics*, 17(3):579–590, 2013.

[10] N.Valkanova, S.Jord'a, and A.V.Moere. Public visualization displays of citizen data: Design, impact, and implications. *International Journal of Human-Computer Studies*, 81:4–16, 2014.

[11] A.S.Hwang, K.N.Truong, J.I.Cameron, E.Lindqvist, L.Nygård, and A.Mihailidis. Codesigning ambient assisted living (AAL) environments: Unravelling the situated context of informal dementia care. *BioMed Research International*, 1–12, 2015.

[12] H.K.Ngankam, H.Pigot, M.Parenteau, M.Lussier, A.Aboujaoudé, C.Laliberté, M.Couture, N.Bier, and S.Giroux. An IoT architecture of microservices for ambient assisted living environments to promote aging in smart cities. In *How AI Impacts Urban Living and Public Health: 17th International Conference, ICOST 2019, New York City, NY, USA, October 14–16, 2019, Proceedings*, Springer-Verlag, 154–167, 2019.

[13] J.Boger, P.Jackson, M.Mulvenna, J.Sixsmith, A.Sixsmith, A.Mihailidis, P.Kontos, J.M.Polgar, A.Grigorovich, and S.Martin. Principles for fostering the transdisciplinary development of assistive technologies. *Disability and Rehabilitation. Assistive Technology*, 12(5):48–490, 2017.

[14] A.Angdresey and J.-Q.Ooi. Analyzing multimodal sensory signals using unsupervised machine learning. In *2023 International Conference on Computer, Control, Informatics and its Applications (IC3INA)*, 301–306. IEEE, 2023.

[15] J.Srivastava, S.Routray, S.Ahmad, and M.M.Waris. Internet of Medical Things (IoMT)-based smart healthcare system: Trends and progress. *Computational Intelligence and Neuroscience*, 1–17, 2022.

[16] L.K.Vora, A.D.Gholap, K.Jetha, R.R.S.Thakur, H.K.Solanki, and V.P.Chavda. Artificial intelligence in pharmaceutical technology and drug delivery design. *Pharmaceutics*, 7(5):1–46, 2023.

[17] A.Fabbrizio, A.Fucarino, M.Cantoia, A.De Giorgio, N.D.Garrido, E.Iuliano, V.M.Reis, M.Sausa, J.V.-Alves, G.Zimatore, C.Baldari, and F.Macaluso. Smart devices for health and wellness applied to tele-exercise: An overview of new trends and technologies such as IoT and AI. *Healthcare*, 11(12):1–20, 2023.

[18] L.A.AlKaabi, L.S.Ahmed, M.F.Al Attiyah, and M.E.A.-Rahman. Predicting hypertension using machine learning: Findings from Qatar biobank study. *PloS ONE*, 15(10):1–17, 2020.

9 Symptom-Based Real-Time Augmented Pattern Detection and Recognition for Healthy Living

Arvik Shah and Hiren Kumar Thakkar

9.1 INTRODUCTION

The integration of symptom-based detection and augmented reality technologies has the potential to transform preventive healthcare through real-time and personalized health monitoring. By combining continuous symptom tracking with context-aware augmented reality interventions, these technologies can promote healthy living and proactive care. Likewise, Figure 9.1 illustrates the conceptual integration of symptom-based detection and augmented reality technologies for proactive healthcare and healthy living.

Real-time symptom monitoring through wearable devices and sensors allows for the early detection of health changes and potential illnesses. Capturing symptoms as they occur provides data that can be analyzed to derive personalized insights.

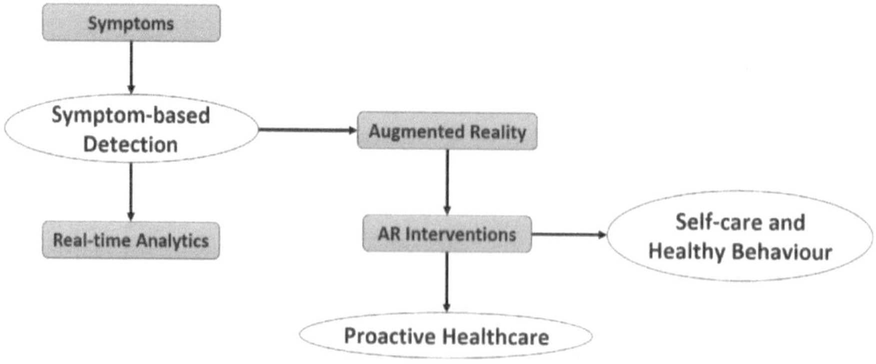

FIGURE 9.1 Integration of symptom-based detection and augmented reality for proactive healthcare and healthy living.

DOI: 10.1201/9781003393498-12

Real-time analytics enable timely interventions based on an individual's evolving health status. Augmented reality further acts on these insights by providing guidance and recommendations. Visual overlays and notifications can nudge users toward targeted actions to preemptively address emerging health issues.

Together, these technologies move healthcare toward an always-on, AI-powered paradigm focused on maintaining wellness. The convergence of symptom tracking and AR bridges physical signals with digital interventions to make health management seamless. It also shifts care from the hospital to daily life by equipping individuals with personalized tools for self-care. Proactive care through real-time adaptation helps prevent minor symptoms from escalating into serious conditions, reducing disease burden.

The integration of these technologies creates an intelligent preventive care loop that connects symptom detection, data analytics, and AR-driven interventions. As symptoms are tracked in real time, analytical engines recognize patterns and customize AR prompts for each user. These prompts activate behavior changes to mitigate emerging health threats based on the specific context. User interactions and compliance feed back data to further tune and personalize this loop. This real-time adaptive system powered by data-driven insights and customizable AR nudges can optimize and tailor preventive care.

Effective integration of real-time symptom analytics and AR faces challenges like privacy, accuracy, user adoption, and managing information overload. As health data collection expands, stringent data governance frameworks are needed to maintain user trust. Sensor accuracy and interpreting multifaceted symptoms also pose technical challenges. Seamless user experience design is essential for adoption. Further, as AR overlays increase information density, interfaces must contextualize prompts smartly to avoid overloading users. A human-centric approach considering these factors is vital for actualizing the promise of these preventive care technologies.

This report provides a landscape analysis of real-time symptom monitoring and AR techniques for preventive care. It discusses emerging wearables and sensors, AI-based health analytics, AR visualization modes, and ethics. The report highlights the potential while also considering the limitations and challenges involved in integrating these technologies. It aims to analyze the current state of the field and to offer insights into future directions for this promising preventive healthcare approach.

9.2 LITERATURE REVIEW

Biometric systems that analyze human physiological and behavioral traits have become essential technologies for identity verification and security in the modern digital era. As discussed by Ghosh et al. (2022) [1], biometrics enable establishing an individual's identity by measuring and analyzing characteristics like fingerprints, faces, irises, voices, or signatures; a person's identity can be established through biometrics. Research in the past decade has successfully applied biometrics in diverse domains, including forensic science, healthcare, financial services, and immigration. The authors present an extensive review of biometric modalities, pattern recognition techniques, and recent technological advances in this field.

TABLE 9.1
Evolution of Symptom-Based Augmented Health Technologies

Timeline	Developments
1903–1936	Early studies in physiological patterns and symptom analysis Initial attempts at manual symptom recognition for health monitoring Development of rudimentary augmented reality for medical visualization
1936–1970	Research on automated symptom-based recognition algorithms begins Introduction of real-time data processing for symptom detection Integration of augmented reality with medical diagnostics First attempts at integrating biometric data for health monitoring
1970–1985	Advancements in computer vision for real-time symptom analysis Early experiments with wearable devices for continuous health monitoring Emergence of AI-driven pattern recognition in medical diagnostics
1985–1995	Development of wearable augmented reality devices for healthcare professionals Integration of biometric sensors in real-time health monitoring systems Pioneering work in voice-based symptom recognition technology Introduction of smart wearables for symptom-based health tracking
1995–2004	Expansion of real-time augmented reality applications in surgery Development of AI algorithms for symptom-based early disease detection Implementation of wearable biometric devices for personalized health insights
2004–2010	Introduction of real-time symptom-based monitoring in mobile health apps Integration of augmented reality in patient education and rehabilitation Advancements in voice and speech recognition for symptom analysis Use of wearable biometric technology for personalized health recommendations
2010–2017	Development of AI-driven augmented reality platforms for symptom visualization Real-time recognition of complex health patterns through machine learning Integration of symptom-based recognition in smart home devices Advancements in voice-controlled virtual health assistants Implementation of real-time augmented reality for remote medical consultations

A key insight from Ghosh et al. (2022) [1] sheds light on the intricate nature of biometric systems. Their findings highlight the importance of sophisticated variable data processing in this context, from gathering biometric information via sensors and preprocessing to feature extraction, identification, labeling, and verification—each step necessitating advanced techniques such as image processing, machine learning, pattern recognition, and artificial intelligence. Ghosh et al. present a comprehensive model of biometric system workflow, emphasizing sensor data collection, preprocessing, dimensionality reduction, and subsequent stages such as the classification, clustering, and validation of biometric patterns. Furthermore, the authors examine fingerprints, facial features, iris patterns, and voices, as well as emerging trends such as biometric integration in smart devices, wearables, e-commerce, and cloud platforms. As depicted in Table 9.1, the various applications of biometrics across distinct time periods correspond to the course of developments for real-time augmented pattern detection for promoting healthy living.

Building upon the discussion of biometric systems, Khan et al. (2022) [2] focus specifically on detecting human activities using hybrid deep learning models that combine convolutional neural networks (CNNs) and long short-term memory (LSTM) networks. The authors highlight that this approach addresses key limitations of previous machine learning techniques for spatial-temporal feature extraction from complex time-series sensor data generated during human activities. On a novel dataset compiled by the authors containing Kinect sensor feeds for 12 different physical activities, the proposed CNN-LSTM model achieves 90.89% classification accuracy, significantly outperforming other techniques. The contributions of this work include generating the new dataset, extensive testing of different machine learning and deep learning models to empirically determine the optimal architecture, and demonstrating the advantages of hybrid deep learning models that integrate CNN-based spatial feature extraction with LSTM networks for temporal sequence modeling—directly suited for human activity recognition tasks.

For enhancing fingerprint biometric systems, Ghosh et al. (2022) [1] put forth mathematical techniques to improve quality assessment and minutiae feature extraction—two crucial steps in fingerprint recognition. The proposed quality assessment approach analyzes ridge and valley slope, thickness, and steepness. For feature extraction, combining 2-D discrete wavelet transforms for dimensionality reduction and support vector machines for classification is suggested. The authors also evaluate an iris recognition model designed for health diagnosis. Here, integrating LL and HL sub-bands from the wavelet decomposition of iris images and using radial basis function kernels gives optimal accuracy of 87.5% and sensitivity of 0.95. Additionally, the merits of deep-learning-based biometric recognition models such as CNNs, LSTMs, and autoencoders that can automatically learn feature representations are discussed.

Focusing on a specific biomedical application, Subasi (2020) [3] provides an in-depth overview of AI techniques for detecting Alzheimer's disease using analysis of medical imaging data. The chapter outlines the key stages in a generalized framework—preprocessing, feature extraction, image segmentation, recognition using machine learning and deep learning models, and ultimately disease detection. A range of machine learning approaches including ANNs, kNN, SVMs that have been employed for AD detection are reviewed. Additionally, deep learning models such as CNNs, LSTMs, and autoencoders that are gaining prominence are discussed. Subasi also underscores the importance of sufficiently large training datasets and avoiding overfitting, both critical factors impacting the real-world performance of AI systems.

Extending the application of AI techniques to other disease domains, Paranthaman et al. (2022) [4] present an extensive literature review synthesizing over 120 research studies that employ AI methods for diverse disease diagnosis applications spanning conditions like cancer, diabetes, neurodegenerative diseases, and cardiovascular as well as respiratory illnesses. The authors distill a generalized AI framework comprising data collection, preprocessing, feature extraction and selection, developing and evaluating classification models, and knowledge discovery. Across the landscape of disease diagnosis research, neural networks, CNNs, SVM, random forests, and ensemble classifiers emerge as the predominant techniques. However, several challenges are highlighted including limited training data, class imbalance, difficulty processing complex high-dimensional feature spaces, and issues with generalizing models trained on single-site datasets. Promising directions identified to advance the field include multi-site data sharing initiatives, transfer learning, and efforts to translate AI systems to clinical practice through close engagements between data scientists and healthcare practitioners.

The detailed analysis in Table 9.2 provides a comparison of disease detection methods, outlining datasets, techniques, and outcomes of contemporary research. Particularly, it showcases the effectiveness of AI, especially deep learning classifiers, in diagnosing diverse diseases, emphasizing the significance of AI-driven approaches in advancing disease detection based on pattern recognition paving the way for healthy living [5].

TABLE 9.2
Comparative Analysis of Different Disease Detection Approaches.

Study	Methodology	Key Insights
Owasis et al. (2021) [6]	Developed an advanced real-time gastrointestinal disease detection system by leveraging innovative deep learning techniques like residual networks and LSTMs to process endoscopic videos.	Pioneers active digestive health monitoring through instant abnormality feedback. Promotes early disease intervention and prevention for healthier living.
Gouda et al. (2022) [7]	Developed a rapid COVID-19 diagnostics using cutting-edge artificial intelligence and CT scans for instantaneous pattern recognition.	Enables prompt COVID-19 symptom assessment, empowering proactive health management and timely precautions for healthier living.
Chatterjee et al. (2020)[8]	Created an AI-powered large vessel occlusion detection algorithm using CTA datasets for instant critical stroke identification.	Ensures urgent medical care, reducing stroke impacts significantly. Fosters healthier lifestyles by enhancing recovery chances.
Bhatt et al. (2021)[9]	Introduced personalized diagnostics for pregnant women using a novel integration of artificial neural networks and random forest models.	Provides tailored thyroid health insights, enabling the prompt addressing of issues for healthier pregnancies.
Hosseinzadeh et al. (2022) [10]	Transformed thyroid disease detection through a robust MRI analysis using a sophisticated artificial neural network.	Enables early subtle thyroid irregularity detection, promoting preventive care for healthier living.
Tang et al. (2022) [11]	Advanced pulmonary disease detection exponentially using deep residual networks and the PanCan dataset.	Enables proactive monitoring and early interventions for healthier living.
Damiani et al. (2021) [12]	Improved squamous cell carcinoma detection using a state-of-the-art artificial neural network analyzing dermatological images.	Empowers early skin issue detection and medical consultations for optimal skin health.

9.3 SYMPTOMS IN HEALTH MONITORING

Health monitoring systems require collecting and analyzing indicators that can provide insight into an individual's health status. Symptoms serve as important signals of medical conditions that need timely interventions. Both physical symptoms like pain, fatigue, neurological signs, respiratory issues, gastrointestinal disturbances and physiological measurements like blood pressure, respiratory rate, heart rate, temperature can be valuable. Mental health monitoring also relies on symptoms like mood, sleep pattern, anxiety, and cognitive decline. Additionally, disease-specific symptoms are utilized in tailored monitoring applications for conditions like diabetes, cardiovascular disease, chronic respiratory illnesses, etc.

Continuous symptom monitoring enables the tracking of disease progression and the effectiveness of treatments and allows early detection of exacerbations so that preventive action can be taken. This is especially important for the management of chronic illnesses, which require frequent observation for changes that would necessitate adjustments in therapy. Wearable sensors allow the real-time collection of physiological metrics indicative of symptoms. Patients can also self-report symptoms through mobile health applications that use prompts and chatbots. The IOT- enabled devices like smart pill bottles, inhalers, and insulin pens also provide adherence monitoring data that gives insight into patient status. Electronic health records can collate information on symptoms from multiple patient encounters to provide the overall profile. Such real-time symptom data from diverse sources provides a holistic view of the patient's condition that can drive timely interventions and personalized care beyond episodic clinical visits.

9.4 AUGMENTED REALITY IN HEALTHCARE

Augmented reality refers to technology that superimposes digital information and virtual objects upon the user's real-world environment in real time. This allows digitally augmented information to be overlaid and interactively used while performing tasks in the physical environment. In healthcare, augmented reality is being explored in applications like performing complex surgery, medical simulation training, guided medical procedures, patient education, and behavioral modifications.

During surgery, CT, or MRI scans can be overlayed on the patient's body to accurately visualize the anatomical structures in context while operating. This improves accuracy and reduces risks of damage to tissues. In medical simulations, augmented reality allows trainees to view detailed anatomical models, visualize blood vessels and nerves, and practice surgical skills. During diagnosis and imaging procedures like needle biopsies, vein punctures, ultrasound, and catheterization, visual guides can be provided via augmented reality to accurately direct the instruments and needles. Complex concepts related to anatomy, medications, and conditions can be explained to patients using augmented reality visualizations and immersive experiences. Augmented reality is also being leveraged in applications like physical therapy, rehabilitation, smoking cessations, and diabetes management by providing behavioral nudges and progress tracking.

Augmented reality has demonstrated benefits in improving procedural accuracy, reducing errors, enhancing training and education, and promoting patient adherence and engagement in healthcare scenarios. However, seamless integration into clinical workflows is important rather than being an external add-on. Interface and interaction design tailored for specific applications is vital for avoiding cognitive overload. There are also concerns regarding distractions caused in critical tasks, especially during complex surgical procedures where focus is paramount.

9.5 PATTERN RECOGNITION TECHNIQUES

Recognizing patterns in health data is crucial for clinical diagnosis, predicting risks, tracking disease progression, and gauging treatment effectiveness. Relevant patterns can exist in diverse forms of medical data like imaging scans, physiological signals, electronic health records, genomic test results, etc. Advanced analytical techniques are required to reliably interpret the large volumes of healthcare data and extract clinically meaningful patterns.

Figure 9.2 presents a system architecture for a symptom-based augmented reality approach. It outlines the various stages involved, including data collection, pre-processing, pattern detection using machine learning techniques, augmented reality interface generation, health recommendation provision, and algorithm refinement based on user feedback. This architecture highlights the integration of different components and the iterative nature of the process, where user feedback and continuous refinement play a crucial role in improving the overall system's performance.

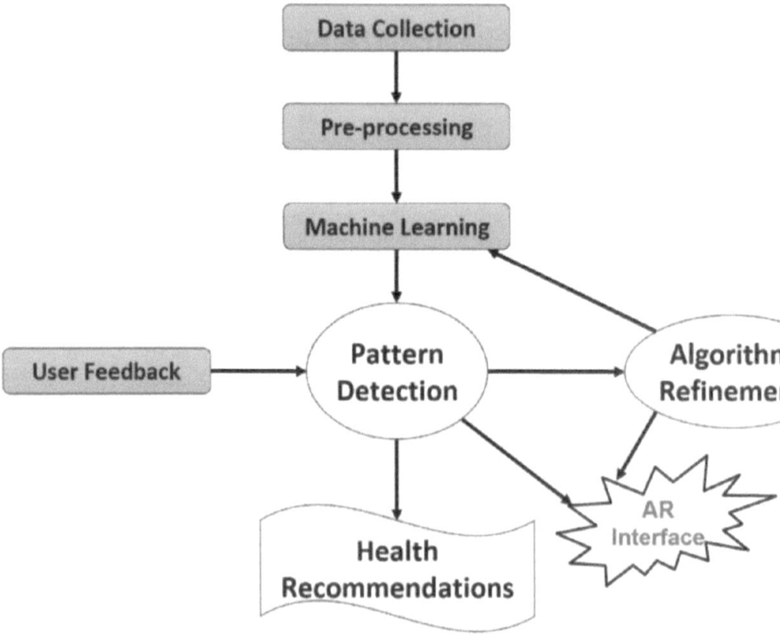

FIGURE 9.2 Comprehensive and detailed system architecture.

Machine learning consists of a range of techniques like neural networks and deep learning models that can automatically detect complex patterns from raw medical data inputs. Algorithms like support vector machines, random forests, and Bayesian networks can enable predictive analytics based on identified patterns. Exploratory techniques like clustering and subgroup discovery can identify subgroups among patients exhibiting similar patterns. Association rule mining and frequent pattern techniques can discover interesting co-occurrence relationships between clinical variables.

Deep learning models like convolutional neural networks excel at finding patterns in medical imaging data and have provided state-of-the-art results in applications like tumor detection, localization, segmentation, and computer-aided screening. Recurrent neural network architectures are suitable for mining temporal patterns from continuous physiological signals. Generative models like GANs can synthesize realistic synthetic datasets exhibiting plausible variations. Self-supervised models are also being developed that can find medically relevant patterns by pretraining based on large volumes of unlabeled medical data.

Apart from machine learning techniques, statistical methods also play a key role in healthcare pattern analysis. Regression modeling can characterize predictive relationships between clinical variables. Hypothesis testing provides the means to determine the statistical significance of observed patterns. Time-series analysis techniques can model seasonal, cyclical, and longer-term sequential patterns in longitudinal health data. Hidden Markov models allow modeling sequential transitions and analyzing chains of dependent events.

Some challenges include high-dimensionality and sparsity of medical data patterns. Feature engineering and dimensionality reduction are important preprocessing steps. Limited availability of large curated healthcare datasets for training models is another issue, addressed through data augmentation and pretraining strategies. Class imbalance is also common, and techniques like sampling and cost-sensitive learning help overcome it. Lack of interoperability between heterogeneous data sources also poses challenges in holistic pattern analysis, which requires standardized representations.

9.6 REAL-TIME DATA COLLECTION AND ANALYSIS

Real-time health monitoring relies extensively on wearable devices and sensors. Modern smartwatches and fitness bands contain sensors that can track heart rate, blood pressure, sleep patterns, and more. Tiny ECG and EMG sensors embedded in skin patches allow continuous monitoring of cardiac and muscle activity. Motion sensors including accelerometers and gyroscopes within wearables can track body movements and activities. Adhesive skin patches with micro-needle biosensors that minimally penetrate the skin allow real-time tracking of metabolites and biomarkers.

Figure 9.3 illustrates the real-time data collection and analysis process for health monitoring. It showcases the various data sources, including wearable devices, skin patches, smart objects, networked devices, and environmental sensors. The collected data is transmitted to cloud-based solutions, where edge computing capabilities enable real-time analysis using machine learning models. End-to-end encryption

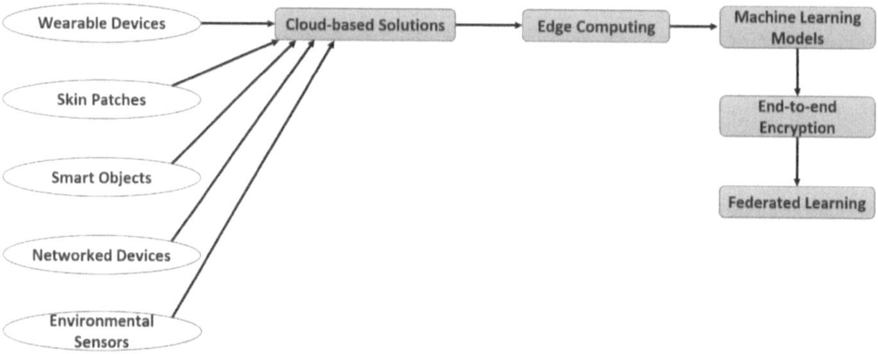

FIGURE 9.3 Real-time data collection and analysis process.

and federated learning techniques are employed to ensure data privacy and security during this process.

The Internet of Things paradigm allows connecting medical devices and everyday objects to aggregate data in real time. Smart inhalers, insulin pens, or pill bottles equipped with sensors provide data on medication adherence patterns. Smart clothing with bio-signal sensors woven into the fabric allows tracking of health metrics seamlessly during daily activities. Networked medical devices like ventilators and infusion pumps capture real-time operational data. Environmental sensors provide contextual information by collecting data on light, temperature, humidity in the patient's surroundings.

The data collected needs to be streamed, aggregated, stored, and analyzed in real time to be clinically actionable. Cloud-based solutions provide the scalable storage and computational capabilities to handle high-velocity heterogeneous health data streams. Edge computing solutions allow real-time analytics and insights at the point of acquisition rather than relying solely on the cloud. The machine learning models deployed on cloud servers can enable low-latency real-time inference on new streaming data.

However, transmitting sensitive health data to the cloud raises privacy concerns. End-to-end encryption provides a mitigating measure. Granular access controls, patient consent, and data anonymization mechanisms are also implemented. Where possible, processing on the wearable device itself rather than transmitting raw data can improve privacy. Federated learning is also an emerging technique that enables collaborative training of shared models without directly sharing the patient data from different sites.

9.7 INTEGRATION OF SYMPTOM-BASED DETECTION AND AUGMENTED REALITY

While significant progress has been made in real-time symptom detection and augmented reality capabilities individually, integrating them offers exciting possibilities

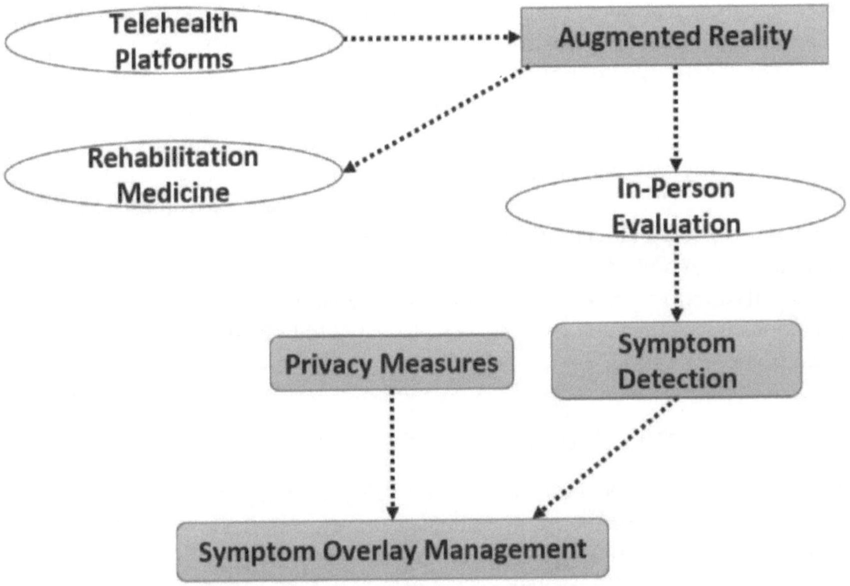

FIGURE 9.4 Integration of symptom-based detection and augmented reality.

for transformational healthcare delivery. Several applications demonstrate initial integrations of symptom monitoring and augmented reality focused on areas like telehealth, multisensory symptom visualization, clinician decision support, and therapy.

As depicted in Figure 9.4, the integration of symptom-based detection and augmented reality technologies across various healthcare domains shows how telehealth platforms can leverage augmented reality for symptom visualization and communication. Symptom detection algorithms can provide input for augmented reality interventions during in-person evaluations and rehabilitation medicine. The integration also involves privacy measures and symptom overlay management techniques to ensure secure and contextualized delivery of augmented reality experiences based on detected symptoms.

In telehealth platforms, augmented reality aids are being developed to guide patients through self-reporting of symptoms, providing an additional communication modality between remote visits. Dynamic visualization of subjective symptoms like pain, fatigue, and anxiety levels through appropriate augmented reality overlays can improve assessments and treatments. During in-person evaluations, clinicians can be provided overlays of patients' historical symptoms data aggregated from wearable passive monitoring and self-reports, giving them rapid insights. In rehabilitation medicine, immersive augmented reality environments are being used for symptom-targeted physical, motor, and neurological therapy programs. During procedures like chemotherapy where patients experience significant symptoms like nausea, distraction using augmented reality has demonstrated benefits.

Key advantages of integrating real-time symptom capture and augmented reality include enabling holistic evaluation within natural environments, continuous unobtrusive monitoring that minimizes reporting biases, improved patient engagement in managing their health, and reduced errors in subjective symptom data interpretation. Just-in-time guidance and care triggered by detected symptoms can be delivered conveniently via augmented reality. However, the accuracy of detection and visualization of subjective symptoms remains a challenge. Care must be taken to avoid cognitive overload and information clutter when presenting multiple dynamic symptom overlays. Patient privacy and ethical implications of using augmented reality to overtly modify perceptions also need to be addressed cautiously. Unrealistic expectations regarding such technologies also need to be managed carefully among all stakeholders.

9.8 CASE STUDIES AND EXAMPLES

Some real-world deployments demonstrate the value emerging from linking symptom-based biometric monitoring with augmented reality. PainScale is an iOS app that uses augmented reality overlays of facial expressions to help patients select the pain intensity level they are experiencing. The quantified symptom data delivers insights into the pain profile. The AMI system developed at Philips Research uses wearable sensors analyzing photoplethysmography signals to identify possible atrial fibrillation and the risk of cardiac arrest in real time, enabling rapid interventions. Magic Leap's MR environment provides multisensory feedback for the rehabilitation of neurological conditions, with symptom tracking to personalize therapy. During chemotherapy sessions, augmented reality headsets have been used to distract patients from symptoms like nausea by immersing them in nature environments, making the experience more tolerable.

Real-world implementations have demonstrated encouraging outcomes on integrating the two technologies. Remote symptom monitoring, along with environmental sensors, reduced COPD exacerbations by 60% in high-risk patients, based on a US study, by enabling preventive care. In a trial by Neuro Rehab VR, stroke survivors showed 35% higher improvement in motor function and 28% in cognitive scores using an augmented reality-based rehabilitation platform monitoring symptom metrics. Smart pill bottles track adherence patterns and link it to symptom surveys, with 74% of diabetes patients reporting they were more adherent due to this digital monitoring. The early detection of cancer-treatment-related symptoms via wearables allows rapid adjustments, with patients experiencing fewer symptoms according to Dana–Farber trial results. Such successful deployments highlight the synergistic potential of real-time symptom tracking and augmented reality.

9.9 FUTURE TRENDS AND INNOVATIONS

Advancements in sensing, monitoring devices, and computing methodologies are expanding the horizons for symptom-based monitoring and augmented reality platforms. Novel ingestible sensors and implantable devices like neural dust will allow access to richer internal biometrics. Electronic skin patches are becoming flexible, with multimodal wearables capable of analyzing sweat, interstitial fluid, and more. Handheld labs on a chip enable rapid quantitative biomarker evaluation from small samples. Smart homes with ambient sensors provide opportunities for contactless monitoring of biomarkers using computer vision and other techniques. With natural language processing advancements, conversational agents are gathering symptom information more effectively through dialog. Digital phenotyping uses smartphone usage patterns and behaviors as indicators for conditions like depression or psychosis. Linking molecular profiling from liquid biopsies to detect early disease signatures before the manifestation of symptoms is also being explored. Computer vision models that can reliably extract symptoms from medical images and videos using deep learning can transform telehealth and remote monitoring.

On the augmented reality side, innovative display technologies like holography and projection mapping allow creating immersive environments. Multisensory augmented reality using auditory, haptic, and other modalities provides comprehensive digital augmentation of real-world healthcare scenarios. Heads-up displays and specialized augmented reality lenses can deliver just-in-time guidance and instructions for clinicians during complex procedures. Seamless integration with electronic health records and medical devices data using standard APIs will enable intelligently contextual augmentation. As augmented reality platforms evolve, they can adapt better to user contexts and create more intelligent and naturalistic healthcare augmented experiences.

9.10 CHALLENGES AND ETHICAL CONSIDERATIONS

While promising, real-time health monitoring and symptom detection using wearables does raise data privacy and security challenges. Granular access controls need to prevent unauthorized access to individuals' sensitive medical data. Third-party cloud services and analytics vendors need oversight to prevent the abuse of real-time health data they may gain access to. Encryption, blockchain-based access mechanisms, on-device processing, and federated learning paradigms are some technological measures that can mitigate privacy risks. But equally importantly, informed consent, allowing user control over data sharing, transparent policies regarding data usage, and ability to retract permissions need to be integral to such systems. The psychological pressures of continuous self-monitoring also need to be evaluated; while useful, it could promote obsessive anxiety in certain individuals. The liability in case of adverse events due to inaccurate symptom detection or recommendations via flawed algorithms and datasets also needs regulatory clarity. The development of safety standards, clinical validation protocols, and mechanisms to incorporate user feedback would be crucial to avoid unintended harm.

Augmented reality experiences can influence human perceptions and behaviors. When used for education or therapy, safeguards need to ensure that accurate, balanced, and clinically validated information is presented. The risks of creating unrealistic expectations of care delivery capabilities also have to be managed. In some cases like symptom distractions during procedures, effects like motion sickness with prolonged immersion also require evaluation. Protecting patient privacy is also crucial; any identifiable information collected, like imaging scans or health records, needs consent and strong anonymization measures before use in multiuser AR scenarios. As healthcare augmented reality applications increase, clinicians would also require training to avoid technology overuse in contexts where human aspects of care are paramount. Adopting a patient-centric approach, allowing user customizations, and implementing ethical-by-design principles for such technologies would help realize their benefits while minimizing potential harms.

9.11 CONCLUSION

The integration of continuous symptom tracking capabilities and augmented reality visualization opens new frontiers in preventive healthcare models. Biosensors woven into wearables, devices connected through the Internet of Things, and nuanced pattern analysis algorithms now permit timely discernment of alterations in an individual's health status, facilitating proactive mitigation before conditions deteriorate. Augmented reality technology superimposes a digital informational layer atop the physical world, rendering an intuitive medium to convey personalized health insights and recommendations to individuals ensconced within their everyday environments.

This interweaving of novel technologies forges an intelligent preventive care cycle, uniting the processes of symptom detection, data processing, and contextualized augmented guidance. Multimodal data streams chronicling an individual's symptom patterns are subjected to advanced analytical techniques, elucidating patterns that trigger visualization of tailored augmented reality interventions. These situated digital prompts catalyze salutary behavioral adaptations, attenuating potential health risks. Propelled by data-derived insights and contextualized interventions, this adaptive system optimizes and individualizes preventive care provision, reorienting the focus from episodic symptom treatment to continuous cultivation of holistic well-being.

Fully actualizing this integrated approach's potential necessitates confronting multifarious challenges. Preserving data privacy and security through robust encryption schemas, granular access control mechanisms, and privacy-safeguarding techniques such as federated learning is necessary. Ensuring accurate symptom pattern discernment, mitigating cognitive overload from visualizations, and fostering a seamless user experience are crucial determinants of adoption and efficacy. Moreover, ethical deliberations surrounding data governance frameworks, transparency in algorithmic decision-making processes, and the judicious deployment of augmented reality must be carefully navigated.

Despite these challenges, the convergence of continuous symptom monitoring capacities and augmented reality harbors exciting innovation prospects for healthcare.

Ongoing advances in sensing modalities, computational techniques, and augmented reality interfaces will inevitably expand the frontiers of feasibility. As these technologies mature through rigorous empirical evaluation, they may well become integral pillars supporting a data-driven, patient-centric, and proactively oriented healthcare ecosystem that empowers individuals to be active custodians of their own holistic well-being and fosters societal progression toward healthier lifestyles.

REFERENCES

[1] Ghosh, U. B., Sharma, R., & Kesharwani, A. (2022). Symptoms-based biometric pattern detection and recognition. In *Augmented Intelligence in Healthcare: A Pragmatic and Integrated Analysis* (pp. 371–399). Singapore: Springer Nature Singapore.

[2] Khan, I. U., Afzal, S., & Lee, J. W. (2022). Human activity recognition via hybrid deep learning based model. *Sensors (Basel, Switzerland)*, 22(1), 323.

[3] Subasi, A. (2020). Use of artificial intelligence in Alzheimer's disease detection. https://doi.org/10.1016/B978-0-12-817133-2.00011-2.

[4] Paranthaman, A. A., Kumar, A., Rao, A. A., et al. (2022). Artificial intelligence for disease diagnosis: A literature review. *Diagnostics*, 12(6), 1182.

[5] Kumar, Y., Koul, A., Singla, R., & Ijaz, M. F. (2022). Artificial intelligence in disease diagnosis: A systematic literature review, synthesizing framework and future research agenda. *Journal of Ambient Intelligence and Humanized Computing*, 1–28.

[6] Arsalan, M., Owais, M., Mahmood, T., Cho, S. W., & Park, K. R. (2019). Aiding the diagnosis of diabetic and hypertensive retinopathy using artificial intelligence-based semantic segmentation. *Journal of Clinical Medicine*, 8(9), 1446.

[7] Gouda, W., & Yasin, R. (2020). COVID-19 disease: CT pneumonia analysis prototype by using artificial intelligence, predicting the disease severity. *Egyptian Journal of Radiology and Nuclear Medicine*, 51(1), 1–11.

[8] Parikh, N. S., Chatterjee, A., Díaz, I., Pandya, A., Merkler, A. E., Gialdini, G.,. . .& Kamel, H. (2018). Modeling the impact of interhospital transfer network design on stroke outcomes in a large city. *Stroke*, 49(2), 370–376.

[9] Bhatt, V. K., & Pal, V. K. (2019, March). An intelligent system for diagnosing thyroid disease in pregnant ladies through artificial neural network. In *International Conference on Advances in Engineering Science Management & Technology (ICAESMT)-2019*, Uttaranchal University, Dehradun, India.

[10] Hosseinzadeh, M., Ahmed, O. H., Ghafour, M. Y., Safara, F., Hama, H. K., Ali, S.,. . .& Chiang, H. S. (2021). A multiple multilayer perceptron neural network with an adaptive learning algorithm for thyroid disease diagnosis in the Internet of Medical Things. *The Journal of Supercomputing*, 77, 3616–3637.

[11] Tang, L. Y., Coxson, H. O., Lam, S., Leipsic, J., Tam, R. C., & Sin, D. D. (2020). Towards large-scale case-finding: Training and validation of residual networks for detection of chronic obstructive pulmonary disease using low-dose CT. *The Lancet Digital Health*, 2(5), e259–e267.

[12] Damiani, G., Grossi, E., Berti, E., Conic, R. R. Z., Radhakrishna, U., Pacifico, A.,. . .& Linder, D. (2020). Artificial neural networks allow response prediction in squamous cell carcinoma of the scalp treated with radiotherapy. *Journal of the European Academy of Dermatology and Venereology*, 34(6), 1369–1373.

Part IV

AI-Enabled Smart Models and Algorithms for IoMT-Augmented Data Analysis

10 OpenCV Algorithm for IoMT-Based Patient Emotion Pattern Analysis

Devshree Jadeja, Priyanka Singh, Hiren Kumar Thakkar, and Vendra Durga Ratna Kumar

10.1 INTRODUCTION

The Internet of Medical Things (IoMT) [1] encompasses a network of medical devices and sensors, including wearable devices like smartwatches, cameras, microphones, and other data-capturing tools, designed to collect and transmit health-related information, including emotional data, over the internet. For example, smartwatches equipped with heart rate monitors can track physiological changes indicative of emotions, cameras can analyze facial expressions and body language, microphones can detect emotional tones in voice recordings, and smartphone apps can enable mood tracking alongside location and activity data. Additionally, specialized sensors such as electrodermal activity (EDA) sensors can measure skin conductance changes linked to emotional arousal. Healthcare providers can enable individualized care, mental health monitoring, and early intervention when emotional distress is detected by utilizing these IoMT technologies and analyzing the data collected, all the while ensuring patient consent and data privacy. A brand-new technology called the Internet of Medical Things (IoMT) combines medical equipment with other wireless devices to give users access to healthcare management systems [2]. The purpose of this chapter is to explore the potential for using machine learning algorithms to provide clinicians and patients with emotional therapeutic suggestions in order to combat the coronavirus disease 2019 (COVID-19) pandemic. The IoMT cognitive model is best adapted to this epidemic since every individual will be connected to and watched over by a cognitive network. However, there are still issues with the COVID-19 pandemic's emotional consideration for infants, young children, the elderly, and people with mental illnesses during the pandemic. In [3], numerous speech feature description methods were put forth in an effort to identify the various sorts of emotional behavior from input data. Figure 10.1 justifies the overall working of the IoMT hierarchy.

10.1.1 Examples of IoMT Devices in Medical Care [3,5]

- **Wearable Gadgets, Such as Smartwatches [6]:** An illustration would be a patient wearing a smartwatch with accelerometers and heart rate monitors.

DOI: 10.1201/9781003393498-14

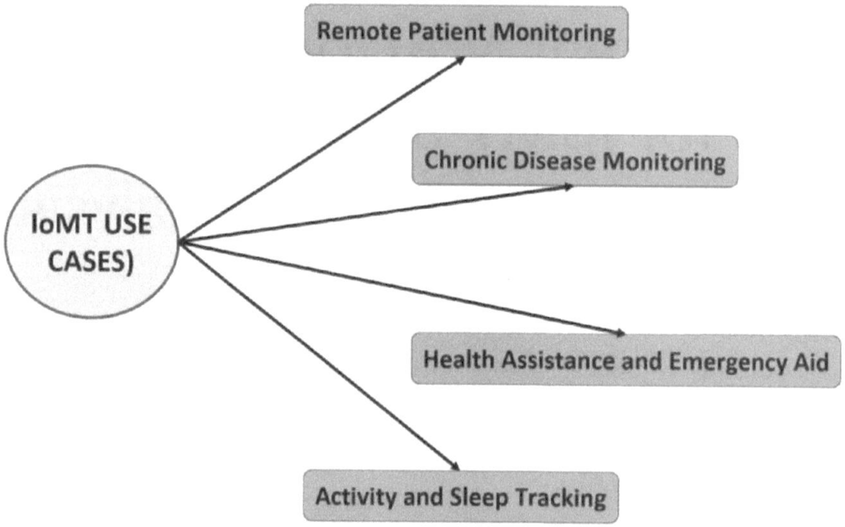

FIGURE 10.1 IoMT application in healthcare [4].

The smartwatch gathers physiological information like heart rate, activity levels, and sleep schedules continually. These factors can change to reflect emotional responses. For instance, a quick rise in heart rate may indicate a more intense emotional state, such as enthusiasm or anxiety.

- **Cameras**: A healthcare facility, for instance, has cameras installed in patient rooms. These cameras record video of the patients, including their body language and facial expressions. These visual data can be examined by computer vision algorithms, such as face expression recognition, to identify emotions. For instance, the camera can detect a patient's smile or frown, which can be used to indicate contentment or sadness.
- **Mics**: As an illustration, voice recordings from microphones can offer insightful emotional indications. Hospitals may have microphones in patient rooms, or patients can wear devices with microphones. Speech analysis can be used to detect emotional undertones in a patient's voice, such as rage or melancholy. For instance, when a patient is stressed or disturbed, their voice may become more aggressive.
- **Apps for Smartphones:** For illustration, patients can monitor their activities and movements using smartphone apps equipped with sensors like accelerometers and GPS. These applications can include tools for tracking mood. Patients can keep track of their emotions throughout the day, and the app can link this self-reported emotional information to information about their physical activities and location.
- **Put-On Biosensors** [7]: An illustration of a wearable biosensor is the electrodermal activity (EDA) sensor, which may detect variations in skin conductance that may signal emotional arousal. EDA sensors may be worn by

patients on their wrists or fingertips. The sensor data can be supplied for examination when changes in skin conductance are brought on by emotional responses.

- **Software for Detecting Emotions**: As an illustration, some IoMT applications might come with specific emotion-detection software that can be used across many platforms. To create a thorough picture of a patient's emotional state, this program may combine data from sensors like heart rate monitors, cameras, and microphones.

10.1.2 Emotion Recognition [8]

A technology called emotion identification seeks to recognize and categorize human emotions, primarily via physiological signs, voice cues, and facial expressions. There are various techniques for identifying emotions, such as facial expression analysis, voice analysis, and physiological monitoring. Physiological monitoring involves keeping track of changes in physiological signals like heart rate, skin conductance, and brain activity to infer emotional responses. Facial expression analysis detects and categorizes emotions like happiness, sadness, anger, and surprise through visual cues. These techniques are widely utilized in a variety of industries, such as healthcare, human–computer interaction, and market research, to enhance user experiences and better understand and respond to human emotions. The integration of the Internet of Medical Things (IoMT) with emotion detection necessitates the use of IoMT devices and data for full emotional well-being assessment. While IoMT sensors, such as microphones and camera lenses, collect visual and audible cues, wearables monitor physiological signs. Facial expression analysis and voice analysis, made possible by systems like OpenCV, classify emotions based on visual and aural data. This integrated technique provides an in-depth understanding of a patient's emotional state by connecting physiological responses to facial expressions and vocal tones. With the use of the information gathered, healthcare practitioners can provide customized care, early intervention, and better mental health support. The data can also be examined and tracked continually to offer real-time insights into a patient's emotional well-being. Ensuring the safety of patient data, protecting privacy, and upholding ethical standards are key to securing sensitive information.

The devices combine these two data streams for real-time analysis, making it possible to look into the connections between emotions and physical responses. The results are shown in real time on a user interface, allowing for further research and insights into the relationships between physiological data and emotions, as well as the possibility of future system development and improvement. Figure 10.2 shows the overall stages at which this work will be implemented or has been implemented till now.

In practice, imagine a hospital room equipped with a camera as part of an IoMT-based patient monitoring system. OpenCV processes the video feed, detecting the patient's face and identifying facial landmarks. It then extracts features related to expressions, and a machine learning model, trained on a dataset of labeled emotional expressions, classifies the patient's emotion as "happy," "sad," or other possibilities in real time. This information is securely logged and integrated into the

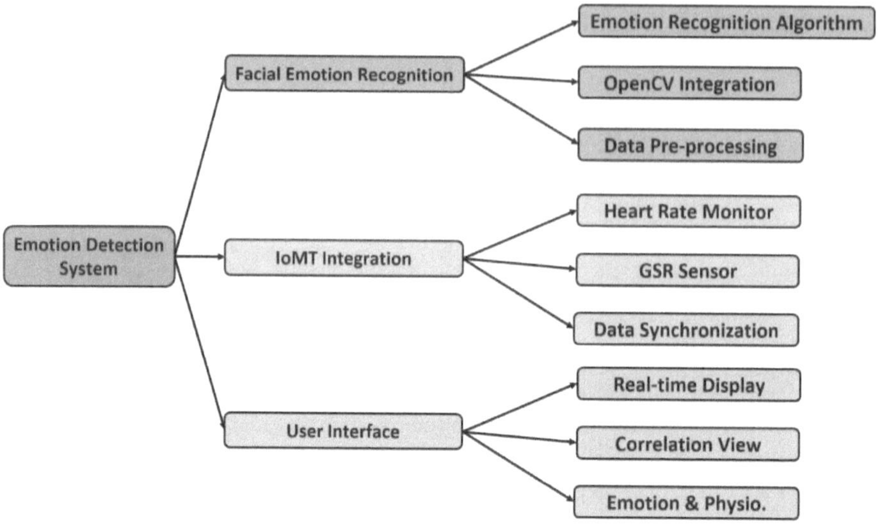

FIGURE 10.2 Emotion detection system.

broader IoMT network, allowing healthcare providers to monitor patient emotions and intervene if significant emotional changes or distress are detected, all while safeguarding patient privacy and data security The two-tier validation method is used by the emotion detecting system. It uses facial image analysis to identify emotions in the first tier. Possibly leveraging OpenCV, computer vision techniques are used to recognize facial expressions and forecast emotions based on visual inputs from the face. To further validate the detected emotions, a second tier of validation includes the use of physiological sensors. These sensors monitor heart rate and galvanic skin response, collecting data that can be correlated with the emotions identified through facial analysis. By combining visual cues with physiological responses, this dual-tier approach enhances the reliability and accuracy of emotion detection, making the system more robust and dependable in recognizing and validating human emotions.

10.1.2.1 Integrating IoMT Techniques

- **Selecting the Right Sensors:** Select the right sensors to gather physiological information. Sensors like heart rate monitors, skin conductivity sensors (GSR), or even facial temperature sensors may be significant in the context of emotion recognition.
- **Data Synchronization:** To link emotions to physiological reactions, make sure the time stamps of the physiological data and the images of the faces are in sync. Using data correlation, investigate the association between physiological indications and facial expressions. Statistical approaches or machine learning models may be used to discover patterns or connections.
- **Data Cleaning and Preprocessing:** Remove noise, outliers, and other artifacts from the physiological data. Apply signal processing methods appropriate for the kind of data collected

10.1.3 Pipeline for the Approach

The technique of identifying facial expressions and classifying them into related emotions such as happiness, grief, anger, fear, surprise, and contempt using OpenCV and Python has been referred to as emotion identification. The goal is to develop a system that correctly identifies facial expressions and categorizes them into matching emotions using OpenCV and Python-type programming languages.

Using OpenCV's face identification techniques, the first step in constructing an emotion detection system is to detect faces in the incoming video input. The location of the face in the image or video needs to be identified initially in order to extract the face region for further analysis. For this purpose, OpenCV provides face recognition models based on deep learning and pretrained Haar cascades. The next stage is to use OpenCV's facial landmark detection techniques to extract the facial features of each detected face, such as the positions of the eyes, mouth, and eyebrows. By indicating the location and shape of the various parts of the face, these facial landmarks make it possible to categorize the various facial expressions.

Once the facial traits have been identified, machine learning methods such as deep learning models or support vector machines (SVM) can be used to categorize facial expressions into the appropriate emotions.

Convolutional neural networks (CNN) and other deep-learning-based models have been demonstrated to produce state-of-the-art outcomes in tests for emotion recognition. It is necessary to train the emotion recognition model using a sizable dataset of labeled facial expressions.

After the facial features have been retrieved, facial expressions can be categorized into appropriate emotions using machine learning methods like support vector machines (SVM) or deep learning models. Convolutional neural networks (CNN) and other deep learning-based models have been demonstrated to perform at the cutting edge in emotion recognition tests. It is necessary to train the emotion recognition model using a sizable dataset of labeled facial expressions. The FER2013 and CK+ datasets, among other publicly accessible datasets, can be utilized for training and evaluation. To enhance the model's performance, it can be trained using a variety of methods, including data augmentation and transfer learning. The pipeline for emotion recognition system is shown in Figure 10.3.

10.1.4 Methodology for the Network of Emotion Detection [9]

The suggested methodology combines OpenCV emotion recognition methods with Internet of Medical Things (IoMT) technology. Gathering training data from multiple sources, such as patient cameras and movies, is the first step. The strategy uses a pipeline that includes face detection using OpenCV, feature extraction from observed faces, and the use of an emotion identification model based on Siemens. The incorporation of IoMT data, such as EEG and ECG signals, improves accuracy and contextual understanding. An emotion prediction that has been validated by the system is produced as a result of cross-referencing facial cues and physiological information. In order to deliver precise and trustworthy emotional insights in a medical setting, a holistic methodology must ensure data privacy, scalability, user-friendly interfaces, rigorous testing, and continuing maintenance. Figure 10.4 shows the emotion classification and how it is followed by the face recognition as an essential step.

10.1.4.1 Steps Involved

- **Data Gathering**: Assemble training data from a variety of sources, including datasets, cameras, and patient footage. The training and validation of your emotion recognition model will both require this data.

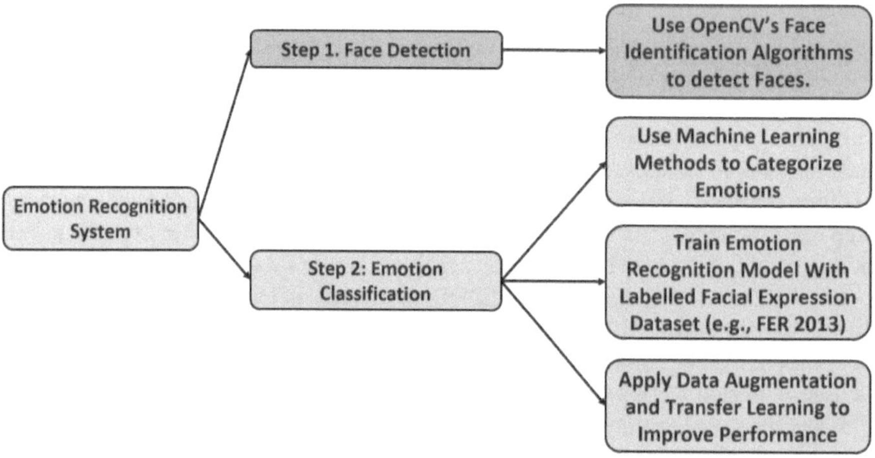

FIGURE 10.3 Emotion Recognition System Pipeline

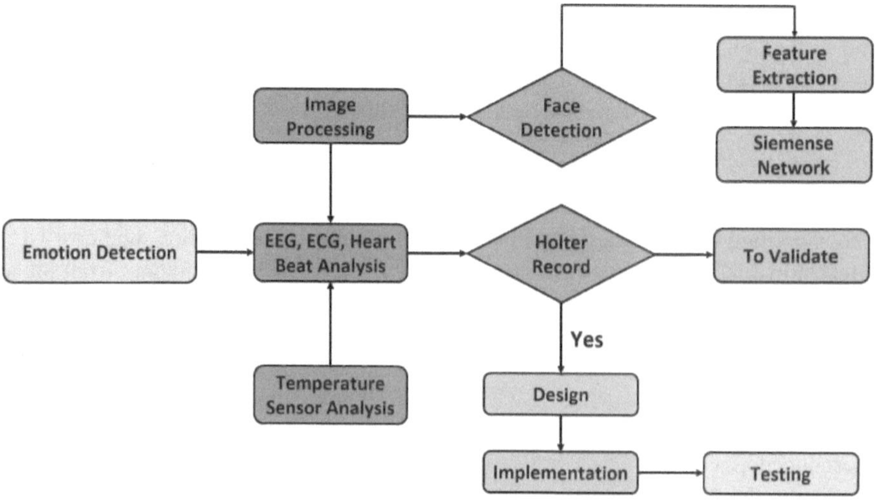

FIGURE 10.4 Emotion detection method.

- **Face Recognition**: Use OpenCV to identify faces. For this use, OpenCV provides pretrained models (based on deep learning or Haar cascades, for example). This stage makes sure that the face is the only object in the picture or video frame.
- **Extracting Features**: From the recognized face, identify the pertinent facial traits. To capture important features on the face, you can utilize OpenCV and deep learning methods like facial landmark detection.
- **Model for Emotion Recognition**: Implement a deep learning architecture for emotion recognition that can be based on Siemens's model or another appropriate deep learning architecture. This model should be able to predict emotions using the extracted facial data as input.
- **Integration of IoMT**: Assemble IoMT sensor data from EEG, ECG, and other physiological sensors. When used in conjunction with facial emotion recognition, these sensors can offer useful context.
- **Validation of Emotions**: Incorporate the sensor data from IoMT with the outcomes of your emotion recognition algorithm. By taking into account both physiological data and facial clues, this integration enables you to validate and improve emotion detection utilizing a comprehensive methodology. Figure 10.5 is the complete flow diagram that highlights the main idea of the work.
- **Feedback Cycle**: Install a feedback loop to help your emotion recognition system get better over time. Gather user feedback to help you retrain and improve your model's accuracy. The feedback cycle and the input process are shown in Figure 10.5.

10.2 FACE DETECTION

What exactly is face detection? And how does it differ from face recognition? Face detection detects the presence of a human face in a photograph, whereas face

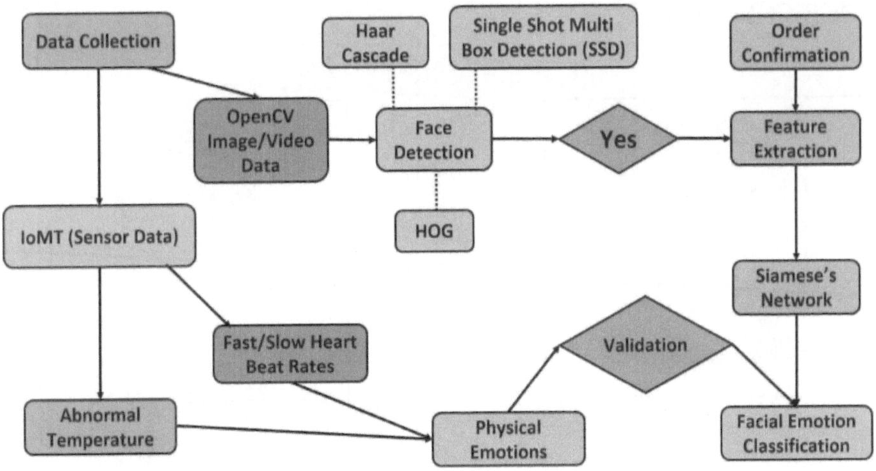

FIGURE 10.5 IoMT and OpenCV integration.

recognition detects the presence of a human face in a photograph while also recognizing the person's identity. So for a face recognition system to work, it must first run face detection to generate a list of all the faces discovered in the photo and then run its authentication process to determine who is/are in the shot. Figure 10.6 presents an example of how both processes are fundamentally different.

Face recognition [10], which identifies and isolates the human face within an image or video frame, is a crucial first step in the development of emotion detection systems. Since facial expressions are the primary means by which emotions are expressed, this process is crucial because it enables the precise localization of important emotional cues, reduces complexity by excluding unrelated areas, and improves the accuracy and overall effectiveness of subsequent emotion recognition steps. The system can identify and crop the face region, preparing it for emotion detection analysis and enabling more precise and reliable emotional assessment by choosing an appropriate face detection method, collecting, or constructing the required models, and preprocessing the input data. Faces are detected using a variety of techniques, with coordinates being collected for each detection, including deep learning models and Haar cascade classifiers. For future emotion recognition, the isolated face region serves as the focal point. This ensures a more accurate and thorough assessment of emotions, which is essential for applications like human–computer interaction and healthcare. The system's overall success depends on accurate and reliable face detection since it makes sure that the subsequent phases concentrate on the right region of interest where emotional cues are expressed. Paper [5] shows the demonstrated methods in the detail of the face recognition task.

Available OpenCV Algorithms for Face Detection

1. LBPH (local binary pattern histogram algorithm [11])
2, Haar cascade detector [12]
3. HOG (histogram of oriented gradients [13]).
4. R-CNN/D-CNN

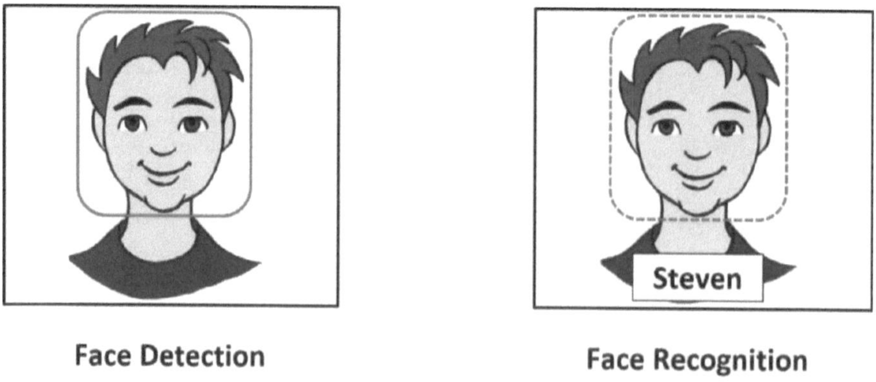

FIGURE 10.6 Difference of face detection and face recognition.

10.2.1 Introduction of LBPH

The LBPH local binary pattern histogram algorithm is a straightforward method for labeling the pixels in a picture by thresholding their surroundings. In other words, LBPH compares each pixel with its neighbors to summarize the local structure in an image, and the result is then transformed into a binary integer. Since its initial definition in 1994 (LBP), it has been discovered to be a potent algorithm for texture categorization.

The primary goal of this method is to extract local information from photos. The fundamental concept is to focus just on the local aspects of an object rather than viewing the entire image as a high-dimension vector. LBPH, in contrast to typical methods that consider images as high-dimensional vectors, concentrates on capturing local properties inside an image, making it particularly suitable for tasks requiring texture and local patterns, such as texture analysis, facial recognition, and object detection [14]. LBPH is a common choice in computer vision and image processing applications due to its effectiveness and simplicity.

10.2.1.1 LBPH Needs the Following Parameters

- **Radius**: Usually set to 1, this parameter represents the radius surrounding the core pixel.
- **Neighbors**: The quantity of sample points used to create the binary circular pattern.

Determine the number of cells in the horizontal and vertical directions for Grids X and Y, as this will affect the feature vector's dimensionality. Using a dataset of facial picture labels—each with a distinct ID—the algorithm is trained. By linking the input image to a particular ID, the system learns to recognize faces. You should include pictures of the individual you want to recognize in the training dataset.

LBP Computation

- A facial-feature-focused intermediate image is produced using the local binary pattern (LBP) operation. The essential steps comprise the following.
- Creating a 3×3 pixel window from the provided grayscale facial image
- Using the intensity of the central pixel as a threshold
- The eight neighboring pixels are assigned binary values (1 or 0) based on whether they are greater or lower than the threshold.
- Concatenating these binary numbers to create a binary string (for example, 10001101)
- This method improves the image's portrayal of face features.

10.2.1.2 Final Steps

Extracting Histograms from the Image: Using the Grid X and Grid Y parameters, the image created in the previous LBP computation stage is divided into various grids in this step. A histogram of 256 places, which represents the occurrences of each pixel intensity, is contained in each grid. These distinct histograms are concatenated to provide a single comprehensive histogram for the entire image. The grids are matched with each of the pixel values of the image, as depicted in Figure 10.7.

Face recognition can be done for a new image if the algorithm has been properly trained and the training dataset's histograms have been extracted to represent each image. Typically, the following steps are involved:

- To create a fresh histogram, run the same LBP operation on the new image.
- Compared the histogram of the new image to the histograms of the photos in the training dataset.
- Find the image in the training dataset with the closest histogram using a similarity measure (e.g., Euclidean distance or chi-squared distance).
- As the recognized individual, return the ID or label associated with the closest matching photograph.

It's worth noting that LBPH is a basic yet successful method for face identification, especially in situations with varying lighting, position, and facial expression. However, when compared to more complex deep learning algorithms, it may have limits when dealing with large-scale datasets and may not attain the maximum recognition accuracy. Following the creation of binary patterns for each cell in the image, you can create a histogram of these patterns. Each histogram bin represents a unique binary pattern. The corresponding bin records the frequency of recurrence of each pattern in the image. The LBPH-based classifier can be used to recognize faces in recent photos after being trained. It determines whether a face is present by computing the LBPH histogram for each area of the image and analyzing the histogram patterns. For specific face recognition applications, LBPH is still a valuable and computationally efficient method, especially when operating in restricted and controlled environments. ConvNets are a deep learning model that can be used when greater accuracy in recognition and scalability is needed but at the cost of more complicated computers and data requirements. The particular application and its needs will determine which approach is better. LBPH may achieve a lower identification accuracy in challenging environments with frequent changes in facial appearance. When trained adequately on various datasets, deep learning models have the potential to be significantly more precise than LBPH. It is also used for tasks that are mostly applied for the task of face recognition or identity recognition.

10.2.2 Haar Cascade Face Detector

A cascade of Haar classifiers is a machine-learning-based method for detecting objects. They are based on Haar-like features, which are basic rectangular patterns that define the contrast between adjacent image regions. These characteristics are used to train a classifier to recognize "object" and "non-object" regions. This classifier is made up of numerous simpler classifiers, called stages, that are applied over the region of interest until the object is rejected or all stages are passed. The decision tree classifiers with at least two leaves are the basic classifiers. The fundamental classifiers use Haar-like features as input. Figure 10.8 highlights its contrast with the HOG method.

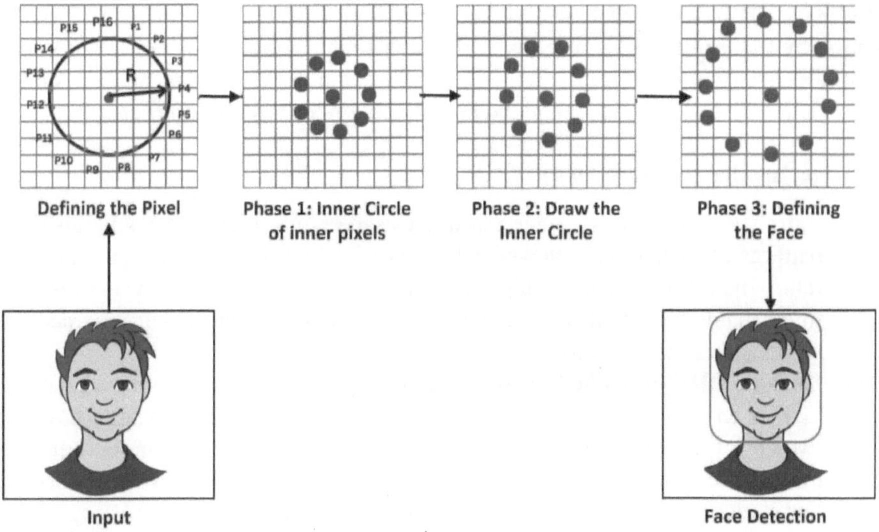

FIGURE 10.7 Pixel picking.

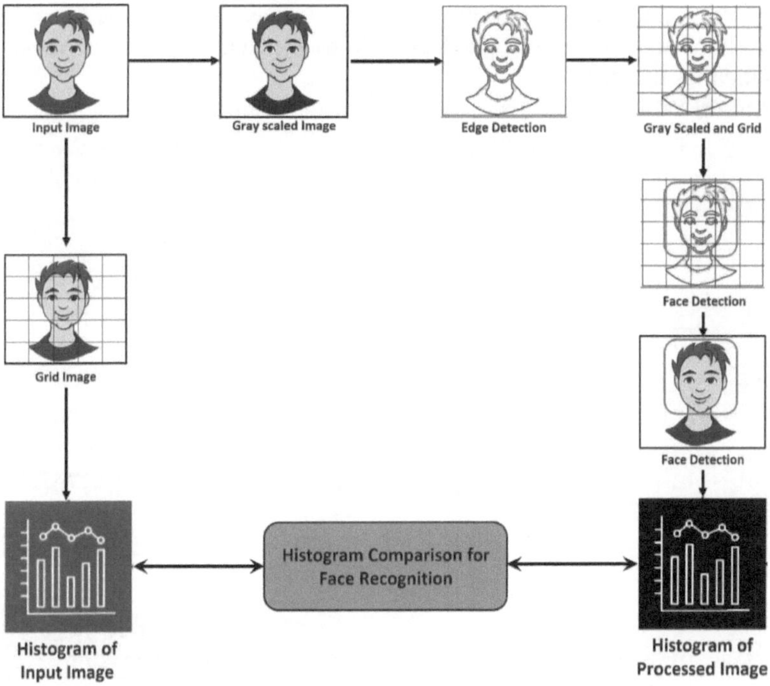

FIGURE 10.8 Histogram plotting.

10.2.2.1 How Do Haar Features Work?

The Alfred Haar wavelet is a series of rescaled square-shaped functions. The concept of using Haar wavelets to create Haar-like features was created by Paul Viola and Michael Jones. They resemble the neural network convolution kernels.

Steps Involved (Figure 10.9)

- **Patterns of Darkness**: Haar cascade classifiers are taught to distinguish patterns of darkness (shadows) and brightness (highlights) inside an image rather than directly identifying face characteristics. These patterns are distinguishable for face detection because they are particular to facial characteristics and configurations.
- **Consider the Haar-like Feature**: The Haar Cascade classifier with the label "1.a" is an illustration of a Haar feature. This feature has the appearance of two dark rectangles over two light rectangles. Because the area around the eyes is often darker than the forehead, this particular feature aids the classifier in recognizing patterns in a picture that belong to that area.
- **Evaluation of the Feature**: The classifier determines whether the pattern it sees in the window corresponds to any of the patterns it has been taught to identify. The classifier designates that area as a potential face if a match is discovered.
- **Grayscale Conversion**: The input image is transformed into a grayscale image in order to evaluate these patterns efficiently. Darker shades in a greyscale image correlate to portions of the image that are less lighted, whereas lighter shades indicate colors in the image. By concentrating exclusively on the amount of light present in each pixel, grayscale conversion simplifies the study.
- **Sliding Window**: The Haar cascade classifier employs a sliding window technique after transforming the image to grayscale. It moves a fixed-size

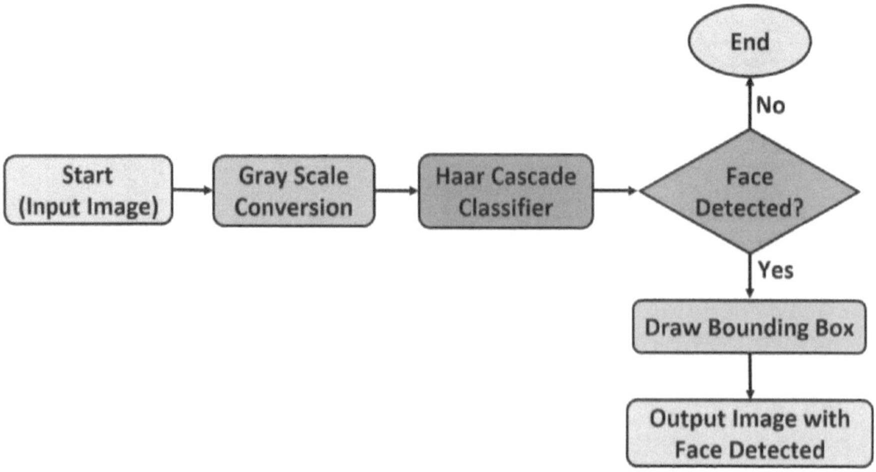

FIGURE 10.9 Haar cascade working for face detection.

window over the grayscale picture, which is commonly a rectangle. It determines whether the pattern or characteristic it is looking for is present at each place of the window.

- **Multiple Stages and Features**: Haar cascade classifiers have several stages, each of which has a number of features. These steps are passed through by the classifier, with each stage becoming more focused and removing false positives. Only if a region successfully completes all steps does the classifier mark it as a face.
- A bounding box is drawn around a region that has been classified as a face in order to show that a face has been found in the image.

10.2.3 HOG (Histogram of Oriented Gradients)

A feature descriptor for object detection in computer vision and image processing is the histogram of oriented gradients (HOG). In particular, for uses like pedestrian detection or general object detection, it is frequently used to identify things in photos. HOG uses mages in grayscale. The gradient of the image, which indicates the variations in intensity and direction of the pixel values, must first be computed. Typically, techniques like the Sobel operator are used for this.

10.3 FEATURE EXTRACTION

CNN, or convolutional neural networks, have changed the way we do face detection [15]. By automating the process of feature learning and object recognition, it became easier to identify faces in images. Designed like the human visual system, it can identify patterns and features by itself. All a model needs is a dataset full of labeled images. The architecture is simple: convolutional layers, pooling layers, and fully connected layers. Convolutional layers scan the image with learned filters to find things like edges and shapes. With those patterns found, pooling layers down-sample them to reduce how much space they take up in memory while also increasing invariance. And last, fully connected layers use these features for predictions. During training, the model minimizes loss function to improve its ability to classify faces by tweaking its internal parameters. You can also employ data augmentation techniques to increase the diversity of training examples so that the model's generalization improves.

Steps

- **Data Preparation**: Gather a labeled dataset containing positive samples (images of faces) and negative samples (images without faces). Annotate the faces with bounding box coordinates.
- **Model Selection**: Choose a pretrained CNN model as the base architecture. Consider that pretrained models already know how to do things like pull a rabbit out of a hat. What I mean by that is that they've already learned to extract features from images through a series of operations, such as image stitching. The earlier layers of the model are responsible for extracting low-level features like edges and textures. Meanwhile, the later layers are responsible for more complex ones.

- **Fine-Tuning**: This is the part where we modify our pretrained CNN model for face recognition. Specifically, we adapt the fully connected layers and output layer for it. While these layers handle making predictions, the feature extraction layers remain unchanged.
- **Training**: When training, our CNN model takes each input image through its series of layers and performs feature extraction on them automatically. You can think of this process as scanning an image in which the model applies a series of convolution and pooling operations to progressively extract relevant features from it. For example, initial layers may recognize things like edges and corners while subsequent ones capture more abstract features, eventually helping it learn how to recognize facial characteristics.
- **Inference**: Once that's done, we move on to using this trained CNN on new images. Given its nature as a detection system, it'll use the same feature extraction process. The way it does this is by sliding through an image with a window at different locations and using them to compute feature maps. These maps represent what the model detects in different parts of an image.

10.3.1 Emotion Detection System for the Detected Face

After detecting the face of the patient and extracting the different features of the face and pixel values for the detected face, we want to use the techniques of OpenCV and predict the emotions of the detected face. For that, we know that we have a classification task; we can use the techniques such as classification models and the CNN ResNet, Unet, AlexNet, etc. networks for efficiently detecting the emotion of the patient. Another technique is to impose the detected face image on the other image of a face with the smiling, or sad, or skeptic look to determine the state of mind of the patient, as we have the data collected through IoMT-based surveillance cameras and the video clips. Now we will examine first how the detected face can undergo the network of emotion detection. The goal is to detect and classify emotions from patients' facial expressions using computer vision and deep learning algorithms. As shown in Figure 10.10, the procedure includes numerous critical stages, the first of which is data collection.

Data Collection: To begin, a thorough dataset containing facial photographs labeled with relevant emotions is necessary. FER-2013, CK+, and AffectNet are examples of publicly available datasets that can be used for this purpose. Scaling the images to a consistent size, leveling the pixel values, and increasing the dataset are all part of this process. Augmentation procedures broaden the dataset's diversity, leading to improved model generalization. Selecting a suitable model architecture is a critical decision. Numerous deep learning models are available.

The reference to the whole process in one shot is given in Figure 10.11. The paper [6] defines the way of the pipeline method just using the library functions that OpenCV provides to the face recognition tasks. The Table 10.1 describes the comparison of face detection methods.

10.3.2 Siamese Network (Sisters Network)

Unconscious emotional responses to intrinsic and extrinsic events that express particular physiological states are produced. Here, making wise decisions and acting

TABLE 10.1
Comparing Face Detection Methods

Method	Key Characteristics	Advantages	Limitations
Haar cascade classifiers	Uses patterns of light and darkness to detect faces and has a quick execution time.	Fast and effective Excellent accuracy in confined spaces	Less precise in situations where changes in stance, lighting, and scale relating to facial frontal views
Histogram of oriented gradients	Captures gradient-based information to depict the structure of the item.	Effective at representing shapes and detecting objects	Fast and effective Excellent accuracy in confined space
(LBPH) local binary pattern Histogram	Captures local textural data using histograms and binary patterns.	Efficiency and simplicity Resistant to changes in lighting and expression	Simplicity and effectiveness Resistant to changes in lighting and emotion
Convolutional neural networks	During training, automatically derives hierarchical characteristics from photos.	Highly precise and capable of adjusting to complicated situations Can adjust to changes in position and illumination	Bigger datasets needed for training Possibly computationally demanding tendency to overfit

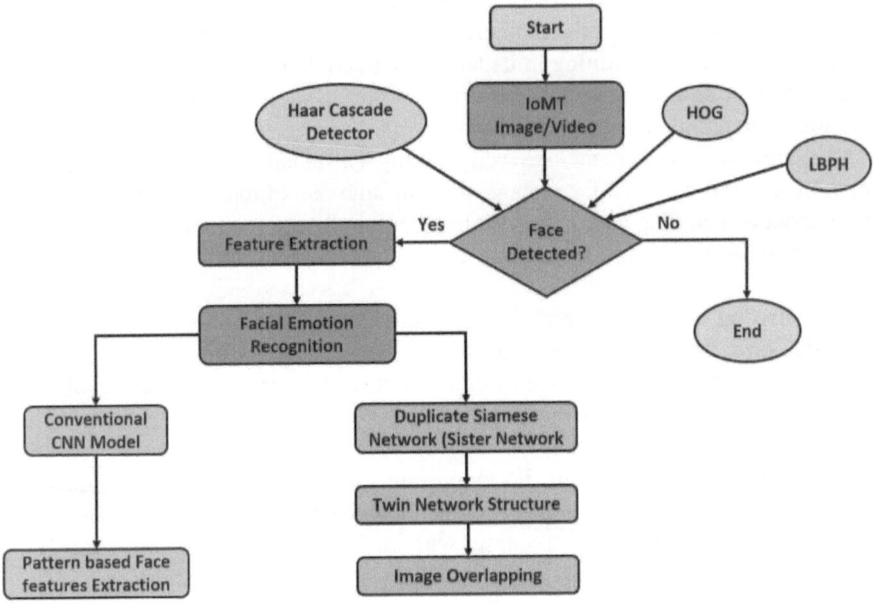

FIGURE 10.10 Methodology for emotion detection.

correctly in life heavily depend on our capacity to comprehend and control our feelings. The kind of data provided to us is always diverse and difficult to handle as the exact match of the features is not always there to map to the correct category. Researchers have been attempting to identify the emotion accurately and precisely from facial expressions using ML models. Even though machine learning (ML) has the potential to simplify difficult computational concerns, issues with business applications like facial expression identification still exist. A Siamese network is made up of twin subnetworks that are the same. These twins are identical in terms of weight and structure. A type of neural network architecture called a Siamese network is used many times for jobs involving determining how similar or dissimilar data pairings are. The term "Siamese" refers to a network that has two identical subnetworks (commonly referred to as "twins") that are connected at their outputs. The weights and designs of these subnetworks are identical, which is the main reason for its ability toaccurately find the common elements. The overview of how the twin design helps to decode the image given in the paper.

A Siamese network's main goal is to learn a similarity measure, which may be used to compare or contrast two input data points When working with the image, we have two sets of pixels and their intensities, and, after detecting the face, we also have the edges of the face. For jobs like face verification, signature verification, image similarity, and other things, this is especially helpful. The conjoined twin brothers Chang and Eng Bunker, who lived from May to January, are credited with coining the phrase. This phrase is used to describe twin children or any kind that are physically combined at the chest, abdomen, or pelvis. The two people came from Thailand, which was historically known as Siam, therefore the name. The term "Siamese Twins" refers to the fact that the neural network we will examine in this article also consists of a pair of networks that are identical.

The main concept is that the Siamese network can learn to capture the emotional parts of a face through training in its learned embedding space. This makes it possible to predict and measure emotions by gauging how similar they are to known emotional exemplars in the dataset. The network doesn't just explicitly classify emotions; it learns to recognize them as well, making it a valuable tool for tasks involving emotion recognition. Each face image goes through one of the twin subnetworks to learn about embedding, where the weights are shared between them. The input face images have to change so that they can create embedding vectors.

- **Learning Emotional Features**: Through a dataset including pairs of faces that have various emotions, the Siamese network gains the ability to map positive pairings of faces with similar emotional expressions closer together in the embedding space and negative ones with differing emotional expressions and further away.
- **Emotion Discrimination**: It's important for a network like this to identify emotional aspects in faces as the face characteristics of one image. It does this by training on a dataset with various pairings of expressions. It then finds what sets apart an angry expression from a neutral one or a sad expression from a happy one. Comparison of the embedding vectors of any two sets of faces assesses how similar or dissimilar they are after the network has been trained. Faces with similar emotional expressions will have embeddings close by in the embedding space, while faces with different emotional expressions will have embeddings spaced further apart.
- **Emotion Recognition**: The trained Siamese network can process a recently discovered face to produce an embedding vector. This embedding vector

can be compared to other recognized embeddings that was previously in the training dataset to determine which emotion is the more comparable.

- **Emotion Prediction**: The emotion label for the closest comparable known sample in the collection can be used to identify the predicted emotion for the identified face.

10.3.3 Approach

10.3.3.1 How Will We Basically Detect Emotions?

As we have integrated the IoMT system for data collection, the system would also capture the tones of images for further real-time processing, and we capture the patient's face with previous techniques of face detection. Now we want the extracted features, ROI (the detected face) and the other images stored on the cloud should be gone through the same two kinds of networks to be decoded and, in the end, to compare the features and the pixel arrangements by using OpenCV and then detecting the main emotion of one of the nine classes using this network. A big part of learning is finding the most effective way to understand and study new information. The same can be said for machines as well, specifically AI. The meta-learning framework was created with this in mind. It is a collection of training tasks and testing tasks that train and teach an AI how to classify information given to it. And then evaluate how well it did using a set of test tasks. Figure 10.11 illustrates the process from the start, and ROI detection is mentioned. Each job in the framework has two attached sets: a support set and a query set. During the training phase, the model checks how effective it is at learning by using the query set. Then it assesses itself using completely different activities during the testing time. "One-shot," "K-shot," and "few-shot" are different terms used in this framework. The one-shot is exactly what you wouldd think when it learns one instance from each class. K-shot takes that up a notch, though; instead of one model learns, K-shot takes examples from *N* classes in *N*-way-K-shot classification, which is a generalization of few shot learning. And the network we are using is one-shot learning because at the same time we provide only one instance or example for each of the class.

After consistently identifying the face and ROI, we cropped only the photos in the pertinent regions. Use (256 × 256) to calculate something more quickly. The next stage is to create a video from the pictures. The grayscale format (.pgm) facilitates easy and practical data administration. Send two facial photos across two connected subnetworks to the Siamese network for facial recognition. The network calculates Euclidean distances between the pictures for image recognition. The Siamese model predicts the similarity score for each test pair. Figure 10.12 is the part where the layer for the each model is thoroughly given.

10.3.4 ConvoNet for the Emotion Recognition

The brain of ConvNet is comprised of convolutional layers. They are in charge of extracting spatial feature hierarchies from the input image. These layers extract local information by convolving across the input image using tiny filters, or kernels. Increasingly complicated features can be captured using many convolutional layers. Figure 10.13 shows the ConvoNet structure that impasses the different layers of the

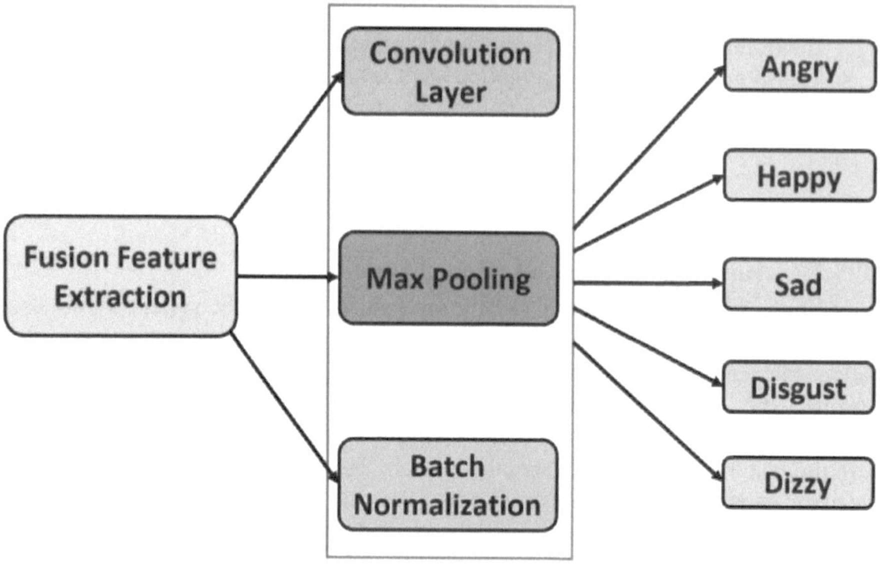

FIGURE 10.11 Main idea.

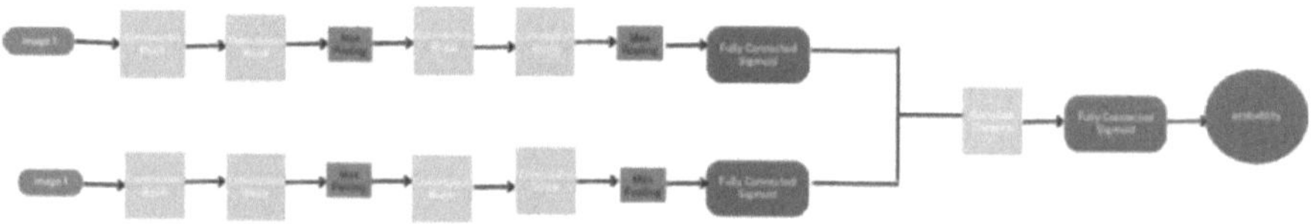

FIGURE 10.12 Duplicate network.

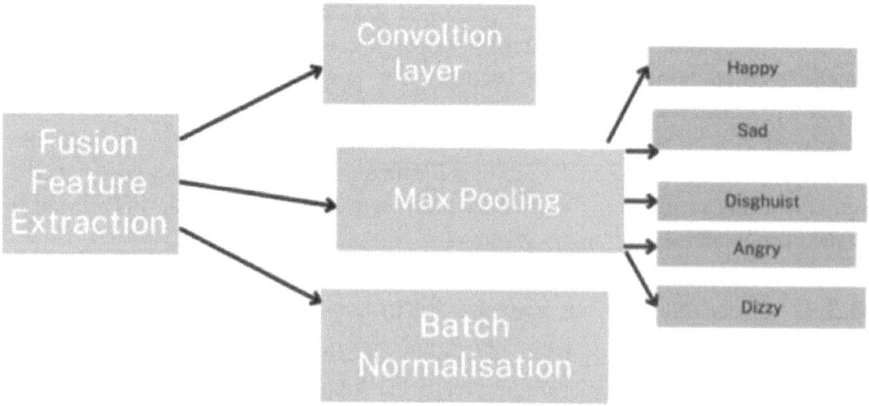

FIGURE 10.13 CovoNet layers for classification.

classification. The main purpose of convolution in convolutional neural networks is to extract features from the input image. Convolution controls the relationship between pixels by learning visual features (i.e., filtering the least squares of the input data). CNN uses the terms "filter," "kernel," and "feature detector." The matrix created by calculating the product of the filter by sliding it over the image is called the "convolution feature," "activate map," or "feature map." In this layer, you can choose the filter size and pitch (the number of pixels that need to be changed). The output of the convolutional process is:,

$$\frac{(W-F+2P)}{S}+1=O \tag{10.1}$$

where *F*, *P*, and *S* represent difference, padding, and step, respectively.

Siamese networks are better suited for tasks like face verification or evaluating facial expressions that require measuring similarity or dissimilarity between inputs. ConvNets are an obvious choice for facial emotion identification since they perform better in challenges where the objective is to classify facial expressions into preset categories. Siamese networks need specific training on pairs of data, which may not be required for conventional emotion recognition tasks. ConvNets are frequently utilized in computer vision tasks and are typically easier to install. A ConvNet is frequently used in facial emotion identification to classify facial expressions into emotions because this fits the typical use-case. However, Siamese networks could be useful if you have a specific similarity-based task that involves emotions. Which solution you should use depends on the precise requirements of your application. Figure 10.13 shows the seven class and the affect that each normalization layer and other layers place on it. Table 10.2 compares the proposed two approaches.

10.3.4.1 Validation with the Results Obtained by IoMT Integration

The emotion detected by our approaches is also validated and cross-verified through the detection of the emotion or the mood of the patient through the temperature, sleep cycle analysis, or the sensorial data of the ECG and EEG.

TABLE 10.2
Comparing the Two Proposed Approaches.

Aspects Relating	Siamese Networks (Twin Networks)	Convolution Networks (ConvoNet)
Purpose and approach	Analyze the degree of similarity or difference between two inputs (such as facial expressions).	Identifying facial features and categorizing emotions based on facial expression in our case
Architecture	This network consists of two identical subnetworks with shared weights. Each input is processed by a single subnetwork, and the feature embeddings are then compared.	Consisting of several layers, including convolutional, pooling, fully connected, and activation layers, all of which are designed to learn hierarchical properties from images

(Continued)

TABLE 10.2 (*Continued*)
Comparing the Two Proposed Approaches.

Aspects Relating	Siamese Networks (Twin Networks)	Convolution Networks (ConvoNet)
Training	Defining whether the pairings of input data are similar or dissimilar throughout training. The network gains the ability to maximize the distance between dissimilar pairs while minimizing the distance between similar ones.	Trained to categorize input photos into predetermined groups (such as emotions) using labeled data. Learns to take information from photos and predict things based on that information.
Use-cases	Useful for applications requiring the comparison of two facial expressions, such as face verification, facial recognition, or similarity-based tasks	Ideally suited for jobs like facial emotion recognition, which involve categorizing facial expressions within predetermined emotion groups using features extracted from the facial expressions
Ease of implementing	Traditional emotion recognition is less widespread and may call very specific training.	Frequently used and simple to implement in computer vision jobs
Data required	We need the pairs of data images to find similarity or dissimilarity.	Requires a dataset of face expressions (emotions) that have been tagged.

REFERENCES

[1] Nassereddine M, Khang A. Applications of Internet of Things (IoT) in smart cities. In: *Advanced IoT technologies and applications in the industry 4.0 digital economy*. CRC Press; 2024. pp. 109–136.

[2] Singh P, Devi KJ, Thakkar HK, et al. Region-based hybrid medical image watermarking scheme for robust and secured transmission in IoMT. *IEEE Access*. 2022;10:8974–8993.

[3] Arefin M, Rahman MM, Hasan M, et al. A topical review on enabling technologies for the Internet of Medical Things: Sensors, devices, platforms and applications. *Micromachines*. 2024;15(4):479.

[4] Thakkar HK, Sahoo PK. IoT based ECG-SCG big data analysis framework for continuous cardiac health monitoring in cloud data centers. In: *Predictive analytics in cloud, fog, and edge computing: Perspectives and practices of blockchain, IoT, and 5G*. Springer; 2022. pp. 177–184.

[5] Joyia GJ, Liaqat RM, Farooq A, et al. Internet of Medical Things (IoMT): Applications, benefits and future challenges in healthcare domain. *Journal of Communications*. 2017;12(4):240–247.

[6] Sahoo PK, Thakkar HK, Lin WY, et al. On the design of an efficient cardiac health monitoring system through combined analysis of ECG and SCG signals. *Sensors*. 2018;18(2):379.

[7] Smith AA, Li R, Tse ZTH. Reshaping healthcare with wearable biosensors. *Scientific Reports*. 2023;13(1):4998.

[8] Krumhuber EG, Skora LI, Hill HC, et al. The role of facial movements in emotion recognition. *Nature Reviews Psychology*. 2023;2(5):283–296.

[9] Edward AS, Jothimani A, Akila V, et al. Smart surveillance system using emotion detection. In: *AIP Conference Proceedings*. Vol. 2427. AIP Publishing; 2023.

[10] Wu H, Xu Z, Zhang J, et al. Face recognition based on convolution siamese networks. In: *2017 10th International Congress on Image and Signal Processing, BioMedical Engineering and Informatics (CISP-BMEI)*, IEEE; 2017. pp. 1–5.
[11] Shakoor MH, Boostani R, Sabeti M, et al. Feature selection and mapping of local binary pattern for texture classification. *Multimedia Tools and Applications*. 2023;82(5):7639–7676.
[12] Sangeetha T, Miruthula V, Kavimalar C, et al. Face mask detection and social distancing using machine learning with Haar cascade algorithm. *Sentiment Analysis and Deep Learning: Proceedings of ICSADL 2022*. 2023:987–999.
[13] Dalal N, Triggs B. Histograms of oriented gradients for human detection. In: *2005 IEEE Computer Society Conference on Computer Vision and Pattern Recognition (CVPR'05)*. Vol. 1. IEEE; 2005. pp. 886–893.
[14] Chandan G, Jain A, Jain H. Real time object detection and tracking using deep learning and openCV. In: *2018 International Conference on Inventive Research in Computing Applications (ICIRCA)*. IEEE; 2018. pp. 1305–1308.
[15] Khan M, Chakraborty S, Astya R, et al. Face detection and recognition using opencv. In: *2019 International Conference on Computing, Communication, and Intelligent Systems (ICCCIS)*. IEEE; 2019. pp. 116–119.

11 Explainable AI Algorithms for Augmented Healthcare Hybridization

Rinkal Jain and Jeet Patel

11.1 INTRODUCTION

In the recent past, the role of explainable artificial intelligence (XAI) in healthcare is gaining popularity due to its combined strength of cutting-edge machine learning and AI. The XAI offers the insight understanding of working of the model, and it seeks to offer the openness, interpretability, and accountability to make informed medical decisions. The XAI models are conceived to help healthcare personnel comprehend the outcome and boost their confidence in the technology. The XAI in healthcare is perceived to reveal the hidden patterns and insights about the way AI models make their forecasts, suggestions, and diagnoses of the healthcare problems. Such aids from XAI models are likely to enhance patient care in the long run. In this introductory section, we will examine the importance, difficulties, and critical ideas of XAI in healthcare.

The very reason for XAI gaining popularity in recent years is due to the model's ability to make the AI systems more trustworthy, dependable, efficient, and robust. XAI describes the techniques and methods employed to design and develop the AI software that offer user friendliness and understandability. XAI is expected to assist all types of users such as end users, data scientists, domain experts, or laypeople without formal AI training. In recent years, few architectures in computer vision are gaining noticeable popularity such as deep learning (DL) in the field of healthcare due to their accuracy outcomes. The robustness and effectiveness of such models has sparked curiosity in healthcare professionals to know the process of their decision-making. Usually, the stakeholders in healthcare like AI systems that offer insights that are simple to comprehend or interpret for making predictions [1].

The XAI process can be explained using three taxonomies: local explanation, global explanation, and counterfactual explanation.

The local explanation of XAI explains the decisions made by AI models by concentrating on specific data points. Local explanation can be useful to comprehend the rationale behind a particular patient's healthcare predictions. On the contrary, the global explanation examines the AI model as a whole and can explain the decisions made by the model. Therefore, it is highly beneficial to understand the local explanation and global explanation to gain insights about the way the model makes

 DOI: 10.1201/9781003393498-15

decisions and spots potential biases. Such insights by the model and data can be helpful to make informed decisions about the patients' health service delivery. Moreover, understanding the model's sensitivity and robustness with regard to the various feature sets can be helped in healthcare industry [2].

11.1.1 Significance of Explainable AI in Healthcare

Several factors play a crucial role for XAI in healthcare:

- **Improved Transparency**: The XAI methods promote transparency and accountability in healthcare processes by explaining the way an AI system produces results. Due to the openness and understanding of XAI models, it increases the level of trust in the system. The explanations provided by XAI techniques can also be used to understand the working of the different components of AI systems and their reasoning behind producing certain outcomes.
- **Model Improvement**: The AI system generates the results from the rules learned from the data. However, sometimes the rules learned from the skewed data may produce incorrect output, leading to false forecasts. XAI may help improvise the model's performance using the XAI-generated explanations.
- **Accuracy Improvement**: XAI methods have the ability to explain the reasoning behind the produced outcome. In the healthcare domain, the accuracy of medical diagnosis and treatment plans can be improved by outlining the way an AI system arrives at its conclusions. This understanding may facilitate communication between doctors and other medical workers, resulting in improved accuracy and effective treatment plans [3].
- **Knowledge Transfer**: The XAI models enables healthcare professionals to access the insights learned by AI systems and apply them to improve patient outcomes such as treatment plans. For instance, an XAI system may detect a correlation between a specific symptom parameter and an unrecognized illness condition. In such cases, the XAI system explanations may help medical experts to learn new insights for prospective diagnoses.
- **Patient Trust**: AI systems usually work as black boxes, and no one gains insight into how results are produced. In AI-supported medical decisions, patients and healthcare providers must have faith in the AI-produced outcomes. In such cases, explainability helps to bridge this trust level by exposing the AI's rule building login more clear and understandable.
- **Clinical Decision Support**: The ability of XAI technology to provide insights potentially assists healthcare professionals in making precise and well-informed judgments, leading to better patient outcomes.
- **Regulatory Compliance**: Each country has well-defined regulatory compliances to be followed by the healthcare industries. XAI potentially assists in meeting these requirements by providing understandable platforms.
- **Error Detection and Correction**: Explainable AI has the ability to understand the reasoning behind the model's biased outcome, and therefore XAI can effectively suggest the corrective measures to prevent potential patient harm.

Figure 11.1 shows Combination of human and AI models can create powerful AI-assisted decision-making.

11.1.2 Challenges in Explainable AI in Healthcare

- **AI Model Explainability**: The foremost challenge of traditional AI models is to describe their functionalities. For instance, the complex deep learning models are very difficult to describe by a doctor considering a huge number of hyper parameters, multiple layers, and complex interconnections among them. Such sophisticated models are difficult to grasp for healthcare professionals to extract insights and interpretations. Contrary to the sophisticated models, simpler models such as decision trees may need less effort for understanding.
- **Data Availability and Quality**: The significant challenge for any healthcare XAI model is to elevate the quality of balanced data by a huge amount. However, it is very challenging to gather reliable and complete data for healthcare studies, for instance heart disease, considering the complexity of data acquisition, diversification, and huge quantity required. Diverse, unbiased, high-quality data is a crucial obstacle to training, validating, and testing XAI systems for orthopedic healthcare.
- **Precision Medicine**: While XAI can advance personalized medicine and care, AI models trained on large datasets can struggle to provide personalized explanations for individual patients. Each patient's unique characteristics, demographics, medical history, and comorbidities may not fully overlap with the training data, making it challenging to develop meaningful explanations at the instance level [2].

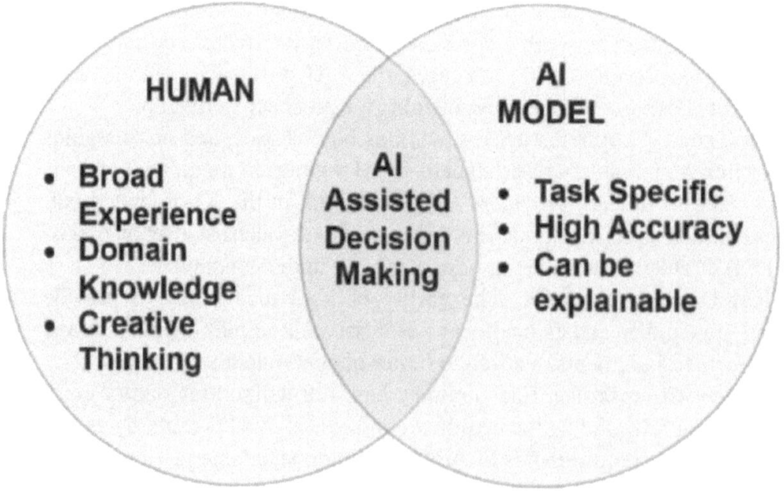

FIGURE 11.1 Combination of human and AI models can create powerful AI-assisted decision-making.

- **Data Privacy**: Protecting patient privacy when describing AI judgments is essential since healthcare data is sensitive.
- **Acceptance and Adoption**: Medical practitioners must be open to accepting and implementing XAI technologies. Education and training are crucial.

11.1.3 Key Concepts in Explainable AI in Healthcare

- **Feature Importance**: Finding the features (variables) in a model that had the most significant influence on a specific prediction or diagnosis is known as determining the feature importance.
- **Model-Agnostic Approach**: Approaches that can be used in any machine learning model, making them valuable in the healthcare industry
- **Visualization**: Creating diagrams, like decision trees or feature significance plots, to demonstrate how an AI model arrived at a particular conclusion
- **Saliency Maps**: Visualizations that highlight the critical areas of X-rays or MRIs that helped make a diagnosis
- **Natural Language Processing (NLP)**: The process of extracting structured information from unstructured medical records to make them machine-readable and understandable [4].

In this context, Figure 11.2 shows the implementation of AI in healthcare.

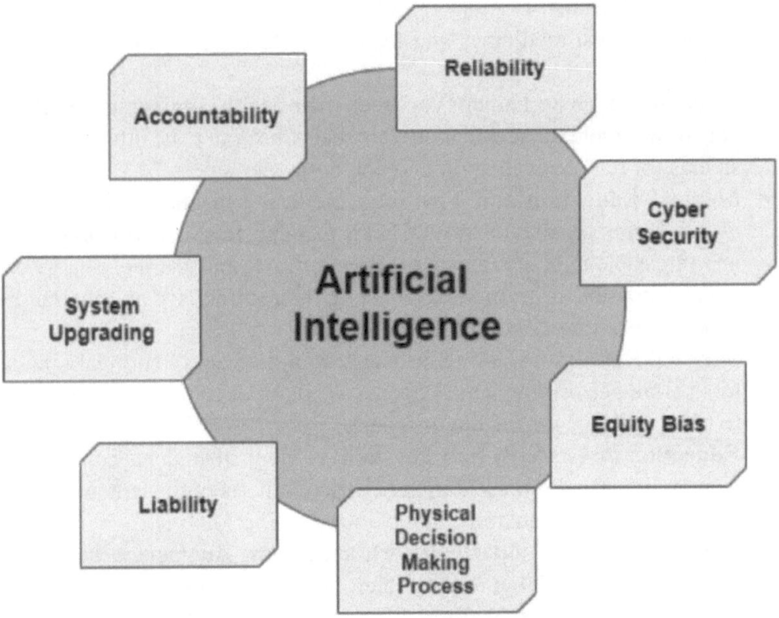

FIGURE 11.2 Implementation of artificial intelligence in healthcare.

11.2 AUGMENTED HEALTHCARE

The augmented healthcare refers to the integration of the state-of-the-arts technologies such as AI, augmented reality (AR), and virtual reality (VR) to improve and support various aspects of medical treatment, patient care, and healthcare management. Augmented healthcare uses these technologies to enhance patient participation, education improvement, diagnosis accuracy, and treatment plan prediction.

The following are the aspects of augmented healthcare:

1. **Medical Diagnosis and Decision Support**: Usually, healthcare professional are provided specific augmented healthcare tools to assist them in diagnosing patients more quickly and accurately.
    - **AI-Assisted Diagnosis**: Recently, smart AI healthcare algorithms have been designed so that they can examine medical images such as X-rays, MRIs, and CT scans to find anomalies and help recognize hidden patterns to increase diagnosis accuracy.
    - **Clinical Decision Support Systems (CDSS)**: CDSS is an AI-driven intelligent system that can suggest multiple alternative therapy options based on information about the patient for health improvement to the healthcare professional [5].
2. **Telemedicine and Remote Monitoring**: Although remote patient monitoring and telemedicine service have gained momentum post-COVID-19, it is becoming more accessible and convenient due to augmented healthcare technology. The following are the examples of augmented healthcare in remote monitoring:
    - **Teleconsultations**: Doctors can diagnose the patient on a virtual meeting and suggest medicines and treatments, leading to convenience and affordability.
    - **Wearable Devices**: Patients can track their health continuously with the help of wearable sensors that provide real-time data to healthcare professionals for remote evaluation and diagnosis.
    - **Medical Education and Training:** Medical education is challenging as it requires practical exposure with real subjects, which is expensive and infeasible in many instances. However, AR and VR technology can make it possible to train students using their immersive and interactive experiences. Some examples are as follows:
    - **Surgical Simulators**: Surgeons can accept the help of surgical simulators before performing actual operations in order to improve their abilities in a risk-free virtual environment.
    - **Education in Anatomy and Physiology**: Medical students can take the help of 3D virtual representation of different parts of the human body to better comprehend anatomy and pathology [5].
3. **Patient Engagement and Health Management**: Augmented healthcare aids patients to control and monitor their health in a flawless manner:
    - **Apps for Health and Wellness**: Several AR- and VR-enabled apps are designed to exercise, eat properly, and manage chronic diseases using gamification.

- **Medication Reminder Systems**: AR apps can also notify patients about the medication instructions with follow-up reminders [6].

4. **Reducing Medical Errors and Enhancing Safety**: The real-time information and decision support provided by augmented healthcare technology can lower the risk of medical mistakes and consequently improve patient safety [7].
   - **Medication Verification**: Augmented healthcare can assist the nurses and doctors in the medication verification and thereby reduces the possibility of mistakes [8].
   - **Fall Prevention**: AI technology, coupled with sensors data analysis, can notify the medical staff of patients in the event of falling and thereby, reduces the number of accidents caused by falls.
5. **Predictive Analytics and Population Health Management**: AI and data analytics can be carefully integrated to design the augmented healthcare to monitor population health and forecast health trends [9]:
   - **Predictive Analytics**: AI algorithms has the potential to predict disease outbreaks, to identify high-risk groups, and effectively allocate resources for the optimization.
   - **Proactive Treatment**: AI can also potentially assist with the proactive treatment of chronic illnesses and the early diagnosis cum treatment of undesirable health conditions.
6. **Methods and Techniques**: Explainable AI (XAI) in augmented healthcare, coupled with artificial intelligence and sensor technology and followed by explanation about the outcome, can provide transparency and interpretability to build systems that healthcare professionals can rely on and comprehend.

11.2.1 Feature Importance and Visualization

Machine learning features also known as the attributes determine and display the key elements that influence the way AI models make decisions. This feature selection and visualization helps the healthcare practitioners to comprehend patient's characteristics those are essential to make predictions. For instance, a feature visualization may emphasize on the certain attributes such as blood pressure, cholesterol levels, etc., while diagnosing heart-related anomalies.

For instance, saliency maps help to highlight areas of an X-ray image that contributed to determining a specific diagnosis. Figure 11.3 shows the implementation of feature visualization method.

11.2.2 Decision Trees

The decision tree is a machine learning algorithm that offers transparency and interpretability, and it is heavily used in healthcare applications and therefore it benefits explainable AI (XAI) in healthcare.

- **Medical Condition Diagnosis**: The decision tree is one of the important machine learning algorithms, and it helps in medical condition diagnosis.

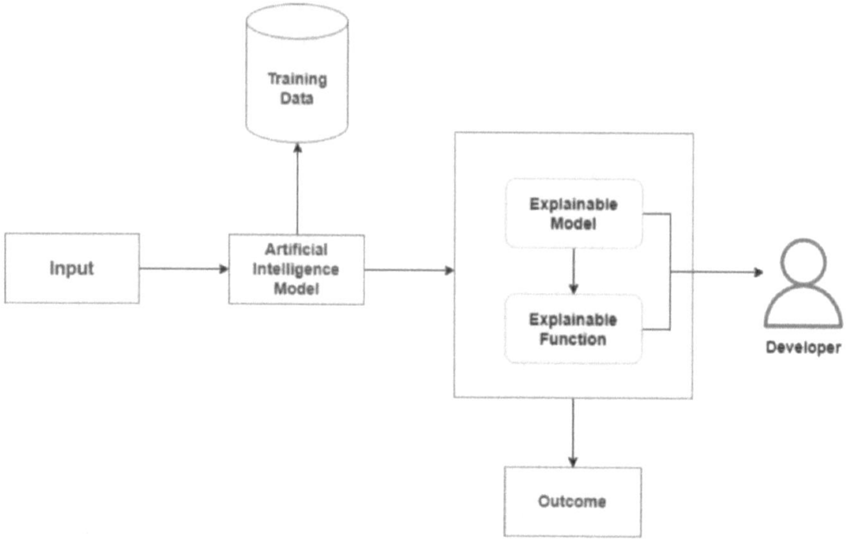

FIGURE 11.3 Implementation of feature visualization method.

Each branch of the tree indicates an outcome based on the unique medical characteristics for the diagnosis. This decision-making process indicates the flow and work of the model and indicates how the model arrived at a specific diagnosis for medical practitioners.

- **Predicting Disease Chance**: The decision tree can make predictions based on the parameters. Considering various patient-specific parameters such as age, genetics, lifestyle, and medical history, the decision tree model may predict a person's chance of contracting a given disease. Model-based prediction makes it evident about the risk assessment's contribution to variables.
- **Treatment Recommendations**: Decision tree models can also assist in direct treatment prediction for the variety of diseases in the healthcare industry. Suchmodels can decide the best suitable customized therapy treatment based on the patient's past medical symptoms, current symptoms, and other important aspects for the healthcare professional to understand and comprehend.
- **Medication dose and Prescription**: The decision tree algorithm can also be trained to identify the correct dose of the medicine or to choose an alternative medicine based on the patient's different parameters such as drug interaction, etc. Alternatively, healthcare professionals may find such dosage predictions helpful to ensure the safety of the patient.
- **Monitoring Disease**: One can also tweak the decision tree algorithm to continuously track the patient's health condition and illness over the period of time while assisting medical professionals to understand how different parameters have a direct or indirect impact on the health of a patient.

- **Early Intervention**: On the contrary, the decision tree algorithm can also be trained to identify individuals with a high risk of developing a specific medical disease. Such early identification can enable early intervention in order to take preventive measures. Early intervention is needed in the healthcare domain for improved patient outcome and to lower the overall healthcare cost. Figure 11.4 shows the Explainable AI use-cases and benefits.

11.2.3 LIME (Local Interpretable Model-Agnostic Explanations)

LIME is a popular XAI method that provides understandable explanations for the predictions made by the complex machine learning models despite the model's complicatedness. LIME is highly useful when working with black box models such as deep neural networks, random forests, and gradient-boosted trees. The fundamental goal of LIME is to provide the candidate decision boundary of complex models such as deep neural networks very close to the data point of interest by employing simpler and more intuitive models.

Similar to SHAP (Shapley additive explanations), LIME also provides explanations in the form of the most important attributes that contribute to the prediction. Different from the cooperative game theory, LIME takes a direct approach and alters

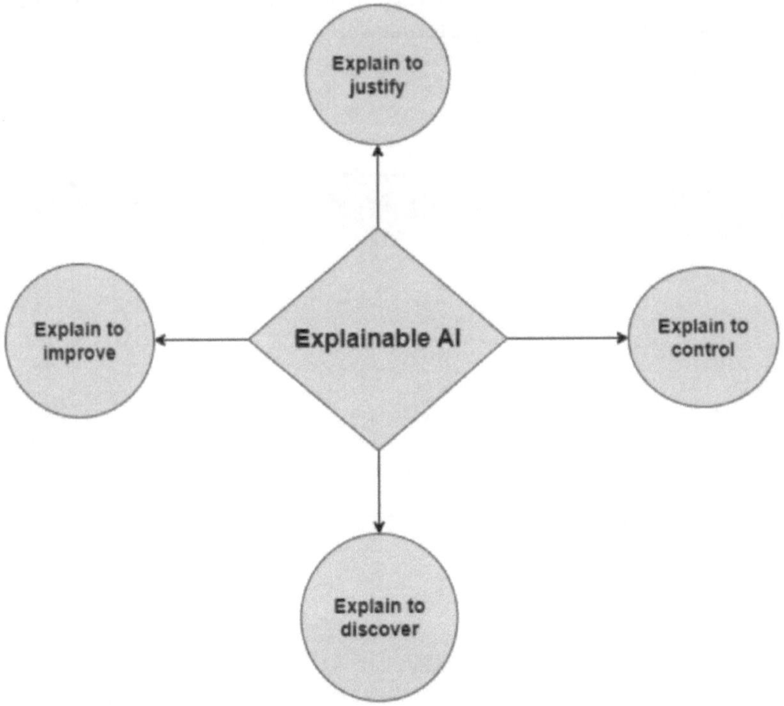

FIGURE 11.4 Explainable AI use-cases and benefits.

the model's input data to see the difference in the predictions. Furthermore, differently from SHAP, LIME explains only a single occurrence and not the entire dataset. To put it in a different way, LIME is used to describe the model prediction for an unknown sample after the model has been trained. The breakdown of how each attribute impacts the model's propensity to predict is how the LIME explanation is laid out [10]. Figure 11.5 shows the development of explainable AI-enhanced AI models.

11.2.3.1 Advantages

- LIME is model-agnostic, meaning that it may be used for any machine learning model, no matter how sophisticated. This makes it adaptable and suitable for a variety of situations.
- It offers instance-level, context-specific explanations, which may be helpful when comprehending the rationale behind a specific model's prediction.
- The interpretable models employed by LIME, such as decision trees or linear regression, are simple to comprehend and communicate to stakeholders.

11.2.3.2 Limitations

- **Sample Dependence**: The performance of LIME is highly dependent on the number of samples and the sampling method. The selection of these parameters can highly impact the effectiveness of LIME explanations.
- **Sensitivity to Hyperparameters**: The number of samples and the local model's complexity are two important hyperparameters in LIME that need to be adjusted for improved performance.

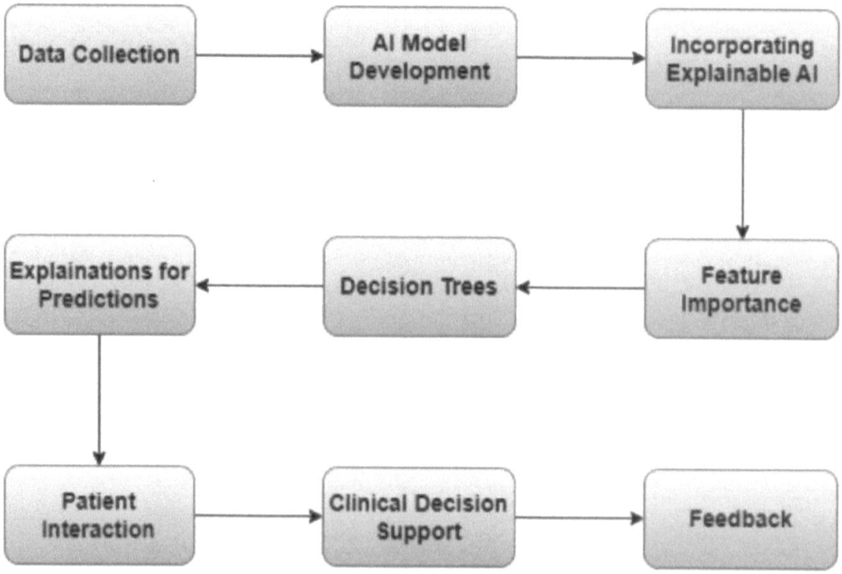

FIGURE 11.5 Development of explainable AI-enhanced AI models.

- **Local Scope**: A fundamental drawback of LIME is that it only offers explanations at the local level and that it is unable to capture global-level behavior [10].

Figure 11.6 shows the implementation of LIME.

11.2.4 SHAP (Shapley Additive Explanations)

SHAP is a practical XAI approach, and it offers a uniform framework that explains the results of any machine learning model. SHAP is designed based on the cooperative game theory concept, and it tries to assign a complicated model's prediction to specific attributes and to estimate the impact of each feature on the model's output. SHAP is a detailed and mathematically solid technique to comprehend the significance of model attributes for a given prediction.

11.2.4.1 Shapley Values

The very foundation of the Shapley values is the underlying cooperative game theory notion. Shapley values provide an equitable distribution of the "credit" for a group achievement among the participating members. When used in the context of feature attribution, Shapley values describe each feature's fair contribution to a prediction.

11.2.4.2 Cooperative Game Theory

Participants work together to accomplish a shared objective in unified game theory. Shapley values fairly and consistently determine how much each participant (feature) contributes to the final result.

11.2.4.3 Properties of SHAP Values

- **Local Interpretability**: SHAP values offer justifications for individual predictions, allowing one to ascertain the reasoning behind a model's choice of prediction for a particular input.

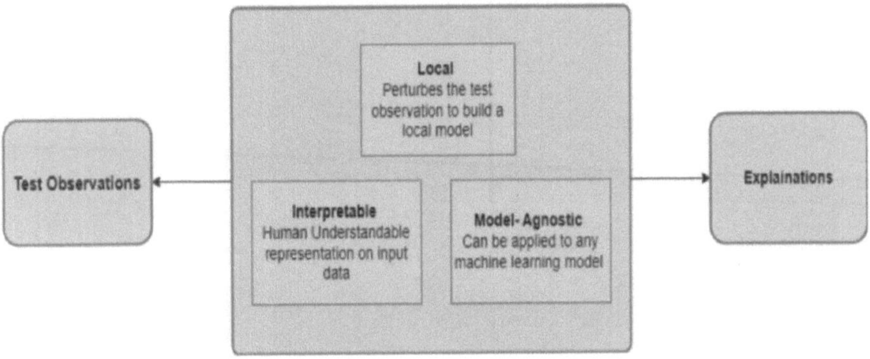

FIGURE 11.6 Implementation of LIME.

- **Global Interpretability**: You can comprehend the overall significance of features and their effect on the model's performance by looking at the distribution of SHAP values over the whole dataset.
- **Model Agnostic**: SHAP may be used with any machine learning model, regardless of complexity, because it is model-agnostic.
- **Additivity**: The SHAP values for every feature are cumulative. In other words, the difference between the model's forecast for an instance and the expected prediction equals the sum of SHAP values for all characteristics [10].

SHAP values are widely used in XAI and machine learning. They may be applied in fields where model transparency and feature significance are essential, including healthcare, to understand why a certain patient was given a particular diagnosis, finance to explain credit risk assessments, etc. Figure 11.7 shows the implementation of SHAP method. Moreover, Table 11.1 shows explainable AI Methods and Techniques for healthcare, Table 11.2 shows Benefits of Explainable AI in Augmented Healthcare, and Table 11.3 shows the application of Explainable AI in Augmented Healthcare.

11.3 CONCLUSION

Explainable AI addresses the crucial requirement for transparency in AI-driven healthcare solutions. It increases confidence among medical practitioners, patients, and regulatory authorities by offering transparent, understandable insights into how AI models make judgments.

Hybridizing augmented healthcare entails combining many technologies, such as artificial intelligence (AI), augmented reality (AR), virtual reality (VR), wearable

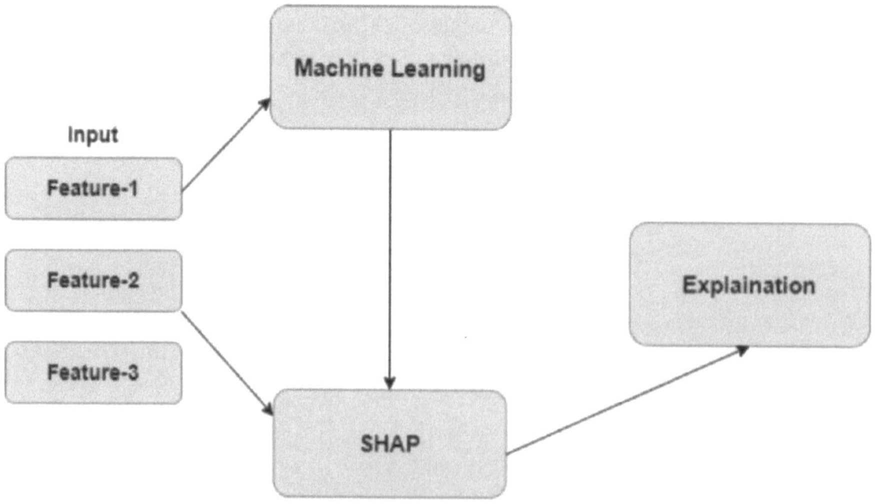

FIGURE 11.7 Implementation of SHAP method.

TABLE 11.1
Explainable AI Methods and Techniques for Healthcare

Sr No.	Method	Description	Application
1	Feature importance	Identifies crucial elements impacting the forecasts of an AI model.	Recognizing the patient characteristics that influence medical diagnosis
2	Decision trees	Represents decision-making logic in a way that is comprehensible.	Clarifying the clinical decisions that some AI models come to
3	LIME (local interpretable model-agnostic explanations)	For particular situations, approximates complicated models with simpler ones.	Supplying regional reasons for specific patient circumstances
4	SHAP (SHapley Additive exPlanations)	Equitably distributes feature contributions to prediction explanations.	Recognizing how various characteristics affect medical forecasts.
5	Model-agnostic approaches	Methods applicable to all machine learning models.	Allowing for adaptability in how predictions are explained across various models
6	Bayesian networks	Illustrates probable connections between several medical factors.	Simulating disease risk variables and their interactions to provide clear risk evaluation
7	Interpretability dashboards	Interactive interfaces let medical practitioners study the results of AI models.	Enabling real-time interaction between models and explanations for use by physicians

TABLE 11.2
Benefits of Explainable AI in Augmented Healthcare

Sr No.	Benefit	Description
1	Enhanced patient outcomes	A more accurate diagnosis and individualized care produce better patient outcomes.
2	Increased trust and adoption	AI systems that are clear and easy to understand are more widely trusted and used in healthcare.
3	Efficient healthcare operations	Process streamlining and AI-driven decision assistance increase operational effectiveness and save costs.
4	Expanded healthcare access	Remote monitoring and telehealth allow for the expansion of healthcare services into rural and underdeveloped areas.
5	Ethical and regulatory compliance	Fairness, transparency, and data security are ensured by commitment to ethical norms and laws.

technology, and more, to produce complete solutions that improve healthcare procedures. By providing thorough reasons and explanations for AI-driven diagnoses, treatment suggestions, and forecasts, explainable AI assists medical practitioners in making wise decisions.

TABLE 11.3
Application of Explainable AI in Augmented Healthcare

Sr No.	Application	Description	AI Contribution
1	Medical diagnosis and decision support	Improving clinical judgment and diagnosis	Describing the rationale behind certain diagnoses or therapy suggestions
2	Medical education and training	Combining AR and VR for immersive training and anatomy instruction	Providing medical students and professionals with open educational opportunities
3	Patient engagement and health management	Encouraging active patient participation in healthcare	Providing clear explanations to inspire patients and maintain their health
4	Robotic assistance in surgery	Assisting doctors as they do less invasive operations	Ensuring that the activities of robotic surgical systems are understandable
5	Big data and predictive analytics	Analyzing huge datasets to control population health	Provide clear explanations of data-driven health projections
6	Augmented reality (AR) and virtual reality (VR)	Improving patient experiences as well as medical education	Offering dynamic and transparent experiences using AR and VR
7	Genomic medicine and personalized treatment	Adjusting medical care based on genetic information	Illustrating the reasoning behind suggestions for individualized therapy

REFERENCES

[1] Sadeghi, Z., Alizadehsani, R., Cifci, M. A., Kausar, S., Rehman, R., Mahanta, P.,. . .& Pardalos, P. M. (2023). A brief review of explainable artificial intelligence in healthcare. *arXiv preprint arXiv*:2304.01543.

[2] Amirian, S., Carlson, L. A., Gong, M. F., Lohse, I., Weiss, K. R., Plate, J. F., & Tafti, A. P. (2023). Explainable AI in orthopedics: Challenges, opportunities, and prospects. *arXiv preprint arXiv*:2308.04696.

[3] https://www.encora.com/insights/the-importance-of-explainable-ai-in-healthcare#:~:text=Explainable%20AI%20in%20healthcare%20has,risk%20of%20developing%20certain%20conditions.

[4] Kose, U., Sengoz, N., Chen, X., Saucedo, J. A. M., eds. (2024). *Explainable artificial intelligence (XAI) in healthcare.* CRC Press.

[5] Bazoukis, G., Hall, J., Loscalzo, J., Antman, E. M., Fuster, V., & Armoundas, A. A. (2022). The inclusion of augmented intelligence in medicine: A framework for successful implementation. *Cell Reports Medicine*, 3(1).

[6] Ramdurai, B. (2020). Growing importance of patient engagement in healthcare. *International Journal of Nursing and Health Science*, 6(3), 1–9.

[7] Almalki, M., Alsehli, F., & Khayyat, M. (2023). Use of technology to reduce medication errors and improve patient safety. *SAR Journal (2619–9955)*, 6(2).

[8] Ahsani-Estahbanati, E., Sergeevich Gordeev, V., & Doshmangir, L. (2022). Interventions to reduce the incidence of medical error and its financial burden in health care systems: A systematic review of systematic reviews. *Frontiers in Medicine*, 9, 875426.

[9] Morgenstern, J. D., Buajitti, E., O'Neill, M., Piggott, T., Goel, V., Fridman, D.,. . .& Rosella, L. C. (2020). Predicting population health with machine learning: A scoping review. *BMJ Open*, 10(10), e037860.

[10] Loh, H. W., Ooi, C. P., Seoni, S., Barua, P. D., Molinari, F., & Acharya, U. R. (2022). Application of explainable artificial intelligence for healthcare: A systematic review of the last decade (2011–2022). *Computer Methods and Programs in Biomedicine*, 226, 107161.

12 Optimized Predictive Algorithms for Augmented Intelligence in Personalized E-Health

Bhargav Limbasia, Hiren Kumar Thakkar, and Hiren Mewada

12.1 INTRODUCTION

A vital component of the healthcare system is medical diagnosis. Computer-aided systems play a vital role in precisely identifying diseases by analyzing the various bodily sections. Fuzzy logic, Genetic Algorithms, artificial neural networks, and other soft computing techniques have been employed to create new, more effective disease diagnosis systems. The development of a potent system of pharmaceutical medications for healthcare solutions has been the focus of precision medicine. It employs several strategies to improve the treatment of current disease symptoms by using medication exercise. It employs state-of-the-art diagnostics and customizes preferred medication based on previous involvement in actions made to improve a medical issue. Through the networking and interoperability of the healthcare system, the diverse features of clinical components—such as analytical tools, technologies, databases, and their application—are required to augment the balance of healthcare. Additionally, using artificial intelligence in inclined systems is a compelling suggestion to lead to the notable improvement of medicine at cheaper prices [1]. As a result, it has concentrated on several AI and machine learning technologies for the updated, data-centric era of the e-healthcare system. Every day, a vast quantity of health data is being collected, making it difficult to extract any kind of meaningful information. Currently, the big data analytics (BDA) approach is employed to carry out the underlying analytical process of disease employing multiple clinical data. Currently, BDA provides numerous satisfied services through the clinical system to quickly identify censorious diseases in their earliest stages and provide all patients with the necessary care. A number of BDA tools are essential for quickly examining large amounts of structured, semi-structured, and unstructured clinical data and creating the appropriate formats for storage and placement.

The development of electronic health records (e-health) has resulted in a heightened need for data analytics of human health and healthcare processes. This section provides an overview of the data analytics methods and techniques employed in e-health systems, including AI methodologies. Data science enables the application of quantitative and

DOI: 10.1201/9781003393498-16

qualitative techniques to address signifiable issues and to predict outcomes. Big data is an integral part of data analysis, as data is seen as the raw material for data science. When using these methods in electronic health systems, the primary objective is to gain knowledge from data to enhance patient care. In addition to being accessible in large quantities, e-health data is characterized by its lack of well-defined structures and its heterogeneous nature, thus necessitating methods that can order, filter, process, extract patterns, and convert data into value. In Van der Aalst's (2016) [2] definition of data science, it encompasses the process of extracting, preparing, examining, transforming, storing and retrieving data, constructing and operating computing systems, all forms of mining and teaching, the presentation of explanations and forecasts, and the utilization of outcomes with regard to ethical, societal, legal, and commercial considerations.

Descriptive analytics techniques are used to detect issues and trends in data. Examples of applications in e-health include diagnosing diseases or providing analysis of medical information from different sources such as mobile apps or medical test equipment. In [3], big data analytics has the following main business capabilities in healthcare:

1. Traceability in patient monitoring including lab results, medication, and historical data, as well as current status
2. Analytic analysis of structured and unstructured data, such as image, voice, text, etc.
3. Speeding up of decision-making with automatic notifications or visual reporting
4. Interoperability with heterogeneous data from various sources.
5. Prediction of patient behavior

These capabilities not only illustrate the potential applications of descriptive analytics in healthcare but also demonstrate the power of big data analytics to improve healthcare processes.

According to authors, i.e., [4,5], predicting future events is one of the capabilities of descriptive analytics. Predictive techniques in electronic health systems can be used to identify individuals who are most likely to develop a disease or to anticipate the development of diseases or viruses, thus aiding in the decision-making process of patients and increasing their likelihood of recovery. Additionally, these techniques can be employed in administrative matters to manage resources in periods of high or low patient volume at medical centers. In summary, predictive techniques can improve the efficiency of healthcare processes.

Prescriptive analytics is a genre that prescribes best practices for operations research and management science, along with machine learning techniques. Generally, these techniques provide valuable insights and support organizations' decision-making, thus providing a competitive edge. Prescriptive analytics is seen as the development of the descriptive and predictive domains of data science because of its ability to provide intelligent recommendations based on analyzed and forecasted data. Because this is still in its early stages, not many papers incorporate this data-driven technique into e-health apps. Table 12.1 lists a few popular predictive techniques used by data science fields and their applications, and Table 12.2 lists the various healthcare applications developed using data science techniques.

TABLE 12.1
Data Science Applications in E-Health

Data Science Fields	Techniques	Examples of E-Health Applications
Descriptive analytics	Data retrieval and retrieval (statistics and data visualization)	Patients diagnostic Epidemic recognition Patient management with mobile apps Visual analysis tools for clinical data Reporting systems Social media analysis Data warehouse tools
Predictive analytics	Machine learning, probabilistic modeling, and statistical analysis	Disease prediction Software as a service Medical decision support system, patient flow, and use of medical resource prediction
Prescriptive analytics	Logic-based modeling, evolutionary computation, mathematical programming, reinforcement learning, and simulation	Decision-making automation Scheduling problems Balanced assignment workload Resources Health management assessment Cloud computing

TABLE 12.2
Recognized Data Science Applications in E-Health

Data Science Techniques	Application Field
Data retrieval and collection (statistics and data visualization)	Epidemiological analysis [6] Computer-assisted surgical skills [7] Preventive health management system [8] Mental healthcare [9] Correlations between clinical medicine subjects [10]
Machine learning	Automatic behavior identification [11] Behavior assessment [12] Symptom classification (cardiology) (Oliver et al., 2018; Spanakis et al., 2017)
Modelling and simulation	Virus propagation risk analysis [13] Disease progression [14] Optimize emergency department operations Human organs simulation (Serra et al., 2021; [15])

12.2 VARIOUS APPROACHES APPLIED FOR E-HEALTH PREDICTION

12.2.1 Fuzzy Systems (FS) for Healthcare

Fuzzy Logicuency (Fuzzy Logic [FL]) is associated with the terms "uncertainty," "vagueness," and "fuzziness," all of which are characterized by their inability to be easily understood by traditional computing methods. Instead of dealing with specific values, Fuzzy

Logic deals with approximate values, which are referred to as "crisp" in the remainder of the chapter. Whereas certain values are cold, Fuzzy Logic values become cold—slightly cold—slightly warm—slightly hot. Examples of fuzzy systems can be found in a variety of applications in real life, such as elevators and razors, subway systems and medical devices, bond rating systems, and bank credit applicant risk analysis systems.

A Fuzzifier is a rule-based system that utilizes fuzzy theory to address ambiguity. Figure 12.1 outlines the components of a Fuzzifier-Inference Engine (Fuzzy Logic) system. The Fuzzifier is responsible for transforming crisp inputs into fuzzy values. The Inference Engine is a human decision-making simulation that provides the engine with the necessary rules for fuzzy output. The Knowledge Base is a collection of knowledge and decision rules that are derived from the expertise of the application domain that manages the relationships between inputs and outputs. The Defuzzifier translates the fuzzy output into a crisp value.

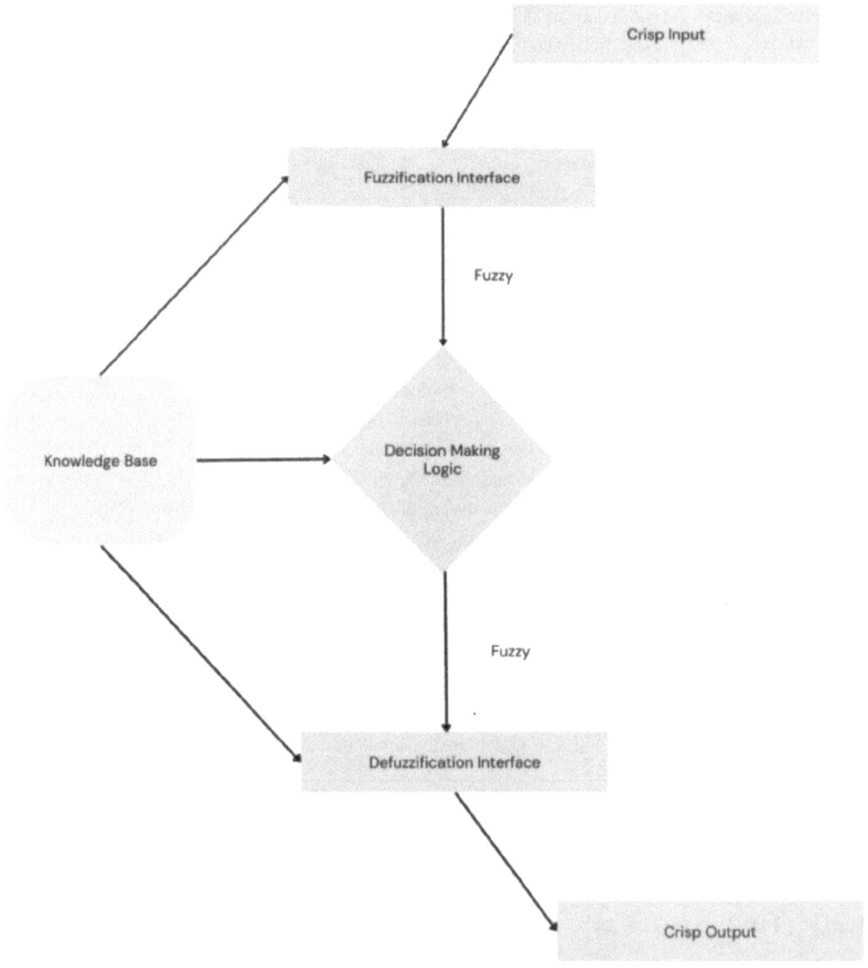

FIGURE 12.1 Fuzzy logic system components.

Fuzzy Logic may be used both alone and in combination with other techniques, such as neuro-fuzzy applications, NN combinations, fuzzy-Bayesian applications, and Bayesian network combinations. Fuzzy Logic is used widely in the medical field. Some of its applications are as follows:

- **Ranking Studies**: Medicine places a lot of importance on ranking studies. For the decision-making process, it is crucial to prioritize tests, risk factors, qualities, medical suppliers, and performance. This can be achieved by optimum means through the application of Fuzzy Logic systems.
- **Clustering Studies**: A data mining approach is clustering. To find meaningful patterns for the goal, it is used to divide the data into groups (referred to as clusters), where items within the same cluster have similar attributes and objects of other clusters have distinct properties. The major applications of clustering in medicine are in the study of tumors, cells, genes, and pictures.
- **Pattern Recognition Studies**: To understand the underlying patterns in the issue under consideration, pattern recognition is a machine learning method. Time-series analysis looks for patterns and laws that change over time; studies of this kind include the identification of medical pictures.
- **Performance Comparison Studies**: In this research, Fuzzy Logic approaches are used to compare the effectiveness of two or more distinct test, diagnosis, treatment, procedure, etc. methods.

The following are some examples of Fuzzy Logic's main medical application areas:

- Clustering cancer cells
- Tuberculosis diagnosis
- Cancer risk prognosis
- Image segmentation for tumors
- Aphasia diagnosis
- Determination of drug dose in pharmacy
- Heart disease diagnosis
- Lung disease diagnosis
- Diabetes care
- Managing malaria disease
- Hypothyroidism diagnosis
- HIV infection cell determination
- Earlier detection of arthritis and treatment
- Anesthesia monitoring
- Diagnosis and treatment of meningitis.

12.2.2 Various Medical Systems Based on Fuzzy Logic

12.2.2.1 Fuzzy Expert Systems in Medicine

The computer-based decision-making tools for healthcare assist medical professionals in identifying illnesses. A fuzzy expert system (FES) is one of several computer-based technologies that facilitate medical decision-making [16]. By ensuring the accuracy of results, FESs have demonstrated their value in the medical diagnostic for the quantitative analysis and qualitative assessment of medical data. The area of greatest interest to researchers is the creation of disease-specific FES applications:

- Knowledge acquisition
- Dealing with inconsistencies
- Treatment planning
- Advisory, monitoring, and control of systems
- Parameters predictions
- Artificial thinking

12.2.2.2 Fuzzy Information Retrieval in Medical Databases

The data in medical databases are presented clearly, just as in all other applications. It takes additional approaches to quickly obtain hazy information from clear databases. Fuzzy searches on medical databases use a significant Fuzzy Logic [17]. Crisp relational query languages' degree of abstraction is insufficient to produce queries that can satisfy the demands of each individual's information needs. When creating a query, such as "Show the low liver enzyme values for children with celiac disease [18]," we should have the chance to include linguistic expressions like "low" or "children." Fuzzy queries are used to cope with complexity and imprecision. A DBMS is extended by a fuzzy relational database management system (FRDBMS), much like the other FL application approaches. In this method, the database's data description is created using fuzzy linguistics.

12.2.2.3 Fuzzy-Logic-Supported Data Mining in Medicine

Medical data mining is another area in which FL is applied in medicine [19]. Data mining is used to extract knowledge and information from the vast amounts of data in healthcare and utilize this knowledge and information to lower costs and improve quality. The following are the two primary issues with data mining:

- Diverse sorts of heterogeneous data, whether numerical or symbolic, exact or approximate, confusing, or having partial files
- The user's request's level of complexity

FL is particularly effective at managing them thanks to its flexibility to represent many types of data, robustness against changes in the user's environment's settings, and distinctive expressiveness. Nearly all data mining methods have a fuzzy form, for example:

- Fuzzy comparison metrics,
- Fuzzy machine learning,
- Fuzzy DTs,
- Fuzzy clustering
- Fuzzy association rules.

The most effective algorithms for diagnosis seem to be DTs, ANNs, and Bayesian algorithms when using data mining approaches for illness diagnosis and prognosis. The most effective algorithms for prognosis were ANNs, Bayesian algorithms, DTs, and fuzzy algorithms. In the same study, research demonstrates that Bayesian algorithms, ANNs, and DTs are the most effective approaches for diagnosing cancer illnesses [20,21], heart disorders [22], and other diseases. ANNs, DTs, and Bayesian algorithms are also the most effective strategies for predicting the prognosis of cancer diseases.

12.2.2.4 Fuzzy Cognitive Maps in Medical Decision-Making

A medical decision support system should be able to conclude a causal knowledge base, which it creates by extracting causal information from the medical database. CMs are a type of knowledge representation that may connect the symbolic method employed by medical ontologies with the unprocessed medical information that describes a patient's health. They provide clear-cut cause-and-effect correlations [23]. FCMs are the fuzzy-directed graph extension of CMs. The primary benefit of FCMs over other approaches is their dynamic features, which may simulate the interactions between ideas. They represent hidden linkages, are dynamic, combinable, and customizable, and they capture more information in the interactions between ideas. FCM uses a strategy comparable to human thinking. The hardest part of modeling an FCM is figuring out how one notion affects the others and to what extent. Historical data are utilized to determine these impacts and their weights. The databases include a vast quantity of medical information. They may be used to build the

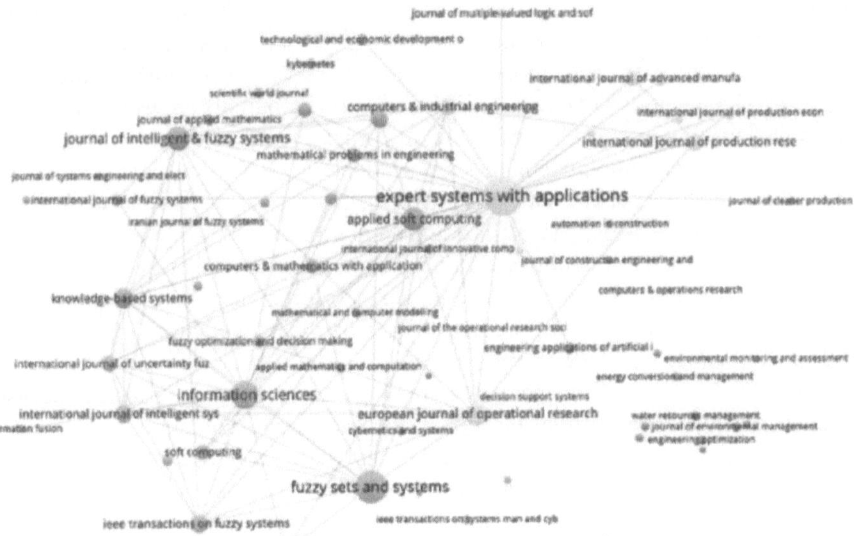

FIGURE 12.2 Relationships between the application of fuzzy expert systems and other relevant systems.

weights and relationships of the FCM models. In the similar context, Figure 12.2 shows the relationships between the application of fuzzy expert systems and other relevant systems.

12.2.3 Fuzzy-Genetic Algorithm Systems (F-GA)

A Genetic Algorithm (GA) is gaining significant attention in recent journal articles due to its capability to explore complex and high-dimensional solution spaces. Fuzzy Rule-Based Classification Systems (FRBCSs) are well established tools in the field of machine learning, valued for their ability to provide interpretable models to end users. These systems have found applications in diverse domains, such as anomaly intrusion detection [24] and image processing. In many of these practical use-cases, the available data often involves a large number of patterns (instances or examples) and variables. However, inductive learning of FRBCSs encounters challenges when dealing with the exponential growth of the fuzzy rule search space in such scenarios. Given the GA's ability to efficiently explore extensive solution spaces, it is apt to treat the routine definition of an FRBCS as an optimization or search problem. Furthermore, GAs can be utilized to incorporate prior knowledge, thanks to their flexible code structure and independent characteristics. In recent years, these capabilities have extended the application of GAs, facilitating the development of various approaches for designing FRBCSs across a wide range of domains. The architecture of the Fuzzy-Genetic Algorithm (F-GA) is shown in Figure 12.3.

Fuzzy Logic and Genetic Algorithms are utilized in this system for diagnosis, specifically for breast cancer disease, and they are regulated with each other throughout disease testing [25]. The fundamental process is created using Genetic and Fuzzy Logic algorithms, as seen in Figure 12.4 for the diagnostic system. Also, other models are designed using the F-GA system. The model is utilized to test brain tumors [26], identify the edge properties of tumors, and validate using a neuro-fuzzy classifier. The methods of GA optimization with fuzzy outputs are used for classification by adjusting parameters and delivering precise test results.

Various soft computing techniques are available, with Fuzzy Logic and Genetic Algorithms standing out as highly significant methods. Fuzzy Logic enables the representation of imprecision, uncertainty, and human-oriented knowledge. However, it lacks the ability for self-learning and rule generalization. On the other hand, Genetic Algorithms are robust general-purpose search algorithms inspired by natural genetics, capable of solving complex problems. They provide adaptability for integration with existing models and are easily hybridized.

In practical applications, especially in intelligent information systems, a successful approach involves combining Genetic Algorithms and Fuzzy Logic. These hybridized techniques have found real-world utility in a wide range of domains, including power systems, data mining, and image processing. Genetic Fuzzy Systems have

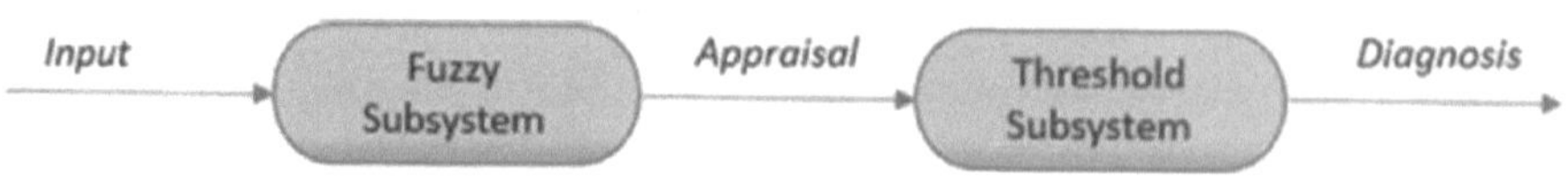

FIGURE 12.3 Architecture of F-GA.

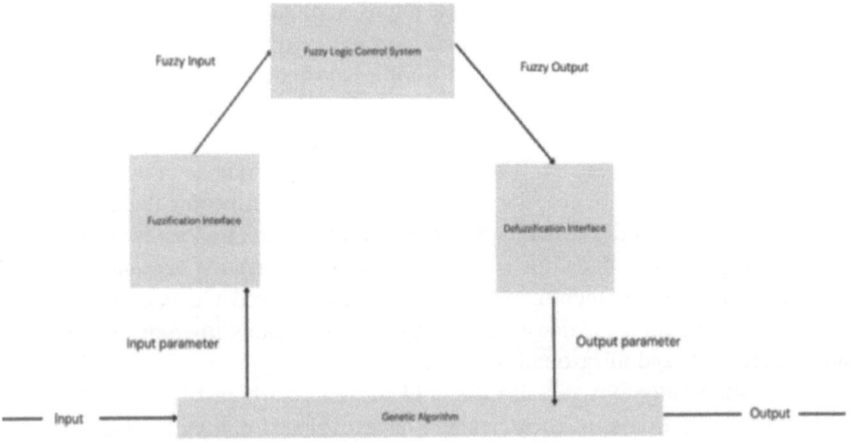

FIGURE 12.4 Automatic fuzzy rules generation using fuzzy Genetic Algorithm.

been applied to address various challenges, and the following list highlights some of the problems they've solved:

1. Diagnostic systems for diseases such as myocardial infarction, breast cancer, diabetes, dental development age prediction, and abdominal pain
2. Trading systems that optimize fuzzy models using Genetic Algorithms
3. Optimization of social regulation policies through these hybrid techniques
4. Development of self-integrating knowledge-based brain tumor diagnostic systems
5. Classification of rules in dermatology datasets for medical purposes
6. Integration of design stages in engineering projects using Genetic Algorithms
7. Multilingual question classification with Genetic Fuzzy Systems
8. University admission processes enhanced through evolutionary computing
9. Genetic mining for topic-based concept distribution
10. Intelligent web mining using a neural-Genetic-Fuzzy approach
11. Extraction of fuzzy classification rules employing genetic expression programming
12. An integrated approach for intrusion detection systems using Genetic Algorithms

In these diverse domains and applications, Genetic Fuzzy systems have proven to be highly effective in addressing complex problems and enhancing decision-making processes. Next, some of the uses of Genetic Algorithms in various fields of medicine are discussed.

12.2.3.1 Radiology

Radiological imaging generates vast amounts of data that require swift and accurate analysis by radiologists. To aid in this process, computer-aided detection and diagnosis technologies have emerged. These interdisciplinary approaches are swiftly advancing, aiming to facilitate quicker and more precise image analysis by identifying, segmenting, and categorizing both normal and pathological patterns across various imaging methods, including X-rays, magnetic resonance imaging (MRI), computed tomography (CT) scans, and ultrasound.

In the field of machine vision, where images of scenes (such as organs in radiological images) are acquired, processed, and interpreted, determining that the shapes and sizes of objects within these images are crucial for a detailed assessment. As a result, the process of edge detection is a fundamental component of automated image processing techniques. Numerous researchers have employed Genetic Algorithms (GAs) for edge detection in images obtained through various imaging modalities, including MRI, CT, and ultrasound.

Screening mammography remains the gold standard for breast cancer detection; however, due to its limitations, researchers have explored computational tools to enhance its sensitivity. Notably, many applications of GAs in radiology have been primarily centered on breast cancer screening, particularly using mammography.

For instance, one study applied GAs to detect microcalcifications in mammograms as potential indicators of breast cancer [27]. Their approach involved enhancing and normalizing mammograms, detecting the breast border and nipple position using GAs, aligning and subtracting the mammogram images, and identifying asymmetry suggestive of breast cancer [28]. Their proposed algorithm achieved a high AZ value, a metric that assesses diagnostic performance.

In another study, a set of computational tools were applied to segment mammograms to enhance breast cancer detection. Their algorithm removed artifacts, denoised images, and enhanced them. Combining wavelet analysis with GAs allowed for the detection and segmentation of suspicious areas with a 95% sensitivity rate. Mewada et al. [29] presented the integration of Fuzzy Logic with wavelet to extract regions of interest from medical images with an accuracy level of 99%. GAs have also been successfully employed for classifying and detecting clustered microcalcifications in digital mammograms.

A treatment strategy must take precise tumor staging into account. For tumor staging, precise measurement of tumor size and volume utilizing noninvasive imaging techniques becomes crucial. A technique for extracting tongue cancer from head and neck MRIs was developed. To decrease the amount of false positive findings, a symmetry-detection technique based on artificial neural networks (ANN) was used after a GA to segment the pictures. This method has a high degree of user independence and was able to accurately extract a tongue cancer diagnosis from an MRI.

12.2.3.2 Oncology

Massive gene expression profiling has been made possible by the development of DNA microarrays, which have the potential to completely change the area of molecular diagnosis and prognosis. Finding important prognostic genes is necessary due to the statistical and analytical difficulties associated with the development of big data sets. GAs have been used to analyze microarray data from various cancer cell lines because of their intrinsic capacity to explore and select the best answer among many different, complicated, and large-scale alternatives.

An investigation was carried out to examine the correlation between soil trace elements and cervical cancer mortality in China [30]. The researchers employed a combination of Genetic Algorithm (GA) and partial least squares (PLS) to select five trace elements out of a total of 25. Subsequently, a model based on the least squares support vector machine (LSSVM), a machine learning technique used for pattern recognition, was developed. The study's findings indicated that the use of GA-PLS in conjunction with LSSVM could effectively predict cervical cancer mortality based on trace elements [30].

Another critical factor influencing the choice of an appropriate treatment approach for cancer patients is the determination of disease prognosis. In a retrospective study involving more than 200 patients, the study compared the performance of four different data mining methods in predicting outcomes for nonterminal cancer patients following hospitalization [31]. Notably, the Genetic Algorithm (GA) was able to achieve accurate predictions while selecting the fewest explanatory variables, including lactate dehydrogenase levels and the reason for admission.

12.2.4 Neural Network and Genetic Algorithm Systems (NNGA)

One of the various analytical methods for data mining that may be used to develop predictions for medical data is neural networks. The best amount of hidden nodes to use, the right input variables, and the right connection weights are just a few of the criteria that go into choosing a model for a neural network. In the realm of medicine, neural networks and Genetic Algorithms are effective instruments with a wide range of uses. Here are some significant uses of Genetic Algorithms and neural network technology in medicine.

12.2.4.1 Endocrinology

Hypoglycemia is a common complication in patients with type 1 diabetes mellitus (T1DM) who undergo insulin therapy. It can lead to changes in electroencephalogram (EEG) patterns. To detect hypoglycemia using EEG signals, Nguyen and colleagues [32] employed a combination of artificial neural networks (ANNs), Genetic Algorithms (GAs), and Levenberg–Marquardt (LM) training techniques. ANNs were utilized to model the relationship between blood glucose levels and EEG signals. They trained the ANN using a combination of GA's global search capability and LM's local search ability. By analyzing data from four EEG parameters obtained from two EEG channels, the system achieved a hypoglycemia detection sensitivity of 75% and a specificity of 60%.

In another study focusing on detecting noninvasive episodes of nocturnal hypoglycemia in children with T1DM, researchers developed a system based on Genetic Algorithms (GA) and multiple regression with a fuzzy inference system [33]. The system used parameters such as heart rate and corrected QT interval to identify hypoglycemia, achieving a sensitivity of 75% and a specificity exceeding 50%.

Regarding cancer prognosis, a retrospective study involving over 200 patients was conducted by Bozcuk and colleagues [34]. The study compared the performance of four different data mining methods in predicting outcomes for nonterminal cancer patients after hospitalization. Notably, Genetic Algorithms (GA) were able to predict patient outcomes with the fewest explanatory variables, specifically lactate dehydrogenase levels and the reason for admission.

12.2.4.2 Surgery

Artificial neural networks (ANNs) are robust mathematical algorithms capable of forecasting system behavior. To enhance predictive accuracy, a Genetic-Algorithm-based ANN (GANN) was devised for forecasting surgical outcomes in patients with non-small cell lung cancer (NSCLC). Genetic Algorithms (GAs) were integrated into the model to optimize the process and avoid getting trapped in local minima [35]. Notably, the GANN model demonstrated superior predictive capabilities compared to logistic regression, particularly when tumor size was incorporated into the calculations. This enhanced the accuracy of predicting outcomes for NSCLC patients.

As the elderly population grows, an increasing number of geriatric patients require cardiac surgeries. Given the prevalence of comorbid conditions in this demographic, accurate prognostication of post-operative morbidity and mortality is crucial. It helps prevent the overestimation of risk, ensuring that deserving patients do not face surgery denials. In this context, the study utilized a Genetic Algorithm (GA) to reveal that a shorter post-surgery stay was associated with younger age, the absence of pre-operative beta blocker use, shorter cross-clamp times, and the absence of congestive heart failure.

Pulmonology

In the field of pulmonology, auscultation serves as the primary diagnostic method for distinguishing between various lung diseases and directing the diagnostic process toward more specialized techniques. To automate the diagnosis of lung sounds, a hybrid Genetic-Algorithm-based artificial neural network (GANN) was created [35]. The Genetic Algorithm (GA) was utilized to fine-tune the training parameters of the ANN, thereby decreasing computational time. This novel system was capable of categorizing lung sounds into three categories: normal, wheeze, and crackle.

12.2.4.3 Infectious Diseases

Tuberculosis is a potentially fatal infectious disease that poses a threat not only in developing regions but also in developed countries, particularly with the advent of the human immunodeficiency virus (HIV). To forecast the diagnosis, distinguishing between tuberculosis and non-tuberculosis patients, a combination of 38 parameters including examination parameters and laboratory data, was employed to construct an artificial neural network (ANN) trained with the assistance of a Genetic Algorithm (GA) [36]. The system achieved an impressive classification accuracy of approximately 95%, surpassing the results obtained through alternative algorithms.

12.2.4.4 Neurology

Multiple sclerosis (MS) is a debilitating inflammatory neural system disorder characterized by the development of white matter scars, known as plaques. Computer-assisted diagnostic methods have been employed to identify pathological features in MS patients. In one study, a Genetic Algorithm (GA) was developed to detect brain lesions associated with MS in MRI scans. The GA-based lesion detection system achieved an 87% similarity index when compared to a radiologist's assessment [37].

Electroencephalography (EEG) serves as a valuable diagnostic tool for identifying abnormal brain electrical activity during seizures. To create an automated system for detecting anomalous EEG signals, various learning algorithms were utilized to train an artificial neural network (ANN) for classifying individuals as epileptic or healthy based on their EEG data. A Genetic Algorithm (GA) was used to optimize the ANN's parameters and architecture. Among the algorithms tested, the combination of the LM method with the GA proved to be the most effective, achieving a 96.5% overall accuracy [38].

There have been suggestions that mitochondrial dysfunction is a significant factor in Parkinson's disease. Given the unique nature of mitochondrial genetics, a straightforward comparison of mitochondrial mutations between healthy and diseased conditions may not provide informative results. Therefore, Smigrodzki and colleagues [39] developed a Genetic Algorithm (GA) to identify biologically significant patterns of mitochondrial mutations in Parkinson's patients. This approach successfully diagnosed Parkinson's disease with 100% accuracy based on mutational patterns in mitochondrial DNA.

12.2.5 Big Data Analysis Tools

These methods are often used to handle the important information from large datasets, which makes it easier to quickly discover approximate data particular to a given patient. A small number of software tools are used with numerous analytical models using predictive analytics, data extraction, text analysis, and statistical analysis to help the healthcare system make timely patient decisions. To address diversity concerns in healthcare, health data analytical techniques are therefore required. A few issues facing the healthcare system are:

1. Identifying many illness aspects through the BDA-inclined system;
2. Creating various BDA tools and a data-analytic environment that aids in advancing the system's performance;
3. Creating BDA diversity stages with essential components;
4. To discuss the various obstacles and diverse disease characteristics with patients in the clinical system to find potential solutions to the character alterations.

12.2.6 Augmented Artificial Intelligence Approach for Disease Prediction

Based on the patient data that is now accessible, artificial intelligence approaches are employed to anticipate illnesses. While doctors and testing facilities are needed for medical diagnosis, artificial-intelligence-based predictive technologies are utilized to identify illnesses before they manifest. Artificial intelligence (AI) is based on biological processes, particularly input processing approaches developed in the human brain. AI is capable of learning, processing inputs, recognizing patterns, predicting, and making decisions. AI techniques are typically classified into supervised and unsupervised learning. In supervised learning, data must be trained on datasets with desired outputs to construct a model that can be used to make predictions in the future. Unsupervised learning involves combining similar data points into clusters, each of which is composed of data points that share similar characteristics. In supervised learning, classification and regression are used to predict final class labels containing positive and negative outcomes. Classification algorithms are employed to construct a predictive model from historical data and classify classes of unlabeled data.

12.2.6.1 Classification-Method-Based Systems

A straightforward data mining technique called classification divides the sample items into target categories to guarantee that each item corresponds to its group or as accurately as possible. The two main categories of classification methodology are binary classification and multilayer classification. The information set for classification is split into training and test sets. The training set is used to create the model, while the test set is used to measure the model's accuracy and verify the training model. One of the often employed models suited to medical data mining is the classification model. Figure 12.5 presents an ANN-based disease classification algorithm.

Classification algorithms can be used for a variety of applications. For instance, instead of using cardiac signals, a system for the automated diagnosis of healthy and coronary artery disease (CAD) situations was developed [40]. Using the discrete wavelet transform (DWT), the cardiac signals are connected to various frequency sub-bands. Three statistical techniques are therefore used with the set of DWT coefficients to extract the cardiac signal from DWT and to decrease the dimension of data. Additionally, a collection of four classifiers, including the support vector machine (SVM), probabilistic neural network (PNN), Gaussian mixture model (GMM), and K-nearest neighbor (KNN), are applied to the normalized data before being used in decision-making. The outcomes show that the GMM model in combination with ICA offers a greater accuracy rate. Researchers [41] have also created a BPSO-, GA-, and SVM-based classification model based on stress testing data to enhance the classification performance of coronary artery disease. To find the appropriate collection of characteristics to forecast coronary artery disease, the BPSO and GA approaches are used. SVM, on the other hand, is used as a classifier method to categorize patients with CAD. The SVM classifier incorporates the 10 cross-fold approach to improve the diagnosis rate. The suggested categorization model, according to the results, has a greater accuracy rate and is less complicated.

Another example of classification-based intelligent systems relates to the advancements achieved in the field of testing one's sugar levels. A hybrid prediction model is developed for diabetic illness to efficiently predict type 2 diabetes and examine the features of diabetic individuals [42]. The diabetes dataset's class labels are validated using the K-means clustering technique [42,43], and the traditional C4.5 approach is used to produce the final classifier utilizing the k-fold cross-validation method. The

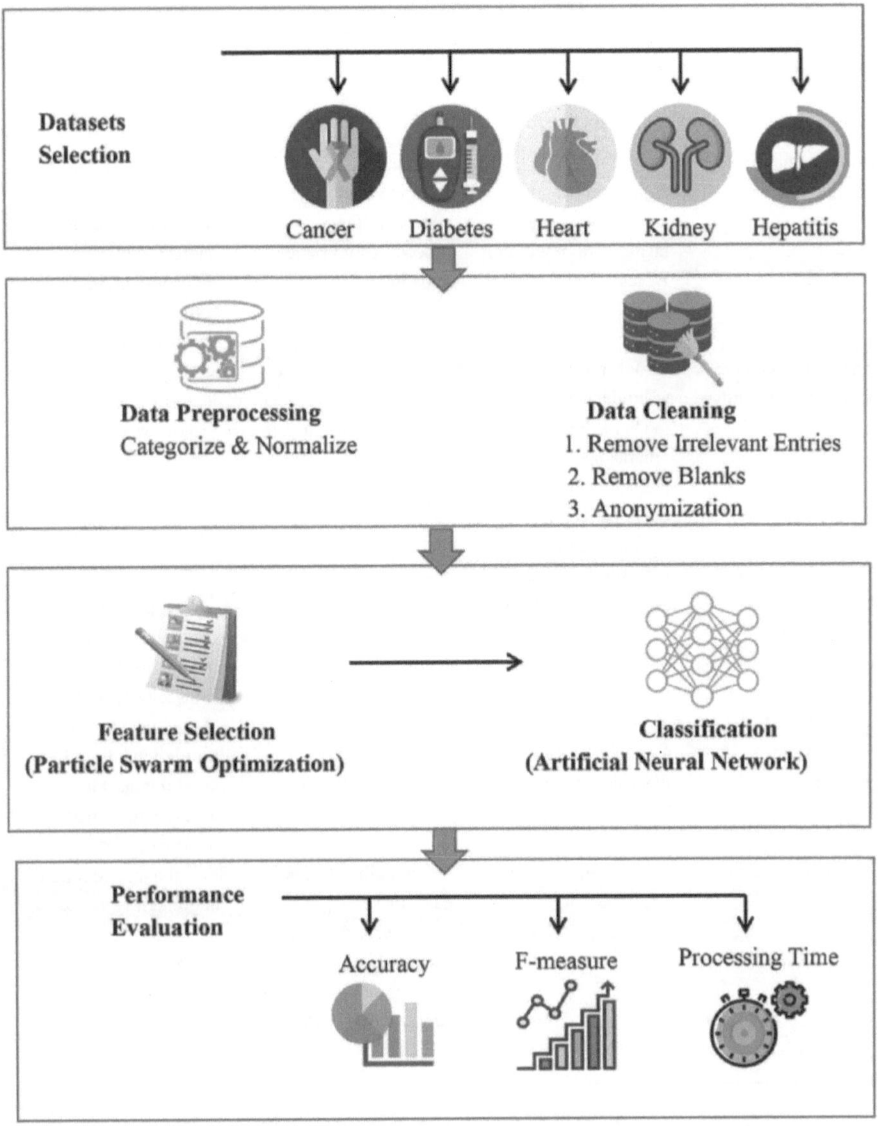

FIGURE 12.5 Augmented artificial intelligence approach for chronic diseases prediction.

suggested approach, according to the results, achieves greater sensitivity and specificity rates than other systems.

Additionally developed is an intelligent hepatitis diagnosis system for the care and treatment of hepatitis patients. Early hepatitis C diagnosis is now achievable without incurring medical costs because of artificial intelligence. The characteristic extraction and reduction portion of the suggested diagnostic system's operation is split into two portions, along with the categorization of the hepatitis illness. First, features are retrieved from the hepatitis database in the feature extraction and reduction

TABLE 12.3
The State-of-the-Art AI Platforms

Technical Items	Objectives	Technical Approach	AI and ML
Artificial intelligent-based medicine	Lessen recurring assignments and troubles with digital health data based on AI and ML	Development of computerization with advanced image procedures for better updating	Use deep convolutional neural network (CNN) for several detection such as skin cancer detection, diabetic retinopathy, oral anticoagulants, etc.
Exactitude medicine with digital records	Use ML for the EHRs to produce individual medicine based on reliable possible predictors and that fits in patient's treatment and prevention of disease	Explain samples of the population for medical phenotypes of intricate disease	Encompasses supervised learning and unsupervised learning
Use knowledge-based ML on ontology in medicine	Test several aspects of medicine such as phenotype categories, statistical analysis	Create database on existing phenotypes, details of patient records	Use ML platform for creating statistical models for phenotype categories and disease
Approaches of AI, BDA on cancer diseases	Use of AI and huge amount of data for identification of cancer and cure	Use the cognitive methodology for cancer identification of cancer and cure	A cognitive approach through the digital system makes for accurate information and treatment procedures
BDA in healthcare	Use BDA in healthcare	The intangible design of BDA makes multisource data input with analysis of existing query language with data extraction	Several data extraction approaches and their analysis

section. Then, using the PCA approach, the more pertinent features are obtained. The LSSVM classifier is used on a smaller collection of features in the classification stage to provide final findings. It has been shown that the PCA-LSSVM-based diagnostic method increases sensitivity and specificity rates as well as the accuracy rate of hepatitis illness [44].

The prevalence of breast cancer is on the rise in Europe and Asia and has become the most common type of cancer among women, resulting in a 15% mortality rate [45]. Diagnosis of breast cancer is a two-step process: screening and early detection. It is essential to accurately predict the presence of breast cancer to provide the necessary medical care and treatment. Many researchers are contributing to the prevention and early detection of breast cancer [46]. Breast cancer has become the second most common cancer among women, necessitating the development of a predictive analysis model to identify the presence of cancer in its earliest stages. Early detection of breast cancer will result in the provision of timely treatment, thus reducing the risk of mortality. Additionally, web-based systems can reduce the cost of laboratory experiments, thus being beneficial to both patients and medical staff. Furthermore, advances in medical database systems enable the generation of vast amounts of data that cannot be processed by humans, along with the utilization of artificial intelligence to extract patterns in vast datasets and to identify labels for patient disease diagnosis. Table 12.3 shows the state-of-the-art platforms for the AI enabled Healthcare.

12.3 CONCLUSION

In healthcare, intellectual approaches play a pivotal role in many clinical breakthroughs through research and analytics. Over the past ten years, several research-based healthcare data management systems have been developed in the business and education sectors. The comprehensive solutions are implemented in the healthcare system's data analytics process, including managing multiple features, updating and distributing EHR forms, automating patient data, appointment scheduling, reporting from multiple lab tests, accurate diagnosis, treatment planning, ongoing testing for improvement, appropriate medication, surgical action plans, and claims, and supporting AI techniques for the creation of classifiers in the medical decision-making process. These days, artificial intelligence is being used more and more to analyze data in the medical field.

REFERENCES

[1] Basu K, Sinha R, Ong A, et al. Artificial intelligence: How is it changing medical sciences and its future? *Indian Journal of Dermatology*. 2020;65(5):365.

[2] Zerbino P, Stefanini A, Aloini D. Process science in action: A literature review on process mining in business management. *Technological Forecasting and Social Change*. 2021;172:121021.

[3] Wang Y, Hajli N. Exploring the path to big data analytics success in healthcare. *Journal of Business Research*. 2017;70:287–299.

[4] Hoekstra O, Hurst W, Tummers J. Healthcare related event prediction from textual data with machine learning: A systematic literature review. *Healthcare Analytics*. 2022; 2:100107.

[5] Pham T, Tran T, Phung D, et al. Predicting healthcare trajectories from medical records: A deep learning approach. *Journal of Biomedical Informatics*. 2017;69:218–229.

[6] Pfeiffer DU, Stevens KB. Spatial and temporal epidemiological analysis in the big data era. *Preventive Veterinary Medicine*. 2015;122(1–2):213–220.

[7] Vedula SS, Ishii M, Hager GD. Objective assessment of surgical technical skill and competency in the operating room. *Annual Review of Biomedical Engineering*. 2017; 19:301–325.

[8] Neubert S, Geißler A, Roddelkopf T, et al. Multi-sensor-fusion approach for a data-science-oriented preventive health management system: Concept and development of a decentralized data collection approach for heterogeneous data sources. *International Journal of Telemedicine and Applications*. 2019;2019.

[9] Neubert P, Weichselbaum A, Reitinger C, et al. HIF1A and NFAT5 coordinate Na+-boosted antibacterial defense via enhanced autophagy and autolysosomal targeting. *Autophagy*. 2019;15(11):1899–1916.

[10] Chen N, Zhou M, Dong X, et al. Epidemiological and clinical characteristics of 99 cases of 2019 novel coronavirus pneumonia in Wuhan, China: A descriptive study. *The Lancet*. 2020;395(10223):507–513.

[11] Crocamo C, Viviani M, Bartoli F, et al. Detecting binge drinking and alcohol-related risky behaviours from twitter's users: An exploratory content-and topology-based analysis. *International Journal of Environmental Research and Public Health*. 2020;17(5):1510.

[12] Liang W, Duan Y, Yang M, et al. Behavioral and mental responses towards the COVID-19 pandemic among chinese older adults: A cross-sectional study. *Journal of Risk and Financial Management*. 2021;14(12):568.

[13] Chatterjee A, Gerdes MW, Martinez SG. Statistical explorations and univariate time-series analysis on COVID-19 datasets to understand the trend of disease spreading and death. *Sensors*. 2020;20(11):3089.

[14] Idrees M, Sohail A. Bio-algorithms for the modeling and simulation of cancer cells and the immune response. *Bio-Algorithms and Med-Systems*. 2021;17(1):55–63.

[15] Quarteroni A, Manzoni A, Vergara C, et al. *Mathematical modelling of the human cardiovascular system: Data, numerical approximation, clinical applications*. Vol. 33. Cambridge University Press; 2019.

[16] Sikchi SS, Sikchi S, Ali M. Fuzzy Expert Systems (FES) for medical diagnosis. *International Journal of Computer Applications*. 2013;63(11).

[17] Srivel R, Kalaiselvi K, Shanthi S, et al. An automation query expansion strategy for information retrieval by using fuzzy based grasshopper optimization algorithm on medical datasets. *Concurrency and Computation: Practice and Experience*. 2023;35 (3):e7418.

[18] Association IRM, et al. *Medical imaging: Concepts, methodologies, tools, and applications*. IGI Global; 2016.

[19] Myrzakerimova A, Kolesnikova K, Nurmaganbetova M. Use of mathematical modeling tools to support decision-making in medicine. *Procedia Computer Science*. 2024;231:335–340.

[20] Shaikh F, Rao D. Prediction of cancer disease using machine learning approach. *Materials Today: Proceedings*. 2022;50:40–47.

[21] Mewada H, Al-Asad JF, Patel A, et al. Multi-channel local binary pattern guided convolutional neural network for breast cancer classification. *The Open Biomedical Engineering Journal*. 2021;15(1).

[22] Mewada H. 2D-wavelet encoded deep CNN for image-based ECG classification. *Multimedia Tools and Applications*. 2023:1–17.

[23] Habib S, Shahzadi S, Deveci M. Pythagorean fuzzy cognitive analysis for medical care and treatment decisions. *Granular Computing*. 2023;8(6):1887–1906.

[24] Subramani S, Selvi M. Intrusion detection system using RBPSO and fuzzy neuro-genetic classification algorithms in wireless sensor networks. *International Journal of Information and Computer Security*. 2023;20(3–4):439–461.

[25] Chaudhari SV, Sasikala T, Gnanamurthy R, et al. Optimizing plant disease prediction: A neuro-fuzzy-genetic algorithm approach. *ICTACT Journal on Soft Computing*. 2023; 14(2).

[26] Barakat T, Elbadwey M, Ibrahim KH. Early classification of brain tumor based on image histogram using fuzzy-genetic algorithm. *Fayoum University Journal of Engineering*. 2021;4(1):166–174.

[27] Kaur H, Virmani J, Thakur S, et al. A genetic algorithm-based metaheuristic approach to customize a computer-aided classification system for enhanced screen film mammograms. In: *U-healthcare monitoring systems*. Elsevier; 2019. pp. 217–259.

[28] Mustra M, Grgic M, Rangayyan RM. Review of recent advances in segmentation of the breast boundary and the pectoral muscle in mammograms. *Medical & Biological Engineering & Computing*. 2016;54:1003–1024.

[29] Mewada H, Patel AV, Chaudhari J, et al. Composite fuzzy-wavelet-based active contour for medical image segmentation. *Engineering Computations*. 2020;37(9):3525–3541.

[30] Tan C, Chen H, Wu T, et al. Modeling the relationship between cervical cancer mortality and trace elements based on genetic algorithm–partial least squares and support vector machines. *Biological Trace Element Research*. 2011;140:24–34.

[31] Diz J, Marreiros G, Freitas A. Applying data mining techniques to improve breast cancer diagnosis. *Journal of Medical Systems*. 2016;40:1–7.

[32] Nguyen HT, Jones TW. Detection of nocturnal hypoglycemic episodes using EEG signals. In: *2010 Annual International Conference of the IEEE Engineering in Medicine and Biology*; IEEE; 2010. pp. 4930–4933.

[33] Ling SS, Nguyen HT. Genetic-algorithm-based multiple regression with fuzzy inference system for detection of nocturnal hypoglycemic episodes. *IEEE Transactions on Information Technology in Biomedicine*. 2011;15(2):308–315.

[34] Bozcuk H, Bilge U, Koyuncu E, et al. An application of a genetic algorithm in conjunction with other data mining methods for estimating outcome after hospitalization in cancer patients. *Medical Science Monitor*. 2004;10(6):251.

[35] Pfeffer MA, Ling SH. Evolving optimised convolutional neural networks for lung cancer classification. *Signals*. 2022;3(2):284–295.

[36] Hrizi O, Gasmi K, Ben Ltaifa I, et al. Tuberculosis disease diagnosis based on an optimized machine learning model. *Journal of Healthcare Engineering*. 2022;2022.

[37] Khotanlou H, Afrasiabi M. Feature selection in order to extract multiple sclerosis lesions automatically in 3D brain magnetic resonance images using combination of support vector machine and genetic algorithm. *Journal of Medical Signals and Sensors*. 2012;2(4):211.

[38] Koçer S, Canal MR. Classifying epilepsy diseases using artificial neural networks and genetic algorithm. *Journal of Medical Systems*. 2011;35:489–498.

[39] Smigrodzki R, Goertzel B, Pennachin C, et al. Genetic algorithm for analysis of mutations in Parkinson's disease. *Artificial Intelligence in Medicine*. 2005;35(3):227–241.

[40] Giri D, Acharya UR, Martis RJ, et al. Automated diagnosis of coronary artery disease affected patients using LDA, PCA, ICA and discrete wavelet transform. *Knowledge-Based Systems*. 2013;37:274–282.

[41] Babaoglu İ, Findik O, Ülker E. A comparison of feature selection models utilizing binary particle swarm optimization and genetic algorithm in determining coronary artery disease using support vector machine. *Expert Systems with Applications*. 2010;37(4):3177–3183.

[42] Patil BM, Joshi RC, Toshniwal D. Hybrid prediction model for type-2 diabetic patients. *Expert Systems With Applications*. 2010;37(12):8102–8108.

[43] Krishna BV, AP B, HL G, et al. A novel application of k-means cluster prediction model for diabetes early identification using dimensionality reduction techniques. *The Open Bioinformatics Journal*. 2023;16(1).

[44] Çalişir D, Dogantekin E. A new intelligent hepatitis diagnosis system: PCA–LSSVM. *Expert Systems with Applications*. 2011;38(8):10705–10708.

[45] Abdel-Rahman O. Incidence and predictors of 1-year mortality among 9236 breast cancer patients referred for adjuvant chemotherapy. *Future Oncology*. 2018;14(23):2335–2341.

[46] Mewada HK, Patel AV, Hassaballah M, et al. Spectral–spatial features integrated convolution neural network for breast cancer classification. *Sensors*. 2020;20(17):4747.

Part V

IoMT Applications and Its Future Trends for AI, Augmented Reality, and Edge Computing

13 Sentiment Analysis and Social Media Analysis for IoMT-Enabled Data

Bhumika Rupchandani, Neel H. Dholakia, Kirtirajsinh Zala, Hiren Kumar Thakkar, and Saurav Mallik

13.1 INTRODUCTION

13.1.1 User Feedback and Product Improvements

One of the main importance of sentiment analysis and social media analysis in the context of IoMT-enabled data is the ability to collect user feedback and opinions and use it to improve the product. This feedback loop is invaluable to IoMT device manufacturers, healthcare providers, and medical application developers. Let me explain what this means in more detail.

13.1.1.1 User-Centric Product Development

IoMT technology is designed to improve patient care, enhance healthcare delivery, and streamline healthcare processes. To effectively achieve these goals, it is important to tailor the development of IoMT devices and applications to the needs and preferences of end users, often patients, healthcare providers, and caregivers [2]. Sentiment analysis and social media analysis provide direct communication with these users.

13.1.1.2 User Experience Capture

Social media platforms, health forums, and online reviews provide users with the opportunity to share their IoMT devices and application experiences. Sentiment analysis allows you to systematically collect this user-generated content and classify it as positive, negative, or neutral. In addition to the atmosphere, you can gain valuable insights from the text: for example, specific features that users appreciate or find problematic, the quality of customer support, and suggestions for improvement.

13.1.1.3 Iterative Development

Leveraging the results of sentiment analysis, IoMT developers can iterate their products to address vulnerabilities and improve popular features. For example, if

DOI: 10.1201/9781003393498-18

sentiment analysis reveals repeated complaints about the usability of a mobile app on a particular IoMT device, developers can focus on improving the app's interface and functionality in subsequent updates.

13.1.1.4 Competitive Advantage

User sentiment analysis not only helps in the further development of existing products but also provides a competitive advantage. By understanding what users value most in their IoMT solutions and what shortcomings they perceive in competitors' products, companies can adapt their marketing strategies and product development efforts to better serve their users. They can more than meet users' expectations.

13.1.1.5 Compliance and Data Security

Aside from product-related feedback, sentiment analysis can also help organizations ensure compliance with healthcare regulations, especially those related to data security and patient protection. Negative sentiment about data breaches [3] and privacy concerns can lead to proactive actions to address the problem and strengthen security measures.

13.2 SENTIMENT ANALYSIS AND SOCIAL MEDIA ANALYSIS FOR IOMT-ENABLED DATA

The Internet of Medical Things (IoMT) is a rapidly growing field that uses connected medical devices and applications to collect and analyze health data. As IoMT technology becomes more widespread, it becomes increasingly important to understand public sentiment and social media discussions about it. Social media analysis [4] and sentiment analysis are useful techniques for learning about the attitudes, feelings, and patterns around IoMT-enabled data.

13.2.1 Sentiment Analysis Methods

Sentiment analysis methods will be discussed next:

1. Rule-based approaches
2. Machine learning algorithms
3. Hybrid approaches
4. Aspect-based sentiment analysis
5. Emotion analysis

13.2.2 Social Media Analysis Techniques

Social media analysis techniques will be discussed next:

1. Natural language processing (NLP)
2. Topic modeling
3. Social network analysis (SNA)

4. Time-series analysis
5. Geospatial analysis
6. User profiling
7. Sentiment propagation
8. Influencer identification
9. Sentiment visualization

13.3 SENTIMENT ANALYSIS METHODS

13.3.1 Rule-Based Approaches

As shown in Figure 13.1, to ascertain the sentiment represented in text data, rule-based techniques in sentiment analysis rely on established sets of rules, lexicons, and patterns. When you have well-defined sentiment indicators and need a clear, understandable technique to assess sentiment, these methods are quite helpful.

Rule-based techniques can assist in extracting sentiments from user reviews, social media posts, or comments regarding medical equipment and healthcare apps in the context of IoMT-enabled data. This discussion will provide a detailed explanation of rule-based sentiment analysis, including examples, diagrams, figures, and tables, along with flowcharts illustrating the process.

13.3.1.1 Rule-Based Sentiment Analysis: Overview

Rule-based sentiment analysis [5] typically involves the following steps:

1. **Text Preprocessing**: In the rule-based text preprocess, the text is converted to lowercase text, followed by word tokenization and punctuation removal. Preprocessing removes the unwanted tokens from the word and thereby reduces the processing requirement and improves the accuracy.

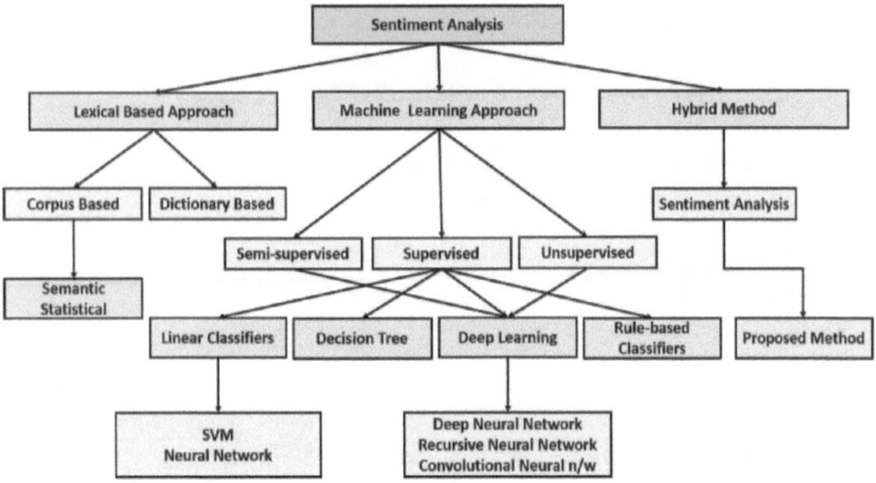

FIGURE 13.1 Sentiment analysis methods.

2. **Lexicon-Based Sentiment Analysis**: In lexicon-based sentiment analysis, the model uses the dictionaries with polarity lexicons that contain words and phrases representing the tones of the words in either neutral, positive, or negative emotions. Depending on the frequency of the words in the text, each lexicon will be given the sentiment score.
3. **Scoring and Aggregation**: In the scoring and aggregations, the overall score is calculated to rank the sentiment ratings of individual words or phrases followed by summing the score to obtain the overall sentiment polarity of the text. Various aggregation techniques can be used to calculate the overall sentiment polarity, such as assigning sentiment rank, and average the sentiment rank across the words and phrases.
4. **Thresholding**: To categorize the sentiment of any text as good, negative, or neutral, a thresholding mechanism can be applied to the overall emotion score. For example, the text can be categorized with a positive, negative, or neutral score against the set threshold value.

13.3.1.2 Example: Rule-Based Sentiment Analysis

An example of rule-based sentiment analysis on a user review of an IoMT-enabled wearable fitness tracker is as follows.

> The fitness tracker app is really awesome and helpful to know the fitness on the regular basis! It's so accurate and has helped me stay motivated to exercise every day.
>
> The battery life is excellent, and the [6] app is user-friendly.

13.3.1.2.1 Step 1: Text Preprocessing

Remove punctuation and convert to lowercase:

> i absolutely love my new fitness tracker its so accurate and has helped me stay motivated to exercise every day the battery life is excellent and the app is user friendly

Tokenize the text into words:

> ["I," "absolutely," "love," "my," "new," "fitness," "tracker," . . .]

13.3.1.2.2 Step 2: Lexicon-Based Sentiment Analysis

Assign sentiment scores using a lexicon:

> "love" → +1
> "accurate" → +1
> "motivated" → +1
> "excellent" → +1
> "user-friendly" → +1

13.3.1.2.3 Step 3: Scoring and Aggregation

Sum the sentiment scores: 1 + 1 + 1 + 1 + 1 = 5

13.3.1.2.4 Step 4: Thresholding

Set a threshold (e.g., 3) to classify sentiment:
Since the score (5) is above the threshold, classify the review as "positive."

13.3.1.3 Summary Table

Table 13.1 summarizes sentiment scores for some example words. In this table, positive words receive positive scores, while negative words receive negative scores.

13.3.1.4 Conclusion

Rule-based methods for sentiment analysis provide clarity and simplicity. Even though they might not be able to catch subtleties in language, they are important for rapid, understandable sentiment analyses, which can be very helpful in IoMT to measure user satisfaction with healthcare tools and services. To increase accuracy and relevance, lexicons must be regularly updated and expanded.

13.3.2 Machine Learning Algorithms

A potent collection of tools for sentiment analysis, machine learning algorithms are capable of autonomously deriving sentiment patterns from data. We'll examine the use of machine learning algorithms for sentiment analysis in this in-depth presentation, which includes examples, graphs, figures, tables, and flowcharts to help [7] with the technical knowledge of the procedure.

13.3.2.1 Machine Learning Sentiment Analysis: Overview

Machine-learning-based sentiment analysis typically involves the steps shown in Figure 13.2.

TABLE 13.1
Words and Their Sentiment Scores

Word	Sentiment Analysis
Love	+1
Accurate	+1
Motivated	+1
Excellent	+1
User-friendly	+1
Dissapointed	−1
Problems	−1
Frustrating	−1
Glitch	−1
Inaccurate	−1

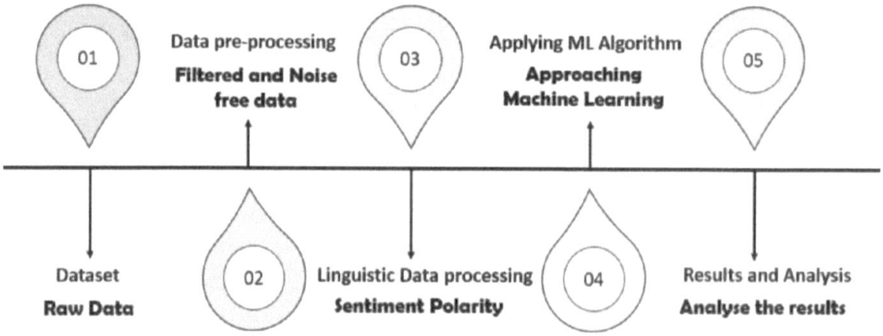

FIGURE 13.2 Steps in machine learning.

- **Data Preprocessing**: Tokenize, remove stop words, and turn words into numerical features by preparing the text data (e.g., using TF-IDF or word embeddings approaches).
- **Feature Extraction**: Identify pertinent aspects in the text data. This could include word embeddings, bag-of-words representations, or more sophisticated techniques like LSTM-based sequences for sequence data.
- **Model Training**: Utilize labeled training data to train a machine learning model, with the labels indicating the text's emotion (positive, negative, or neutral).
- **Model Evaluation**: On a different validation or test dataset, assess the performance of the trained model using measures like accuracy, precision, recall, F_1-score, and confusion matrices.
- **Inference**: To predict sentiment, apply the trained model to fresh, unlabeled input.

13.3.2.2 Example: Machine Learning Sentiment Analysis

Let's take a look at a scenario where sentiment analysis is performed using a machine learning model, more precisely an SVM. We'll make use of a condensed dataset containing the categories "positive" and "negative."

13.3.2.2.1 Step 1: Data Preprocessing

Tokenize the text and remove stop words:

"I love this product" → ["love," "product"]
"This is terrible" → ["terrible"]

13.3.2.2.2 Step 2: Feature Extraction

Convert words into numerical features [7] using a bag-of-words representation:

"love" → [1, 0]
"terrible" → [0,1]

13.3.2.2.3 Step 3: Model Training

Train an SVM classifier on the labeled training data as shown in Table 13.2.

13.3.2.2.4 Step 4: Model Evaluation

Calculate measures like accuracy and produce a confusion matrix to assess the model using a validation dataset.

13.3.2.3 Diagrams and Flowcharts

A simplified flowchart is shown in Figure 13.3, illustrating the process of machine-learning-based sentiment analysis.

13.3.2.4 Model Performance Table

Let's create a table as shown in Table 13.3 showcasing the model's performance on a validation dataset.

TABLE 13.2
Labeled Training Data

Text	Features	Sentiment
"I love this product"	[1,0]	Positive
"This is terrible"	[0,1]	Negative

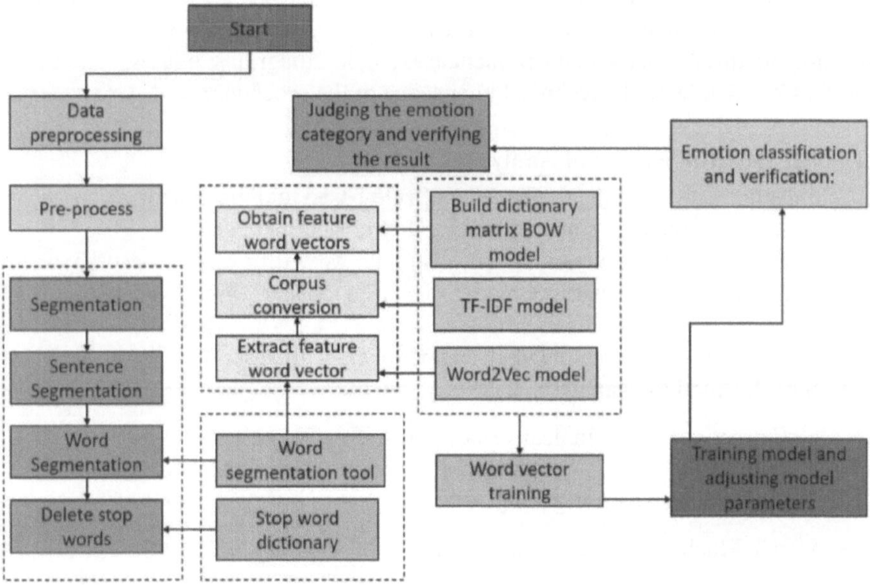

FIGURE 13.3 ML sentiment analysis.

TABLE 13.3
Model's Performance on a Validation Dataset

Metric	Value
Accuracy	0.85
Precision	0.88
Recall	0.82
F_1-score	0.85

13.3.2.5 Conclusion

The capacity of machine learning algorithms to recognize intricate patterns and context in text data has made them the state-of-the-art technique for sentiment analysis. The preceding example showed how to utilize an SVM model, but other algorithms can also be used, including logistic regression, naïve Bayes, and deep learning models like recurrent neural networks (RNNs) and transformers (for example, BERT).

Although machine learning has a high degree of accuracy, it can be difficult to comprehend models because it needs a lot of labeled data for training. However, it continues to be a reliable method for sentiment analysis in the context of IoMT, where it is crucial to comprehend user sentiment toward healthcare applications and devices in order [3] to enhance patient experiences and healthcare results.

13.3.3 Hybrid Approaches

To provide more accurate and nuanced sentiment analysis results, hybrid methodologies combine the benefits of rule-based techniques and machine learning algorithms. We'll examine the use of hybrid methodologies for sentiment analysis in this in-depth discussion, which will include examples, diagrams, figures, tables, and flowcharts to help with the technical knowledge of the procedure.

13.3.3.1 Hybrid Sentiment Analysis: Overview

Hybrid methods [8] combine the benefits of rule-based and machine learning techniques to improve the precision and adaptability of sentiment analysis.

Hybrid Sentiment Analysis: In this example, we will use rule-based keyword extraction and a machine learning model, such as a logistic regression classifier.

- Step 1: Data preprocessing to clean and tokenize the user reviews
- Step 2: Rule-based analysis
  - Extract sentiment-indicative keywords, e.g., "excellent," "poor," "user-friendly," "buggy." Assign sentiment scores to these keywords (e.g., +1 for positive, −1 for negative).
- Step 3: Machine-learning-based analysis
  - Train a logistic regression model using labeled data, where labels indicate sentiment categories (positive, negative, or neutral).

- Step 4: Integration
  - Combine the sentiment scores from the rule-based analysis with the predictions from the machine learning model. Apply a weighting scheme if necessary to prioritize one source of sentiment over the other.
- Step 5: Model evaluation
  - Evaluate the hybrid sentiment analysis model's performance using metrics like accuracy, precision, recall, F_1-score, and confusion matrices [2].

13.3.3.2 Diagrams and Flowcharts

A simplified flowchart is shown in Figure 13.4, illustrating the process of hybrid sentiment analysis.

13.3.3.3 Model Integration Table

Let's create a table as shown in Table 13.4, showcasing how sentiment scores from the rule-based and machine-learning-based analyses are integrated. In this table, sentiment scores from rule-based analysis are combined with predictions from the machine learning model to determine the final sentiment.

13.3.3.4 Summary of Hybrid Approaches

With the use of both rule-based and machine learning techniques, hybrid approaches provide a well-rounded answer to sentiment analysis. When working with complicated text data and when rule-based procedures alone might not be sufficient, they

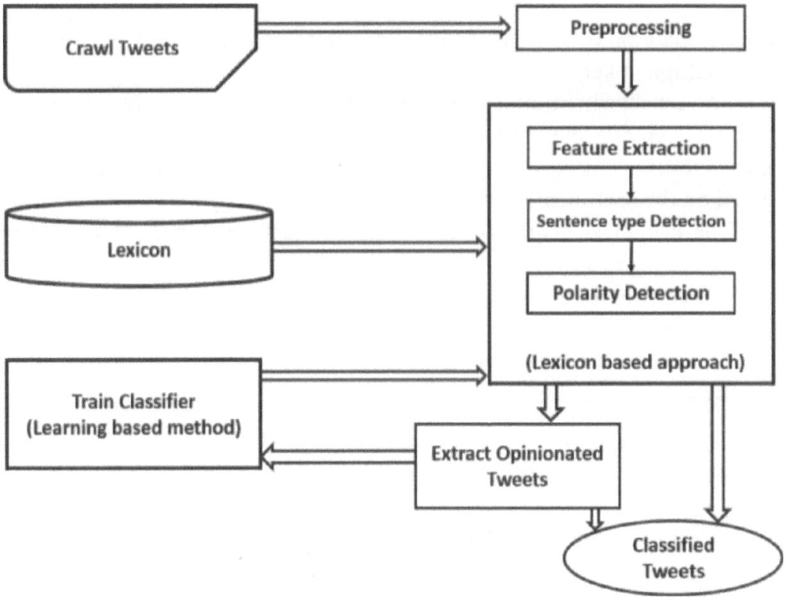

FIGURE 13.4 Workflow for sentiment analysis.

TABLE 13.4
Model Integration Table

Review Text	Rule-Based Score	ML-Predicted Sentiment
"Excellent app"	+1	Positive
"Buggy and Slow"	−1	Negative
"Easy to Use"	+1	Positive

are especially helpful. In the context of IoMT, where healthcare applications and patient experiences are tightly tied to sentiment, hybrid approaches are essential because they combine the capabilities of various methodologies to deliver a more accurate assessment of sentiment.

13.3.4 Aspect-Based Sentiment Analysis

Aspect-based sentiment analysis (ABSA) [9] is a specialized sentiment analysis technique that goes above and beyond traditional sentiment categorization to offer insights into the sentiment expressed toward particular elements or parts of a good, service, or entity. ABSA can be extremely helpful in determining user sentiments toward specific features or elements of healthcare devices and applications when used in conjunction with IoMT-enabled data.

13.3.4.1 Example: Aspect-Based Sentiment Analysis

The following are the steps for aspect-based sentiment analysis:

- Step 1: Data preprocessing cleans the text and tokenizes the user reviews into multiple tokens.
- Step 2: Aspect extraction extracts the specific aspects available in the user reviews such as accuracy, battery life, and user interface.
- Step 3: Sentiment classification involves the classification of each aspect based on the sentiment expressed in the text.
  1. "The accuracy of this tracker is impressive!" → Aspect: Accuracy → Sentiment: Positive
  2. "Battery life drains too quickly." → Aspect: Battery Life → Sentiment: Negative
  3. "The user interface is intuitive and easy to navigate." → Aspect: User Interface → Sentiment: Positive
- Step 4: Aggregation aggregate a sentiment score for each aspect to obtain an overall sentiment assessment for the healthcare application.

13.3.4.2 Diagrams and Flowcharts

A simplified flowchart is shown in Figure 13.5, illustrating the process of aspect-based sentiment analysis:

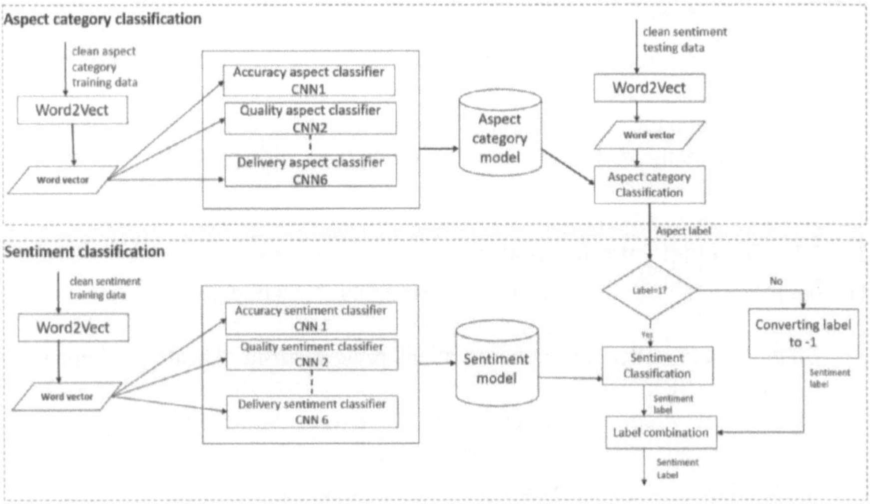

FIGURE 13.5 Flowchart illustrating the process of aspect-based sentiment analysis.

13.3.4.3 Aspect Sentiment Summary Table

Let's create a table as shown in Table 13.5, summarizing the sentiment analysis results for each aspect.

This table provides a clear breakdown of sentiment across different aspects, offering valuable insights into which aspects of the healthcare application are well received and which need improvement.

13.3.4.4 Conclusion

Particularly in the context of IoMT-enabled data, aspect-based sentiment analysis is a useful technique for assessing user sentiment at a detailed level. Organizations can identify areas for improvement, organize development efforts, and enhance user experiences with healthcare applications and devices by concentrating on particular features [3] or elements. ABSA is an effective method for precise sentiment analysis, enabling data-driven choices in the healthcare industry.

TABLE 13.5
Sentiment Analysis Results

Aspect	Positive Reviews	Neutral Reviews	Negative Reviews
Accuracy	30	10	5
Battery life	5	10	20
User interface	25	5	2

13.3.5 Emotion Analysis

Emotion analysis is a method for locating and examining particular emotions represented in text or audio data. It is often referred to as sentiment analysis or affective computing. Emotion analysis [10] offers important insights into the emotional states of patients or users interacting with healthcare devices and applications in the context of IoMT-enabled data.

13.3.5.1 Example: Emotion Analysis

The goal is to classify the emotional state expressed in each review.

- **Step 1**: Data collection gathers patient reviews from a healthcare app's feedback section.
- **Step 2**: Text preprocessing cleans and tokenizes the text data, removing punctuation and stop words. It also performs stemming or lemmatization to reduce words to their base forms.
- **Step 3**: In emotion classification, a machine learning model, such as a deep learning model (e.g., LSTM or BERT), trained on emotion-labeled data, is used to classify each review into specific emotions. For example, a review might be classified as [7] "happy," "neutral," or "sad."

13.3.5.2 Diagrams and Flowcharts

A simplified flowchart is shown in Figure 13.6, illustrating the process of emotion analysis.

13.3.5.3 Emotion Distribution Pie Chart

Let's create a pie chart as shown in Figure 13.7, representing the distribution of emotions in patient reviews. The pie chart in the figure visually displays the prevalence

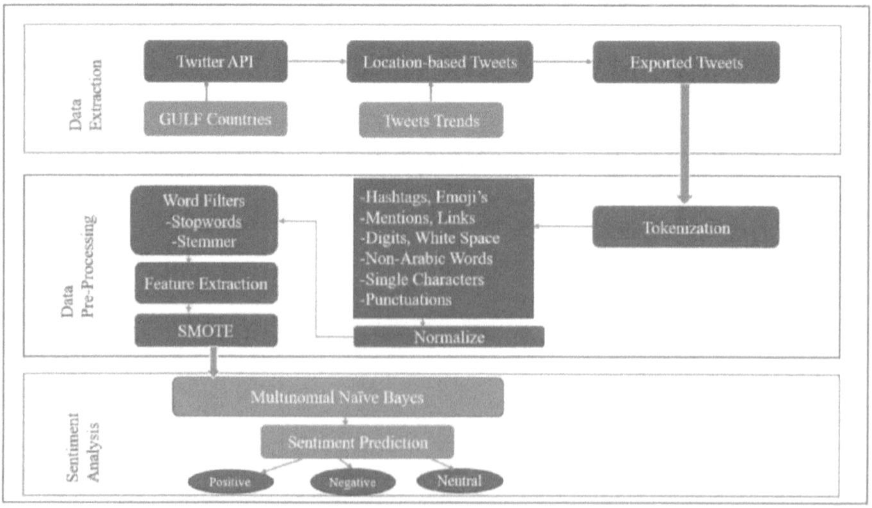

FIGURE 13.6 Flowchart illustrating the process of emotion analysis.

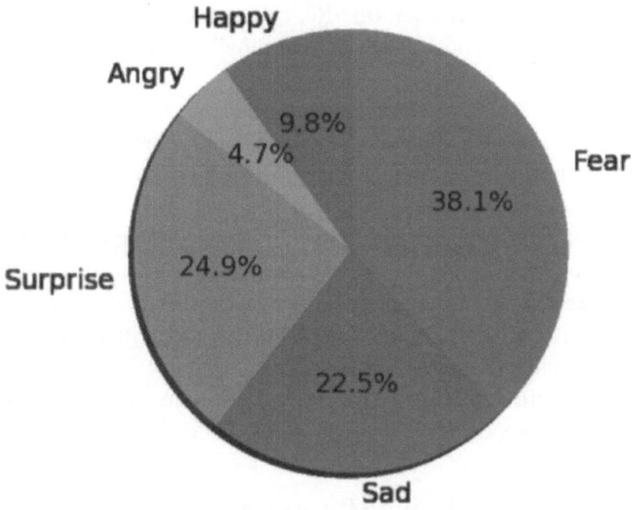

FIGURE 13.7 Patient reviews.

of different emotions among the patient reviews, providing a clear overview of the emotional states expressed by users.

13.3.5.4 Conclusion

Understanding the emotional reactions of patients and users interacting with healthcare devices and applications in the IoMT ecosystem is possible through the use of strong emotion analysis techniques. Organizations can learn a lot about user experiences, spot opportunities for development, and better serve the emotional requirements of their patients by classifying and visualizing the emotions represented in text data. The interpretation of user sentiments in healthcare situations is improved by the addition of emotion analysis to sentiment analysis.

13.4 SOCIAL MEDIA ANALYSIS TECHNIQUES

13.4.1 Natural Language Processing (NLP)

An essential tool for social media analysis, natural language processing (NLP), enables the processing and comprehension of human language in textual information from multiple social media platforms. Insights, mood, and trends can be gleaned from user-generated material and social media interactions thanks to NLP. This in-depth presentation will cover NLP, using examples, diagrams, figures, tables, and flowcharts to help with the technical [5] comprehension of this approach.

13.4.1.1 Natural Language Processing (NLP): Overview

NLP encompasses several techniques and processes used in social media analysis:

1. **Tokenization**: The process of separating text into tokens, or individual words, to enable further analysis

2. **Stemming and Lemmatization**: Reducing words to their root or basic form to manage variations (such as "running" to "run") by stemming and lemmatization
3. **Part-of-Speech Tagging (POS)**: Labeling words in a phrase according to their grammatical parts of speech, such as nouns, verbs, and adjectives
4. **Named Entity Recognition (NER)**: The process of locating and categorizing names, places, and dates in the text
5. Sentiment Analysis: The process of identifying the emotions present in a text and categorizing them as positive, negative, or neutral
6. **Topic Modeling**: Using techniques like latent dirichlet allocation (LDA) or non-negative matrix factorization (NMF), the identification of themes or subjects in a collection of documents
7. **Entity Sentiment Analysis**: Examining the attitudes held toward particular entities (such as goods or businesses) in text data

13.4.2 Example: Social Media NLP Analysis

Let's consider an example of using NLP to analyze Twitter data related to a new IoMT wearable device. We want to understand public sentiment and identify key topics of discussion.

- **Step 1: Data Collection**: Collect a dataset of tweets related to the IoMT device.
- **Step 2: Text Preprocessing**:
    - Tokenize tweets to extract individual words.
    - Perform stemming or lemmatization to standardize words.
    - Remove stop words and punctuation.
- **Step 3: Sentiment Analysis**:
    - Apply sentiment analysis to determine the overall sentiment (positive, negative, or neutral) of each tweet.
    - Classify each tweet as per the sentiment result.
- **Step 4: Topic Modeling**:
    - Apply topic modeling techniques to cluster tweets into common topics or themes.
    - Visualize the topics with word clouds or bar graphs.

13.4.2.1 Diagrams and Flowcharts

A simplified flowchart is shown in Figure 13.8, illustrating the NLP process for social media analysis.

13.4.2.2 Conclusion

NLP is a fundamental method for social media analysis that enables businesses to glean insightful information from textual data. It assists in tracking trends, acquiring a thorough understanding of user preferences and opinions, and interpreting public mood in the context of IoMT. Organizations may improve their IoMT solutions and customize them to user needs by processing and analyzing social media data. Effective social [6] media analysis is built on the flexible tool of NLP.

13.4.3 Topic Modeling

In social media analysis, topic modeling is a potent method for finding underlying themes, topics, or patterns in massive collections of textual data. Understanding the major topics of conversation and finding hidden insights in social media chats are particularly advantageous uses of it. Topic modeling will be covered in detail in this in-depth talk, along with examples, diagrams, figures, tables, and flowcharts to help with the technical understanding of this technique.

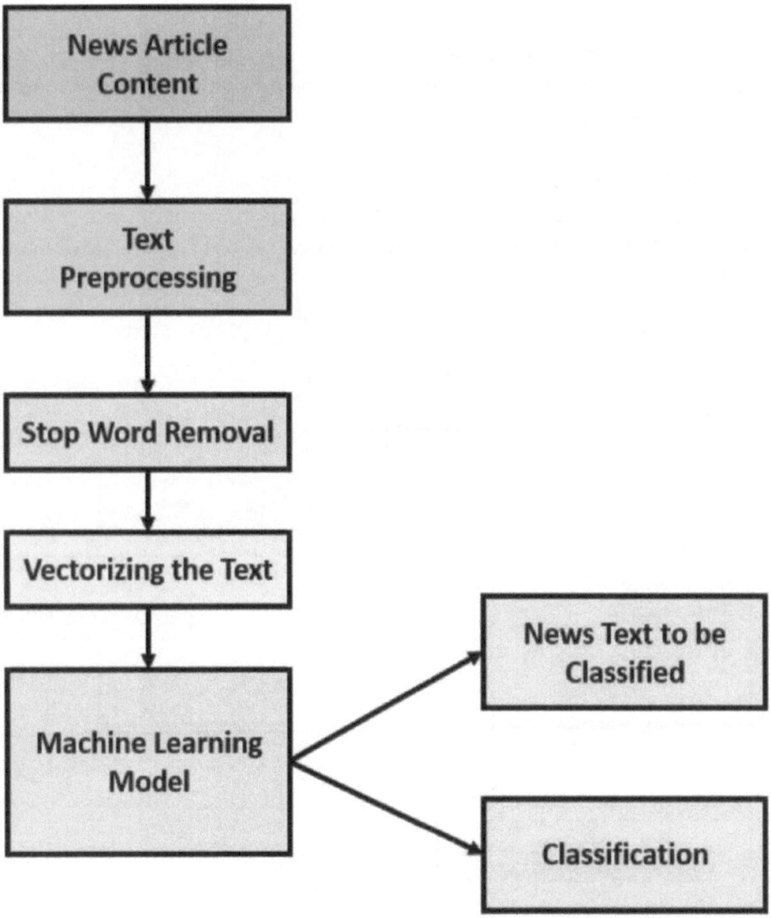

FIGURE 13.8 Flowchart illustrating the NLP process for social media analysis.

13.4.3.1 Topic Modeling: Overview

We aim to identify the main topics of conversation.

- **Step 1: Data Collection**: Collect a dataset of tweets and social media posts discussing the smart health device.
- **Step 2: Text Preprocessing**: Preprocess the text data by tokenizing the text, removing stop words, and standardizing words.
- **Step 3: Topic Extraction**:
  - Apply topic modeling, such [7] as latent dirichlet allocation (LDA), to uncover the underlying topics within the dataset.
  - Identify the top terms associated with each topic.
- **Step 4: Topic Visualization**:
  - Visualize the topics using word clouds that display the most frequent terms within each topic.
  - Create a bar graph showing the distribution of topics in the dataset.

13.4.3.2 Diagrams and Flowcharts

A simplified flowchart is shown in Figure 13.9, illustrating the process of topic modeling for social media analysis.

13.4.3.3 Conclusion

A useful method for locating significant themes and patterns in vast amounts of social media data is topic modeling. In the context of IoMT, it enables businesses

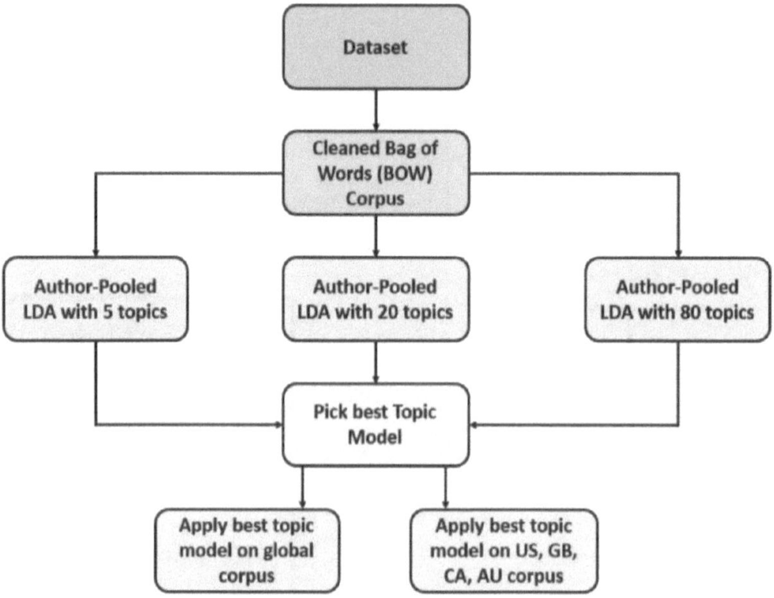

FIGURE 13.9 Flowchart illustrating the process of topic modeling.

to better comprehend their interests, keep track of trends, and unearth insights that can guide product development, marketing plans, and user engagement. Social media analysis is made more structured and understandable through the use of topic modeling, making it a crucial tool for data-driven decision-making in the IoMT ecosystem.

13.4.4 Social Network Analysis (SNA)

In order to comprehend the relationships, interactions, and structures inside social networks, such as those on social media platforms, social network analysis (SNA), a potent approach, is applied. SNA [11] assists in locating user connection patterns, locating important influencers, and analyzing information flow. The technical understanding of social network analysis will be supported by examples, graphs, figures, tables, and flowcharts in this in-depth presentation.

13.4.4.1 Social Network Analysis (SNA): Overview

Social network analysis typically involves the following key components:

1. **Data Collection**: Compile information from social networking sites, such as user profiles, posts, comments, and interaction information.
2. **Network Construction**: The data should be represented as a network, with users acting as nodes (vertices) and interactions (such as follows and mentions) and acting as edges (links) between nodes.
3. **Centrality Measures**: To find influential users within the network, analyze network centrality metrics including degree, betweenness, and eigenvector centrality.
3. **Community Detection**: Utilize algorithms to find communities or clusters of users who are related to one another closely [5].
5. **Visualization**: Use graphs or network diagrams to visualize the network structure in order to understand the relationships and information flow.

13.4.4.2 Example: Social Network Analysis

Let's consider an example of social network analysis for a healthcare-related social media platform. We want to identify key opinion leaders and analyze user interactions.

- **Step 1: Data Collection**: Gather user profiles, posts, comments, and interaction data from the social networking platform.
- **Step 2: Network Construction**: Construct a network graph in which users are the nodes and interactions (such as follows, mentions, and comments) are the edges.
- **Step 3: Centrality Measures**: To determine who the influential users are, calculate centrality scores for each user:
  - Measures a user's network of connections, or degree centrality.
  - Measures a user's significance in promoting communication among other users through betweenness centrality.

- Considers a user's connections and the value of those relationships using eigenvector centrality.
- **Step 4: Community Detection**: Use community detection algorithms to identify user communities or groups with shared interests or interactions.

13.4.4.3 Diagrams and Flowcharts

A simplified flowchart is shown in Figure 13.10, illustrating the process of social network analysis:

13.4.4.4 Summary of Social Network Analysis

Understanding the dynamics of social connections within social media platforms in the IoMT ecosystem requires the use of social network analysis, which is a useful technique. Organizations can use it to locate user communities, track the information flow, and identify important influencers. Businesses and healthcare professionals can improve patient care and healthcare outcomes by utilizing social networks by making informed decisions, engaging with their audience efficiently, and understanding the structure and interactions within the network.

13.4.5 User Profiling

We want to create profiles based on user interests, behavior, and demographics.

- **Step 1: Data Collection**: Obtain from the social media platform any user-provided data, including age, gender, location, and interests, as well as user-generated content and engagement data (likes, comments, shares).
- **Step 2: Data Preprocessing**: The data should be cleaned up and preprocessed to extract pertinent information and to guarantee data consistency.

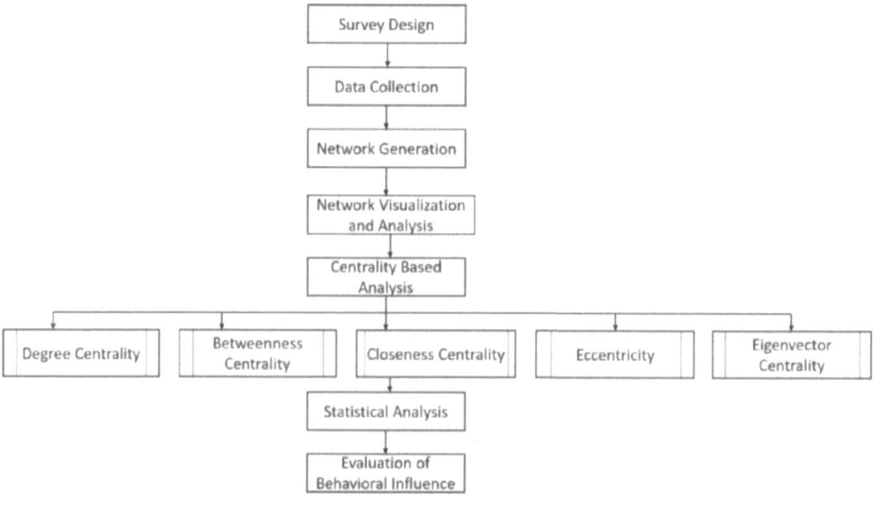

FIGURE 13.10 Flowchart illustrating the process of social network analysis.

- **Step 3: Feature Extraction**: Develop tools that record user [5] activity, content choices, and demographics. The quantity of health-related posts, the regularity of interactions, and self-reported interests are examples of features.
- **Step 4: Machine Learning Models**: Apply classification or clustering algorithms to divide consumers into distinct user profiles. Users with varied profiles can be those who are interested in making nutritious meals, fitness, or mental health.

13.4.5.1 User Profile Example

Let's create an example of a user profile as shown in Table 13.6.

- **User Profile: Health Enthusiast**: This user profile represents a health enthusiast, providing information about age, gender, location, interests, and online behavior.

13.4.5.2 Summary of User Profiling

User profiling is an effective method for social media analysis that helps businesses understand their consumers better. Businesses and healthcare providers can adjust their content, marketing plans, and user engagement initiatives to fit the unique needs and interests of various user segments by developing thorough user profiles. User profiling improves the user experience, results in more successful social media marketing campaigns, and ultimately aids businesses within the IoMT ecosystem in connecting with their target market. It is a crucial tool for social media decision-making based on facts.

13.4.6 Influencer Identification

Let's create an example of an influencer profile as shown in Table 13.7. This influencer profile provides key information about Jane Doe, who is an industry expert in IoMT security and privacy.

13.4.6.1 Summary of Influencer Identification

Organizations in the IoMT ecosystem can identify influential people within a specialty or industry by using the useful technique of influencer identification for social

TABLE 13.6
Health Enthusiast Profile

Attribute	Value
Age	30–40
Gender	Female
Location	Los Angeles, CA
Interests	Fitness, yoga, healthy cooking, meditation
Behavior	Posts daily workout updates, engages with fitness-related content and recipes, participates in wellness challenges

TABLE 13.7
Influencer Profile Example

Attribute	Value
Follower count	50,000
Engagement rate	7% (likes, comments, shares)
Domain expertise	IoMT security and privacy
Content relevance	Posts on IoMT cybersecurity topics
Influencer category	Industry expert
Key contributions	Organizes IoMT security webinars

media analysis. These influencers can be crucial in raising awareness, offering [7] knowledgeable commentary, and increasing brand reputation. Businesses and healthcare providers can use influencers' reach and knowledge to successfully engage with their target audience by recognizing them and forming partnerships with them. For strategic efforts in influencer marketing and engagement, influencer identification is a crucial tool.

REFERENCES

[1] Angelika Dohr, Robert Modre-Opsrian, Mario Drobics, Dieter Hayn, and Günter Schreier. The Internet of Things for ambient assisted living. In *2010 Seventh International Conference on Information Technology: New Generations*, pp. 804–809. IEEE, 2010.

[2] Muhammad Farrukh Khan, Taher M Ghazal, Raed A Said, Areej Fatima, Sagheer Abbas, MA Khan, Ghassan F Issa, Munir Ahmad, Muhammad Adnan Khan, et al. An IoMT-enabled smart healthcare model to monitor elderly people using machine learning technique. *Computational Intelligence and Neuroscience*, 2021, 2021.

[3] Shams Forruque Ahmed, Md Sakib Bin Alam, Shaila Afrin, Sabiha Jannat Rafa, Nazifa Rafa, and Amir H Gandomi. Insights into Internet of Medical Things (IoMT): Data fusion, security issues and potential solutions. *Information Fusion*, 102:102060, 2024.

[4] Ferdaous Benrouba and Rachid Boudour. Emotional sentiment analysis of social media content for mental health safety. *Social Network Analysis and Mining*, 13(1):17, 2023.

[5] Fadl Dahan, Roobaea Alroobaea, Wael Alghamdi, Mustafa Khaja Mohammed, Fahima Hajjej, Kaamran Raahemifar, et al. A smart IoMT based architecture for e-healthcare patient monitoring system using artificial intelligence algorithms. *Frontiers in Physiology*, 14:1125952, 2023.

[6] Laavanya Rachakonda, Saraju P Mohanty, and Elias Kougianos. Stress-lysis: An iomtenabled device for automatic stress level detection from physical activities. In *2020 IEEE International Symposium on Smart Electronic Systems (iSES)(Formerly iNiS)*, pp. 204–205. IEEE, 2020.

[7] Tao Zhang, Minjie Liu, Tian Yuan, and Najla Al-Nabhan. Emotion-aware and intelligent Internet of Medical Things toward emotion recognition during COVID-19 pandemic. *IEEE Internet of Things Journal*, 8(21):16002–16013, 2020.

[8] Jiahui Wen, Anwen Huang, Mingyang Zhong, Jingwei Ma, and Youcai Wei. Hybrid sentiment analysis with textual and interactive information. *Expert Systems with Applications*, 213:118960, 2023.

[9] Ganpat Singh Chauhan, Ravi Nahta, Yogesh Kumar Meena, and Dinesh Gopalani. Aspect based sentiment analysis using deep learning approaches: A survey. *Computer Science Review*, 49:100576, 2023.

[10] Lai Po Hung and Suraya Alias. Beyond sentiment analysis: A review of recent trends in text based sentiment analysis and emotion detection. *Journal of Advanced Computational Intelligence and Intelligent Informatics*, 27(1):84–95, 2023.

[11] Xianyong Li, Jiabo Zhang, Yajun Du, Jian Zhu, Yongquan Fan, and Xiaoliang Chen. A novel deep learning-based sentiment analysis method enhanced with emojis in microblog social networks. *Enterprise Information Systems*, 17(5):2037160, 2023.

14 Deep Learning for Augmented Medical Image Data Analysis

Hemant Maravaniya, Hiren Kumar Thakkar, and Chinmaya Dehury

14.1 INTRODUCTION

Deep learning plays a pivotal role in the field of augmented medical image data analysis, it uses the power of negative electronic data to improve the processing and interpretation of medical images, playing a key role in improving medical data analysis and ultimately transforming the way healthcare diagnoses and treats patients. Convolutional neural networks (CNN) and other deep learning methods are well-suited to this task because they are good at extracting complex and blurry patterns from complex image data. They help clarify image segmentation, allowing the body or structure to be identified and measured. Deep learning also provides valuable support to radiologists by facilitating computerized diagnosis by detecting diseases such as tumors or bones. It also makes it easier to save images by creating different images from different models or time points for clear comparison. It also helps rebuild the image by improving the image quality of bad or missing data. Deep learning will improve healthcare performance by providing faster and more accurate diagnosis, reducing human error and potentially detecting diseases earlier. Despite challenges related to data privacy, regulatory oversight, and the need for large amounts of data, deep learning continues to evolve, and research continues to focus on elucidating the skills and training in government to ensure that the health of the patient is more important.

14.1.1 Medical Imaging

Medical imaging is a cornerstone of modern healthcare, playing a pivotal role in the diagnosis, treatment, and monitoring of various medical conditions. It involves the use of various imaging modalities and technologies to visualize the internal structures of the human body. Common modalities are shown in Figure 14.1 and are described as follows:

- **X-ray**: Uses electromagnetic radiation to create images, commonly used for bone fractures and lung examinations.

DOI: 10.1201/9781003393498-19

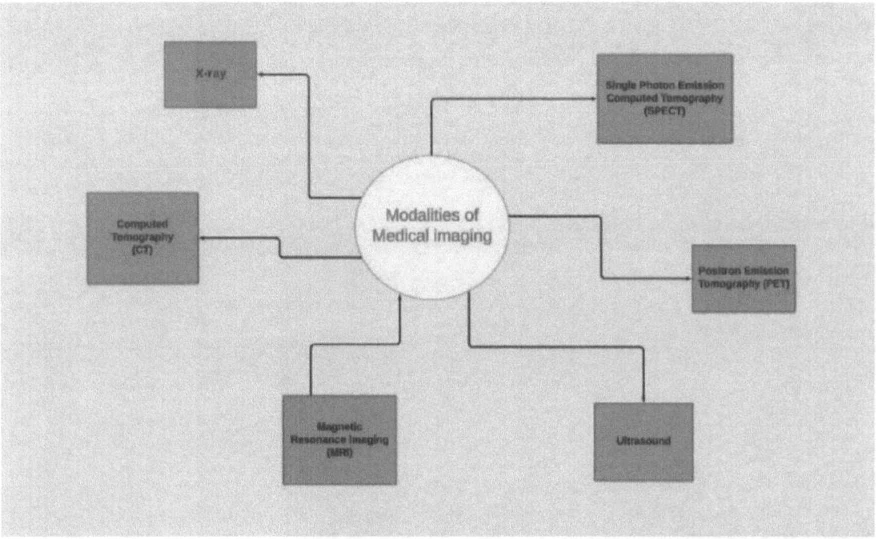

FIGURE 14.1 Modalities of medical imaging.

- **Computed Tomography (CT)**: Combines X-rays from different angles to create cross-sectional images, suitable for detailed anatomical examinations.
- **Magnetic Resonance Imaging (MRI)**: Uses strong magnetic fields and radio waves to create detailed images of soft tissues, organs, and the brain.
- **Ultrasound**: Employs high-frequency sound waves to create images, commonly used in obstetrics and cardiac imaging.
- **Positron Emission Tomography (PET)**: This involves injecting radioactive tracers to visualize metabolic processes in the body.
- **Single Photon Emission Computed Tomography (SPECT)**: This is similar to PET but uses different tracers and techniques.

The importance of medical imaging is shown in Figure 14.2 and can be comprehensively understood through the following aspects.

- **Early Disease Detection**: Medical diagnosis provides early detection of diseases and conditions. For example, mammograms are important for early diagnosis of breast cancer, and computed tomography (CT) scans can detect lung cancer and other abnormalities. Early diagnosis of the disease often leads to better treatment and better patient outcomes [1].
- **Accurate Diagnosis**: Imaging technology provides doctors with a noninvasive way to obtain detailed information about a patient's internal organs. This information is important in diagnosing a variety of diseases, from abnormalities in the bones and body to dementia and heart disease. Correct diagnosis is the basis of a good treatment plan.
- **Treatment Planning and Guidance**: Usually, the clinical diagnosis is considered relevant and important before planning and directing treatment to

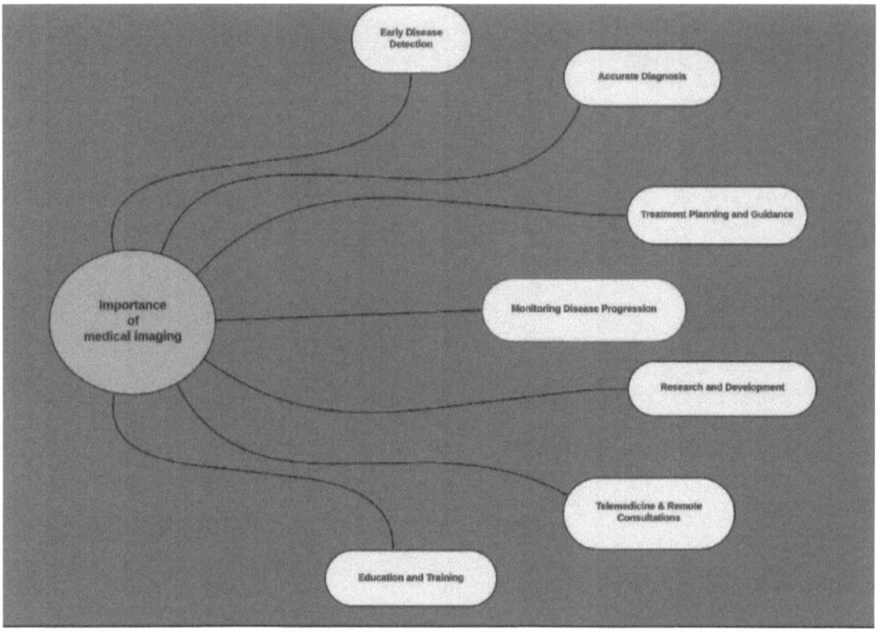

FIGURE 14.2 Importance of medical imaging.

the patient. The surgeons are expected to use the preliminary images to plan for the surgical procedures. However, the radiologists heavily rely on the visual aids such as fluoroscopy and ultrasound to decide going for the minimally invasive treatments for the patients. Nevertheless, imaging plays a vital role to decide on the radiation therapy, and it also helps doctors to plan for the radiation therapy for cancer patients.

- **Monitoring Disease Progression**: In a patient healthcare monitoring, the clinical diagnosis plays a pivotal role in monitoring the progression of the disease and helps to decide on an effective treatment. For example, in a healthcare treatment, magnetic resonance imaging (MRI) can help the doctors to monitor the progression of multiple sclerosis. On the contrary, positron tomography (PET) scans can help the doctors to measure the response to the cancer treatment.
- **Research and Development**: For several diseases, the medical imaging is a vital tool for the diagnosis and monitoring of a disease. Based on the outcome of such tools and imaging, researchers use them to study the human body, its functions, and the effects of the planned treatments on diseases. The continuous progression of research and development helps the medical sciences to employ medical technologies to diagnose for the patient and decide on effective treatment strategies.
- **Education and Training**: Medical imaging is an essential component of medical education and training. Medical students, radiologists, and healthcare professionals use images to learn about anatomy, pathology, and clinical

practices. Simulation training using medical images helps improve the skills of healthcare providers.

- **Telemedicine and Remote Consultations**: Advances in technology have made it possible to transmit medical images to remote locations for expert consultation. Telemedicine and teleradiology enable healthcare providers to receive specialized input, even in areas with limited access to specialized medical services.

14.2 CHALLENGES IN MEDICAL IMAGE

The challenges associated with medical image acquisition are inherent to various imaging modalities, and they can significantly impact the quality and diagnostic utility of the images. Addressing these challenges is vital for healthcare professionals to make accurate diagnoses and treatment decisions. Recent advancements in medical technology and the development of effective image processing techniques have drastically improved the quality of medical images. However, there is a lot of scope and challenges in the field of medical imaging for research and development. For the effective treatment of a patient, the accurate diagnosis is essential. In this regard, the correct and reliable acquisition of medical images is a very critical component that enables clinicians and healthcare professionals to make accurate diagnoses and treatment decisions. However, medical images obtained from diversified imaging modalities such as MRI, CT, ultrasound, etc., often face several challenges such as low resolution, high noise levels, low contrast, geometric deformations, and the presence of imaging artifacts. Next we discuss the five main challenges in detail.

14.2.1 Low Resolution (in the Spatial and Spectral Domains)

- **Spatial Resolution**: The low spatial resolution captured by the MRI, CT, or any healthcare device for medical imaging refers to the inability of the imaging system to capture details of the disease in the image. The low spatial resolution of images can result in a blurry or pixelated outcome, which makes it very challenging for a healthcare professional to identify small lesions and structures.
- **Spectral Resolution**: In some imaging modalities such as spectral, imaging has a limited ability to distinguish among different wavelengths and energy levels in a medical imaging. The limited ability of imaging modalities may affect the differentiation of tissue types or contrast agents in the image, leading to poor diagnosis.

14.2.2 High Level of Noise

Noise is another challenging concern, and it is induced by variety of factors such as sensor noise, body movement of the patient, exposure to the radiation, etc. While capturing the medical imaging data, the presence of a high level of noise may reduce the clarity of the image, which makes it very challenging to correctly identify the relevant and important features. Therefore, it is very crucial to apply noise reduction techniques to further improve the image quality.

14.2.3 Low Contrast

Several image capturing modalities lack state-of-the-art image capturing sensors, and therefore the captured images have low contrast. Usually, the low-contrast images do not offer the ability to differentiate between various tissues and structures with similar intensity levels. This is often considered a major problem in modalities such as X-rays and CT scans. Low contrast can lead to difficulties in detecting abnormalities and lesions within the body image.

14.2.4 Geometric Deformations

Generally, geometric deformations are induced in the captured image due to the movement of the patient and sometimes due to the positioning error of a patient. Such geometric deformations change the anatomical structures, leading to inaccurate measurements, which makes it challenging for healthcare professionals to correctly assess the patient's overall health condition.

14.2.5 Presence of Imaging Artifacts

The artifacts are considered external features that are not part of the original entity. In medical imaging, artifacts are considered any undesired features, also called distortions, that are not the representative features of the actual patient's anatomy. The artifacts may comes from a variety of sources such as metal implants, beam hardening in CT scans, and motion artifacts in MRI. The presence of artifacts in a diagnosis image can potentially mislead doctors to make an incorrect diagnosis, and therefore it needs to be corrected or minimized to ensure accurate interpretation [2,3].

14.3 ROLE OF THE DEEP LEARNING TECHNIQUES E-HEALTH

In the field of automation and artificial intelligence, deep learning is considered subfield of machine learning, which specifically focuses on employing artificial neural networks to model the problem in order to correlate the complex hidden patterns in data. In the context of medical image analysis, several deep learning techniques are described next.

14.3.1 Convolutional Neural Networks (CNNs)

- CNNs are considered a type of neural network specifically designed to process the data arranged in a grid-like structure, such as images. Nowadays, CNNs have become one of the important frameworks for several medical image analysis applications due to their ability to learn the features automatically and predict the output. The predicted output is expected to aid the healthcare professional to get the hidden insights [4].

- CNN frameworks are comprised of several layers, and each layer is designed to perform a specific task. For example, convolutional layers are expected to extract the important features, and pooling layers are expected to down-sample the image size. On the contrary, the final layers are often fully connected for the classification or regression tasks.
- Usually, the CNN layers are coupled with the specific filters to detect the relevant features from an image hierarchy. In addition to the filters, weight sharing and transfer learning are common techniques employed with CNN for training robust models.

In the following, we describe each layer and its role in making predictions.

14.3.1.1 Convolutional Layers

- Convolutional layers play an important role in the CNN architecture and are applied with kernels to identify local patterns and features from the medical images. For example, convolutional layers can help to identify edges, textures, and small structures in the medical images.
- Generally, the convolutional layers are followed by the nonlinear activation functions such as Sigmoid, ReLU, leaky ReLU, etc., to introduce the nonlinearity into the model [5].

14.3.1.2 Pooling Layers

- Pooling layers reduce the spatial dimensions of the feature maps created by the convolutional layers. The example of pooling layers are max-pooling, min-pooling, and average-pooling. However, in many medical applications, max-pooling is commonly applied as it retains the maximum value in a local region and reduces information loss.
- Pooling layers are expected to help make the network translation-invariant. Moreover, pooling layers also reduces sensitivity to small shifts and distortions in the input, which is essential to retain the original image structure for subsequent processing.

14.3.1.3 Hierarchy of Features

- CNNs are designed to learn features hierarchically. Lower layers typically capture simple features like edges, while deeper layers capture more complex features, such as shapes, object parts, and textures.
- The hierarchy of features empower CNN models to identify the complex hidden pattern from the images, which make these models more suitable for medical image analysis with complex structure and anomalies.

14.3.1.4 Weight Sharing

- One of the key characteristics of the CNN models is the ability to share weights across the layers. In CNN architecture, the convolutional layers use the same set of filters for a given input, which allows the CNN network to learn and recognize the complex features present in the different parts of the image, and thereby it may improve the efficiency.

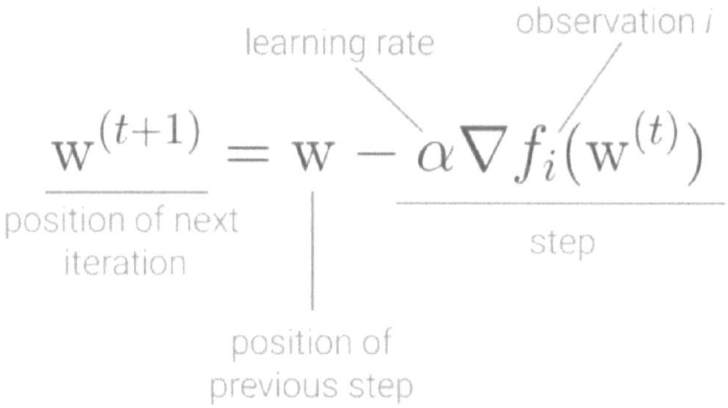

FIGURE 14.3 Gradient descent update rule for step $t + 1$.

- Weight sharing is especially advantageous in medical image analysis, where data can be limited, and generalizing from a smaller dataset is essential.

14.3.2 Feature Learning

One of the key strengths of deep learning, especially CNNs, is their ability to automatically learn hierarchical features from the input data. In the context of medical images, this means that the model can learn to detect relevant structures or patterns (e.g., tumors, organs) without the need for handcrafted feature engineering.

14.3.3 Training Process

- Deep learning models, including CNNs, are trained on labeled data. In the case of medical image analysis, this typically involves pairing images with their corresponding diagnoses or annotations (e.g., tumor masks).
- During training, the model's parameters are adjusted to minimize the difference between its predictions and the ground truth labels. This process is often done using optimization algorithms like stochastic gradient descent (SGD).

14.3.3.1 Stochastic Gradient Descent (SGD)

Stochastic gradient descent (SGD) is an optimization algorithm commonly used to train machine learning models, including neural networks in deep learning. It's especially useful for large datasets. In short, it updates model parameters (weights) in small, random batches of data rather than the entire dataset, which makes training faster and more efficient. The formula for updating model parameters in SGD is shown in Figure 14.3. In each iteration, a random batch of training data is used to calculate the gradient, and the weights are updated accordingly. This process repeats until the model converges to a solution, meaning it finds the weights that minimize the loss function. SGD is computationally efficient and is a cornerstone of deep learning training [6].

14.3.4 Transfer Learning

- Given the limited availability of labeled medical image data, transfer learning is frequently employed. This approach involves using pretrained deep learning models as a starting point.
- Pretrained models, often trained on large, diverse datasets like ImageNet, have already learned valuable low-level features and can be fine-tuned for specific medical image analysis tasks.
- Transfer learning can significantly reduce the amount of the labeled medical data needed to train an effective model.

14.3.5 Architecture Choices

- Different deep learning architectures can be used for various medical image analysis tasks. For instance:

  1. **U-Net**: Widely used for image segmentation tasks, such as tumor delineation
  2. **ResNet**: Known for its depth and skip connections, which help avoid vanishing gradient problems and improve feature learning
  3. **VGG (Visual Geometry Group)**: Known for its simplicity and effectiveness in various image analysis tasks

The choice of architecture depends on the specific task and the available data.

14.3.6 Hyperparameter Tuning

Like any machine learning models, deep learning models have hyperparameters that must be tuned to achieve optimal performance. These include learning rates, batch sizes, and the number of layers or filters in the network.

14.3.7 Overfitting and Regularization

- Overfitting is a common concern in deep learning. Techniques like dropout and weight decay are used to regularize models and prevent them from fitting noise in the data.
- Augmented data, as mentioned in the original point, can also help reduce overfitting.

14.3.8 Interpretability

Understanding how a deep learning model makes its predictions is crucial in medical applications. Techniques like Grad-CAM (Gradient-weighted Class Activation Mapping) can highlight the regions that are most influential for the model's decision in an image, aiding in clinical interpretability.

14.3.9 Validation and Evaluation

Deep learning models for medical image analysis need thorough validation. Techniques like *k*-fold cross-validation can assess model performance. Evaluation metrics are chosen based on the specific task, such as sensitivity, specificity, or the Dice coefficient for segmentation tasks [7–9].

14.4 METHODOLOGY

The augmentation of medical images using deep learning involves various steps that help to generate additional, diverse, and realistic training data for training machine learning models. The comprehensive methodology for the augmentation of medical images is shown in Figure 14.4.

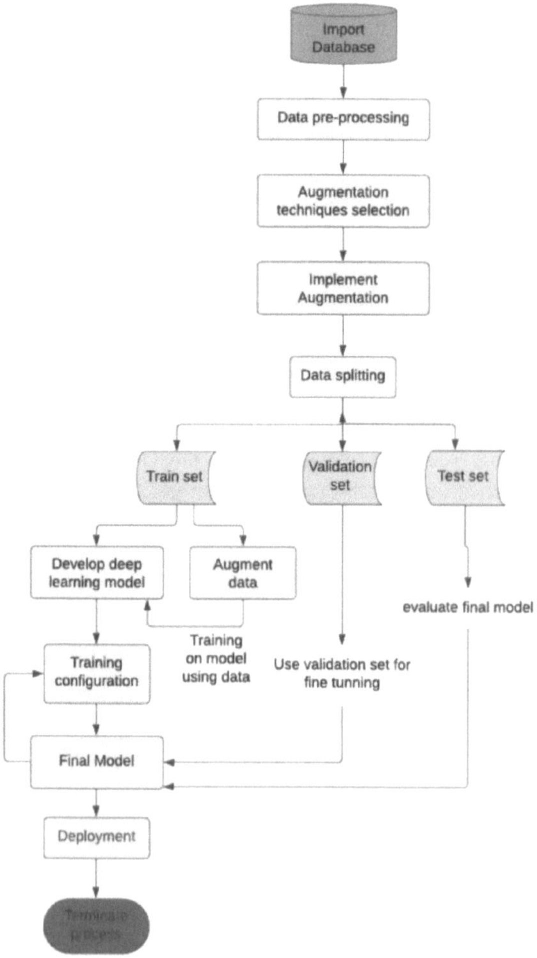

FIGURE 14.4 Data-augmentation-supported expert system design for healthcare applications.

14.4.1 Step 1: Data Collection and Preprocessing

- **Collect Medical Image Data**: Gather a substantial amount of medical image data that is representative of the clinical scenarios you want the deep learning model to work in. Ensure that the data is properly anonymized and complies with data privacy regulations.
- **Data Preprocessing**: Preprocess the collected data to ensure uniformity and quality. This may include resizing images to a common resolution, normalizing pixel values, and handling missing or corrupted data.

14.4.2 Step 2: Selection of Augmentation Techniques

Select the augmentation techniques that are relevant to your specific medical imaging task. Common augmentation methods include rotation, translation, scaling, flipping, brightness adjustments, noise injection, and elastic deformations. More specialized techniques may be used for 3D medical images.

14.4.3 Step 3: Implement Augmentation

Develop or use software libraries to implement the selected augmentation methods. You can use deep learning frameworks like TensorFlow or PyTorch to incorporate augmentation into your data pipeline.

14.4.4 Step 4: Data Splitting

Divide your dataset into three subsets: a training set, a validation set, and a test set. The training set is used for model training, the validation set for hyperparameter tuning, and the test set for final model evaluation.

14.4.5 Step 5: Augment the Training Data

Apply the selected augmentation techniques to the images in the training set. For each training sample, create multiple augmented versions by randomly applying one or more augmentation methods, varying the parameters if applicable.

14.4.6 Step 6: Model Training

- **Deep Learning Model**: Develop a deep learning model architecture suitable for your medical imaging task. This may include convolutional neural networks (CNNs) for image classification, segmentation, or other tasks.
- **Training Configuration**: Configure the training process with suitable hyperparameters, such as learning rate, batch size, and optimization algorithms. Implement techniques like early stopping and learning rate schedules to prevent overfitting.
- **Train on Augmented Data**: Train the deep learning model using the augmented training data. The augmented data should be used in conjunction with

the original, non-augmented data. Figure 14.4 shows the data-augmentation-supported expert system design for healthcare applications and Figure 14.5 shows the data augmentation techniques.

14.4.7 Step 7: Validation and Fine-Tuning

Use the validation set to monitor the model's performance and identify the optimal hyperparameters. Fine-tune the model as needed.

14.4.8 Step 8: Model Evaluation

Assess the model's performance on the test set to evaluate its real-world effectiveness. Measure relevant metrics, such as accuracy, sensitivity, specificity, and other domain-specific indicators.

14.4.9 Step 9: Interpretation and Validation

Analyze the model's predictions and its ability to generalize to unseen data. Interpret the model's decision-making process and validate its performance against clinical standards.

14.4.10 Step 10: Deployment

If the model performs well, integrate it into clinical workflows for use by healthcare professionals. Ensure compliance with regulatory requirements and maintain vigilance for ethical and quality control considerations [4,5,10].

14.5 MEDICAL IMAGE AUGMENTATION TECHNIQUES

The different data augmentation techniques are shown in Figure 14.5 and can be explained as follows.

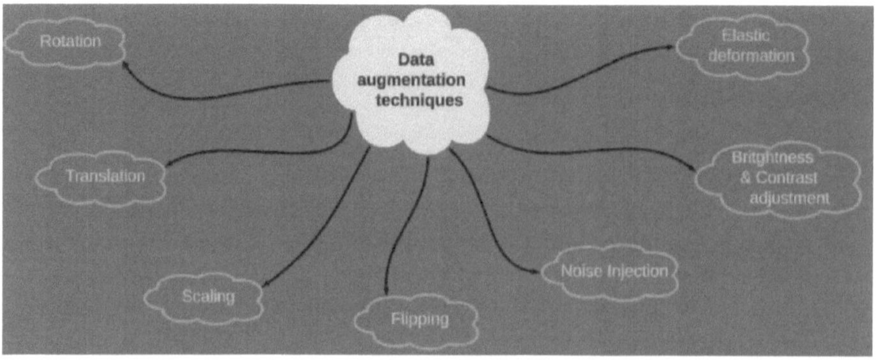

FIGURE 14.5 Data augmentation techniques.

14.5.1 Rotation

- Rotation involves changing the orientation of an image by a specified angle, typically within a defined range, like ±15 degrees. This technique simulates variations in patient positioning during imaging. In medical imaging, even a slight angle change can result in variations in the position and shape of anatomical structures.
- Rotation augmentation is particularly important for X-ray and CT scans, where a patient's positioning can vary slightly between scans. Training on rotated images makes the deep learning model more adept at recognizing features from different perspectives, making it robust with respect to patient position variability.

14.5.2 Translation

- Translation refers to shifting an image horizontally and/or vertically by a certain number of pixels. This technique emulates slight changes in the patient's position during imaging. It helps the model adapt to variations in the location of anatomical structures within the image.
- Translation augmentation is beneficial in all modalities but is particularly relevant in MRI, where small shifts due to patient motion or repositioning can occur. By training on translated images, the model becomes more resilient to variations in patient and organ location.

14.5.3 Scaling

- Scaling involves resizing the image by a specific factor, either enlarging or reducing its size. The resizing can simulate variations in image resolution and field of view, which are common in medical imaging.
- This augmentation is crucial for creating models adaptable to image size variations. In radiology, for instance, imaging protocols and resolutions may differ, and the scaling augmentation helps the model accommodate these changes.

14.5.4 Flipping

- Flipping entails mirroring the image horizontally or vertically. This technique helps the model recognize anatomical structures and abnormalities from different perspectives. It's often used in medical image analysis to introduce diversity.
- Flipping is applicable across various medical imaging modalities. For instance, in ultrasound, flipping can simulate changes in probe orientation, leading to more comprehensive training of the model.

In summary, the advantages of various augmentation techniques in healthcare can be described as shown in Table 14.1.

TABLE 14.1
Advantages of Various Technologies in Healthcare

Advantage	Description
Improved robustness and generalization	The image augmentation provides the much needed exposure to the deep learning model such as a wider range of variations, patient positioning, varied illumination, etc. This exposure makes the models more robust and the least sensitive against the little noise, inconsistencies, and artifacts in a medical image. As a consequence, the models become more and more robust with improved performance, leading to the generalization on the unseen data.
Increased data availability and size	The deep learning models require exposure to a sufficient number of images for model generalization. However, medical imaging datasets are often limited in size. Such limitations poses a challenge for effective deep learning model training. On the contrary, data augmentation techniques can expand the effective size of the dataset by generating additional variations and samples from the same set of images, and it allows for detailed training of the model.
Reduction in overfitting	Deep learning models are prone to overfitting, where they memorize training data rather than learning meaningful features. Augmentation helps in reducing overfitting by introducing diversity into the dataset. The models trained on augmented data are less likely to learn noise, which improves their performance with real-world data.
Transfer learning and adaptability	Augmented data can be used to fine-tune pretrained models, making them more adaptable to specific medical imaging tasks. Transfer learning with augmented data allows models to leverage knowledge learned from a broader range of data sources and domains.
Time and cost Efficiency	To create large annotated medical imaging datasets is a highly complex, labor-intensive, and resource-intensive task. However, data augmentation is a handy toll that offers a cost-effective and efficient alternative to increase the size of the dataset without much of a hurdle, leading to reduced time and cost for data collection.

14.5.5 Brightness and Contrast Adjustments

- Adjusting brightness and contrast levels in an image helps the model become more adaptable to variations in lighting conditions. This augmentation is especially useful for radiographic images.
- In X-ray and mammography, image quality can vary due to differences in imaging equipment and settings. The deep learning model learns to recognize anatomical structures under different lighting conditions by training on images with varying brightness and contrast.

14.5.6 Noise Injection

- Noise injection involves adding various types of noise to the image, such as Gaussian noise or speckle noise. It replicates the inherent noise in medical imaging equipment and enhances the model's resilience with real-world data.

- Noise injection is critical in all imaging modalities, particularly in MRIs, where images can be susceptible to artifacts and noise. This augmentation helps the model generalize better and make accurate predictions, even in noisy clinical images.

14.5.7 Elastic Deformations

- During ultrasound, sometimes the elastic deformations introduce the random and localized distortions in the image, which simulates tissue deformation and organ motion. The elastic deformation technique is specifically useful for ultrasound and MRI images.
- In ultrasound, sometimes the tissue deformations may occur due to external factors such as pressure from probe. In such situations, the elastic deformation augmentation technique may allow models to learn to handle images with the nonuniform distortions and subsequently to improve its robustness.

These augmentation techniques are essential in training deep-learning models for medical image analysis. The selection and customization of these techniques depend on the specific challenges and characteristics of the imaging data, ensuring that the models are well prepared to handle the complexities of real clinical scenarios [11–13].

14.6 APPLICATIONS

The summary of applications and algorithms, technique used, and future scope is shown in Table 14.2.

14.6.1 Tumor Detection and Classification

In the field of medical image data analysis, deep learning models such as convolutional neural networks (CNNs) are extensively used to detect a tumor followed by its classification into categories. These trained deep learning models can analyze MRI images, CT images, and mammography images to identify tumors and to subsequently distinguish them as benign or malignant. Moreover, recent advancements such as transfer learning, data augmentation, and semantic segmentation can also help to enhance the accuracy of these models.

14.6.2 Brain Image Analysis

Deep learning models can also be designed to analyze brain images obtained from MRI and fMRI scans to analyze the severity of brain damage. The deep learning models may help to identify the brain structures, to study the neural connectivity among the neurons, and to detect various brain-related anomalies such as tumors, lesions, etc. Moreover, the advanced techniques such as 3D CNNs and recurrent neural networks (RNNs) are also applied for detailed investigation using 3D image analysis and time-series data.

TABLE 14.2
Summary of Applications and Algorithms

Application	Technique Used	Algorithm Used	Future Scope
Tumor detection and classification	Convolutional neural networks (CNNs)	Deep residual networks (ResNets), DenseNets, U-Nets	Improved accuracy and sensitivity in tumor detection and classification, development of algorithms for early tumor detection, and personalized treatment planning
Brain image analysis	CNNs, 3D CNNs, graph neural networks (GNNs)	ResNets, DenseNets, U-Nets, graph convolutional networks (GCNs)	For early detection of neurological disorders such as Alzheimer's disease and Parkinson's disease; for the personalized treatment planning for brain tumors
Cardiac image analysis	CNNs, 3D CNNs, GNNs	ResNets, DenseNets, U-Nets, GCNs	For early detection of heart disease such as coronary artery disease and heart failure; for the personalized treatment planning of heart conditions
Skin lesion classification	CNNs, transfer learning	ResNets, DenseNets, VGGNets	For an early detection of skin cancer and other skin diseases; for monitoring the progression of skin diseases
Ophthalmology image analysis	CNNs, 3D CNNs	ResNets, DenseNets, U-Nets	For eye disease detection such as glaucoma and diabetic retinopathy. To monitor the progression of eye diseases
Endoscopy and pathology	CNNs, 3D CNNs, transfer learning	ResNets, DenseNets, U-Nets	To detect cancer and other diseases in endoscopic and pathology images in an early stage to improve the accuracy of diagnosis and prognosis
Multimodal data fusion	CNNs, 3D CNNs, GNNs, transformers	Late fusion, early fusion, deep fusion	Development of algorithms for fusing multimodal medical data, such as MRI, CT, and PET images, to improve the accuracy of diagnosis and prognosis

14.6.3 Cardiac Image Analysis

In the field of heart disease analysis, the deep learning is utilized to analyze cardiac images such as echocardiograms and angiograms. Such deep learning models can work on the multiple cardiac functions such as to detect heart diseases and to segment the heart's chambers. The ConvNets coupled with the attention mechanisms are often used to capture intricate details and subtle changes in heart images.

14.6.4 Skin Lesion Classification

Deep learning models are also helpful and applicable in the field of dermatology to classify skin lesions, which aids in the early diagnosis of skin cancers. For deep learning models to provide improved accuracy, the pretrained models need to be fine-tuned on a given dataset. This process of fine-tuning the pretrained model on a new dataset is called transfer learning, which leverages the benefit of large datasets and improves the model's accuracy.

14.6.5 Ophthalmology Image Analysis

The one of the finest transformations in healthcare data analysis is in the field of ophthalmology by means of deep learning that analyzes retinal images to provide the early detection of eye diseases such as diabetic retinopathy and glaucoma. In the field of ophthalmology, the retinal scans, optical coherence tomography (OCT) images, and fundus images are processed using deep learning models, CNNs, and sequential deep learning models such as recurrent networks to provide accurate diagnoses and disease progression tracking.

14.6.6 Endoscopy and Pathology

In endoscopy, deep learning models assist in identifying polyps, lesions, and abnormalities in gastrointestinal and other medical procedures. These models, combined with image segmentation techniques, help clinicians make real-time decisions during procedures. In pathology, deep learning is used for the automated analysis of histopathological slides, helping pathologists detect cancer cells and classify tissues accurately.

14.6.7 Multimodal Data Fusion

Multimodal data analysis involves combining data from various sources such as medical images, clinical notes, drug prescriptions, and genomics. The deep learning techniques such as fusion models and recurrent networks are the most suitable for integration with diversified data types, processing them, and providing analytical insights, which enable a more comprehensive assessment of a patient's condition and creation of a personalized treatment plan [14].

14.7 CONCLUSION

Deep learning for augmented medical image data analysis represents a transformative frontier in healthcare. By leveraging advanced neural network architectures and a diverse array of data augmentation techniques, deep learning empowers clinicians and researchers with sophisticated tools to interpret, diagnose, and plan treatments based on medical images. It enhances the robustness and generalization of models, mitigating challenges posed by variations in imaging conditions, patient positioning, and equipment differences. Through augmentation, deep learning models adapt to the intricacies of clinical data, enabling earlier disease detection, accurate diagnosis, and personalized treatment strategies. Moreover, these advancements contribute to increased data availability, reduced annotation burden, and the potential for cost-effective solutions in a field where large, labeled datasets are often scarce. As the synergy between deep learning and augmented medical image analysis continues to evolve, the future holds promise for more precise and efficient healthcare delivery, ultimately benefiting patients and healthcare providers alike by advancing the capabilities of diagnostic and prognostic tools in the medical field.

REFERENCES

[1] Adler TJ, Ardizzone L, Vemuri A, et al. Uncertainty-aware performance assessment of optical imaging modalities with invertible neural networks. *International Journal of Computer Assisted Radiology and Surgery.* 2019;14:997–1007.

[2] Deng J, Dong W, Socher R, et al. ImageNet: A large-scale hierarchical image database. In: *2009 IEEE conference on computer vision and pattern recognition*; IEEE; 2009. pp. 248–255.

[3] Sun J, Darbeha F, Zaidi M, et al. SAUNet: Shape attentive U-Net for interpretable medical image segmentation. *arXiv.* 2020. https://doi.org/10.48550/arXiv.2001.07645.

[4] Stano M, Benesova W, Martak LS. Explainable 3D convolutional neural network using GMM encoding. In: *Twelfth international conference on machine vision (ICMV 2019)*; Vol. 11433; SPIE; 2020. pp. 507–513.

[5] Shrikumar A, Greenside P, Kundaje A. Learning important features through propagating activation differences. In: *International conference on machine learning*; PMLR; 2017. pp. 3145–3153.

[6] Bento C. Stochastic gradient descent explained in real life. [https://towardsdatascience.com/stochastic-gradient-descent-explained-in-real-life-predicting-your-pizzas-cooking-time-b7639d5e6a32]; 2020.

[7] Solawetz J. Why and how to implement random rotate data augmentation. 2020. [https://blog.roboflow.com/why-and-how-to-implement-random-rotate-data-augmentation/]

[8] Shorten, C., & Khoshgoftaar, T. M. (2019). A survey on image data augmentation for deep learning. *Journal of big data*, 6(1):1-48.

[9] Monigatti L. Image augmentation techniques for audio data in Python. 2023. [https://towardsdatascience.com/data-augmentation-techniques-for-audio-data-in-python-15505483c63c].

[10] Sayres R, Taly A, Rahimy E, et al. Using a deep learning algorithm and integrated gradients explanation to assist grading for diabetic retinopathy. *Ophthalmology.* 2019; 126(4):552–564.

[11] Yeche H, Harrison J, Berthier T. UBS: A dimension-agnostic metric for concept vector interpretability applied to radiomics. In: *Interpretability of machine intelligence in medical image computing and multimodal learning for clinical decision support.* Cham, Switzerland: Springer; 2019. pp. 12–20.

[12] Graziani M, Andrearczyk V, Müller H. Regression concept vectors for bidirectional explanations in histopathology. In: *Understanding and interpreting machine learning in medical image computing applications.* Cham, Switzerland: Springer; 2018. pp. 124–132.

[13] Codella N, Lin C, Halpern A, et al. Collaborative Human-AI (CHAI): Evidence-based interpretable melanoma classification in dermoscopic images. In: *Understanding and interpreting machine learning in medical image computing applications.* Cham, Switzerland: Springer; 2018. pp. 97–105.

[14] Badar M, Haris M, Fatima A. Application of deep learning for retinal image analysis: A review. *Computer Science Review.* 2020;35:100203.

Index

U

V

W